BELLY WOMAN

Benjamin Black

Dr Benjamin Black is a consultant obstetrician and gynaecologist in London and a specialist advisor to international aid organisations. His focus on sexual, reproductive and maternal healthcare for populations in times of crisis has taken him to many countries. Benjamin has supported the response to various infectious disease outbreaks since the West African Ebola epidemic. Throughout the COVID-19 pandemic he provided frontline healthcare to pregnant women and helped develop international guidelines. Benjamin also teaches medical teams around the world on improving sexual and reproductive healthcare to the most vulnerable people in the most challenging of environments.

PRAISE FOR *BELLY WOMAN*

From Sierra Leone to London, from 2014 to 2020, Benjamin Black's account of helping pregnant women in the midst of an Ebola epidemic and a Covid-19 pandemic is heartbreaking and terrifying. Black has done a stellar job of narrating what it is like to be on the frontline of a crisis as it enfolds and then engulfs. Death waits in the shadows of the delivery room, not just for the mother or her child, but for the medical staff, too. A needle prick or a slipped mask can mean the end. The parallels between the two outbreaks are evident, the range of human response not much different: fear, desperation, denial, anger, stoicism, compassion and courage all take their turn. Belly Woman is a must-read for our times. It is riveting, illuminating and humbling.

**Aminatta Forna, author of *The Memory of Love*
and *The Devil That Danced on the Water***

Moving, kind, eye-opening, terrifying and inspirational – this book will stay with me for years.

Adam Kay, author of *This Is Going To Hurt*

This is an inspirational story of compassion and dedication in the face of a brutal epidemic, and Benjamin Black is the one to tell it.

Leah Hazard, author of *Hard Pushed: A Midwife's Story*

Brave, moving, and vital. A unique account of battling the Ebola outbreak while providing maternity care in Sierra Leone, and of the incredible women, families, and health workers Dr Black encountered. Read it.

Damien Brown, author of *Band-Aid for A Broken Leg*

Belly Woman is a jaw-dropping, mind-expanding read, a work of vast compassion and delicate insight into the bracing reality of giving birth in today's Africa. At times it's hard to read on without wanting to weep — at the mistakes made and the sheer implacability of death. But like the author himself, you never become numbed or unaffected by the women we encounter, such is their courage and the vividness of Black's writing in capturing their experiences.

Michela Wrong, author of *Do Not Disturb: the story of a political murder and an African regime gone bad*

Black has penned a reflective account of providing obstetric care during and after the 2013-16 Ebola outbreak in Sierra Leone. He writes with sensitivity and is attentive to his own positionality, avoiding the problematic tropes so typical of "humanitarian memoirs". Black offers profound insight into the many medical, ethical and political challenges that characterise the pursuit of health equity in times of crisis

James Smith, co-editor of *Humanitarian Action and Ethics*

Oh my goodness, I could not put the book down. Benjamin Black has the most amazing gift for telling a story. Belly Woman transports you to Sierra Leone, to the compounds, to the hospital wards, to the villages ravaged by Ebola. As Dr Black and his colleagues fought for better care and to improve maternity services, you feel every drip of sweat inside their PPE, you hold your breath as they too wait for the newborn to cry, and you weep at every life that could have been saved but for the lack of facilities and equipment.

Victoria MacDonald, Health and Social Care Editor at *Channel 4 News*

BELLY WOMAN

BIRTH, BLOOD AND EBOLA

THE UNTOLD STORY

Belly Woman (pronounced 'be'leh 'uman') – Krio for pregnant woman

BENJAMIN BLACK

This is a work of nonfiction. It reflects the author's recollections of memories and experiences. Some names and characteristics have been changed; some conversations have been recreated and certain characters may be composites to protect the privacy of the people involved.

Belly Woman is a title created by the author. It has no specific meaning in English or Krio. The pronunciation, 'be'leh 'uman', is the Krio word for a pregnant woman.

Published by Neem Tree Press Limited 2022
Neem Tree Press Limited
95A Ridgmount Gardens, London, WC1E 7AZ
info@neemtreepress.com

A catalogue record for this book is available from the British Library
ISBN 978-1-911107-56-9 Hardback
ISBN 978-1-911107-57-6 Paperback
ISBN 978-1-911107-58-3 Ebook

For everyone within these pages, named and unnamed

'I was devastated and restless when I looked at the pregnant women.'
— Fatmata Jebbeh Sumaila, Sierra Leonean
midwife and colleague

CONTENTS

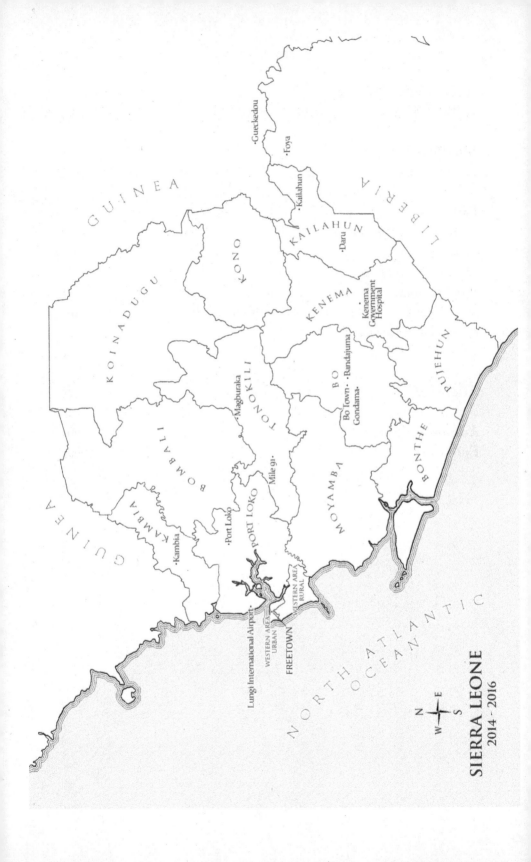

EBOLA TREATMENT CENTRE (ETC)
2014

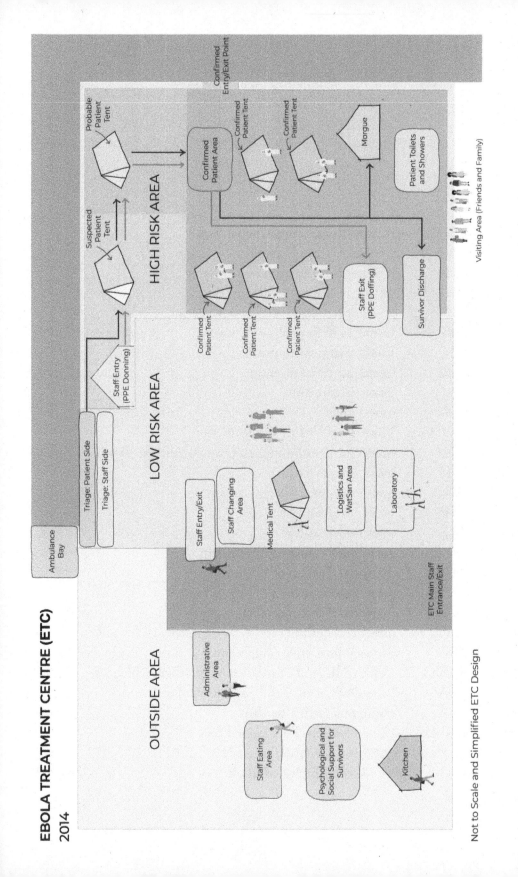

Not to Scale and Simplified ETC Design

ACRONYMS

BBC	British Broadcasting Corporation
CAR	Central African Republic
CHO	community health officer
DHMT	district health management team
DIC	disseminated intravascular coagulation
DRC	Democratic Republic of Congo
ETC	Ebola treatment centre
GRC	Gondama referral centre
ICU	intensive care unit
IV	intravenous
MOHS	Ministry of Health and Sanitation
MSF	Médecins Sans Frontières/Doctors Without Borders
MTL	medical team leader
NGO	non-governmental organization
NHS	National Health Service
OC	operational centre
OCA	operational centre of Amsterdam
OCB	operational centre of Brussels
PC	project coordinator
PCR	polymerase chain reaction
PHU	peripheral health unit
PPE	personal protective equipment
RCOG	Royal College of Obstetricians and Gynaecologists
SOAS	School of Oriental and African Studies
TBA	traditional birth attendant
UNFPA	United Nations Population Fund
WatSan	water and sanitation specialist
WHO	World Health Organization

AUTHOR'S NOTE

Person, Position and Purpose

I was in Sierra Leone in January 2020, when I read about a new illness reported to be spreading in Wuhan, China. It was my first time in the country since March 2016, where this book ends.

I had been thinking a lot about epidemics, as I often do. A phrase had been playing in my mind as I travelled: *with a flick of the wrist, we are brought to our knees.* This was my feeling about the 2013–2016 West African Ebola epidemic.

Like dust from a rug when it is shaken, we are thrown tumbling through the air. How nature reminds us of our frailty; her power immense, our control limited.

In that same month, January 2020, I had published, with two colleagues, Gillian McKay and Alice Janvrin, an advocacy paper for sexual and reproductive health rights to be integrated into epidemics. We had gathered data and interviews from the Democratic Republic of Congo (DRC), where another Ebola epidemic stubbornly continued to fester. We had questioned whether any lessons had been learnt. Was there hope for the next epidemic?

I first went to Sierra Leone in June 2014, deployed as an obstetrician and gynaecologist with Médecins Sans Frontières (MSF). It was to be the beginning of a journey like no other. I returned home, in October, several months into that journey. As I jogged around the leafy streets of north-west London there were visions of the Ebola camps coursing through my mind, along with the memory of two young brothers I had promised not to forget.

It was then, that I made a personal commitment to write this book. I began collecting these memories eighteen months later, in April 2016, as I re-entered the UK National Health Service (NHS).

As 2015 drew to a close, the embers of the Ebola outbreak of West Africa continued to glow. There were already committees, conferences and congratulations underway; conclusions being drawn; knighthoods bestowed; medals and prizes awarded. The epidemic simmering, the underlying causes remaining unresolved, and the world's attention predictably shifting.

I wrote *Belly Woman* to open the door to a battle for life many people are unaware of. I want to take the reader behind the Ebola headlines to meet the people on the ground, so they can face the dilemmas with them. My hope is to add to the narrative of one of the greatest public health crises in history, to explore what it is to be pregnant with limited access to emergency care, and to consider the choices we make in extremis. This is a raw account, at times distressing. There are descriptions of suffering, medical procedures and emotional turmoil (I advise caution, or guidance from a friend, for readers with pregnancy-related trauma). But it also depicts moments of joy, camaraderie and the hope for better.

The intertwining circumstances which fed and led to the West African epidemic demand far more analysis than is possible here. This book is a taster; a small addition to the wealth of papers and texts available on the epidemic, humanitarian systems and maternal healthcare.

Contexts change, policies are revised and, sometimes, lessons *are* learnt. Our approach to Ebola virus disease has changed too. Since the times described in this book, there have been effective vaccines produced and large multidrug trials undertaken, discovering treatments and cures. Perhaps, by the time you read this, a simple pill will solve the ailment. Progress, though, does not equal forgetting. The emergence of COVID-19 brought us back to the start: the search for solutions renewed, ethical conundrums unanswered and our faith in humanity shaken.

This book is not a critique of Médecins Sans Frontières, the governments of affected countries or the international response. I have been honest in sharing my opinion, and accept that, inevitably, not everyone will agree with my point of view. This is an unaffiliated piece of work, written in my own time. This is my story, my experience and my reflections. It is through the nature of being my recollections that I play the central character; in reality, though, I was a peripheral figure to the events witnessed. Above all, it was the people who lived in the countries where I was welcomed who worked longest and hardest, and it was they who paid by far the highest price for doing so.

I am acutely aware that I am a man in a high-income country writing about maternity care and events in African countries. There is no intention for my voice or perspective to represent or replace anyone else's, say, a woman from a rural village in Sierra Leone. While I was writing *Belly Woman*, the humanitarian sector was reflecting on its structures and how they perpetuate racist and colonial approaches to the work. Though not the focus of this book, the events described took place in an era when aid work was in need of reform. The terminology used is reflective of the period of writing. International staff, also referred to as expatriates or *expats*, lived and socialized together. The time working abroad was called a *mission* and the location was always the *field*. A part of my journey has been the growth in my awareness of the inequalities and imperfections of the modern humanitarian approach.

In writing this memoir, I have balanced the risk of being accused of playing the 'white saviour'. If I have presented myself as *that* person – possessing a superiority complex, patronizing tone or patriarchal stance – I apologize for my naivety and for any offence caused, but not for recording these events.

Some names have been changed and some events altered to maintain confidentiality and avoid collateral damage. Names of patients, if given at all, have been changed as have identifying and medical case details, with the exception of those already in the public domain. Memories are my own; no doubt they are far from perfect. Time and trauma can play many tricks on the mind, and, where these have resulted in errors, I take full responsibility and apologize.

In statistical terms, maternal deaths are often described as being the tip of an iceberg. For each death, approximately thirty women are severely or permanently disabled through complications of pregnancy. A large mass hidden below the water's surface, but no less significant.

Similarly, in writing this book, I could not tell every patient's story, nor do justice to all the people with whom I had the privilege of working or interacting. For each individual, there are at least another thirty, and where names or actions are not present in the pages that follow, it is no reflection of worthiness, but merely the result of the limitations of my mind and the confines of book writing.

The people and organizations I've written about faced stresses and circumstances at the extremes of human experience. Where my writing exposes failure, the failure is mine for inadequately portraying the complexities and nuances of the situation. I remain a proud member of the MSF movement, fiercely supportive of their incredible work, while accepting that they (which includes me and my actions) have faults.

Crises expose our resilience. The change in circumstance lays bare our personal and collective investment in social structures, trust and access to resources. It is no accident the Ebola epidemic swept through communities in the countries with some of the world's highest maternal and child death rates. It is no coincidence the worst-affected populations in epidemics are in neglected regions, conflict-affected areas, the poorest and most crowded districts. The disease moves within human suffering. The spread of disease is symptomatic of the status quo. Whether it be cholera in famished Yemen, diphtheria in an overcrowded Rohingya refugee camp of Bangladesh, or hepatitis E spreading in the unsanitary conditions of the displaced South Sudanese, the illness is opportunistic to the conditions we have handed it.

Through 2020, as the COVID-19 pandemic surged, I worked as an obstetrician and gynaecologist in London, joining my colleagues in the struggle to provide complex maternal healthcare to women with COVID-19, women without, and the many for whom we had no result, all while negotiating safety for health workers and pregnant women alike. In the evenings, I supported international humanitarian responses to the pandemic, considering dilemmas from across the world. How will women with pregnancy emergencies access care if all facilities shut down? How can we treat rape survivors? What if our supply of contraception burns out?

Over a hundred epidemics unified into one, the COVID-19 pandemic overwhelmed in spread and volume. As the dominoes fell, I asked, Could we have predicted what was coming?

When Ebola struck West Africa, the international community should have done better.

COVID-19 is not Ebola, but, like a circus mirror, there is enough to recognize within its distorted reflection.

Through my public catharsis, I am sharing the journey and decisions of the past. I hope you, the reader, will join me in questioning the events, their roots and the ramifications for the present. To ask: What does it mean to be humanitarian? How can we strive to prevent unnecessary deaths and needless suffering? Is it possible to avoid repeating previous errors?

Part 1

1: BIRTH COMPLICATIONS

GONDAMA, SIERRA LEONE

JULY 2014

The woman is lying on the floor outside the maternity department; her large pregnant belly slopes to one side as her back arches, face muscles clench and a violent, jerking convulsion resumes. It's past midnight, the air is warm and humid, hanging heavily around us. The two men who had squeezed her on to the back of their motorbike stand silently, staring; everyone is staring.

If this is an eclamptic seizure, her life, and that of her unborn child, can be saved. Take her inside the hospital, begin treatment and deliver the baby. The husband is watching us with red, pleading eyes. Every day, women come with emergencies; they come to us trusting we will treat them. But now we stand, frozen, contemplating the woman and the life lying on the floor in front of us.

Blood is round her nose and mouth.

'She fell forward on to her face with the first seizure,' says the weary looking husband.

Around the world, a woman dies every two minutes from a pregnancy-related complication, eclampsia being one of the leading causes. Virtually all maternal deaths are preventable. It is the reason we are here, and why she has come to us. Her death will be tragic, not only for herself and her children, but for her whole community. It will mean the loss of all the functions she, as a woman, brings to society.

Almost all maternal deaths occur in poor countries, affecting the most vulnerable, with the least resilience. A disparity so large is humiliating in our modern world, representing social, political and economic failures. Will we fail her, and her family too? An unseen force is holding us back;

the life-saving medicine is behind the door, in a room with other women in labour.

The seizure stops, her arms flop to her sides and her chest rises with rapid shallow breathing.

'What is your address?' a nurse in green scrubs shouts from several metres distance to the husband. Small beads of sweat shine on her forehead, reflecting the headlight of the motorbike.

They have travelled far. Their journey began in a town six hours away – a town with a recent cluster of Ebola cases. If this is Ebola, it changes everything.

Ebola, or Ebola virus disease, strikes fear into the public and healthcare workers alike. In 2014, no vaccine existed. There were no medical treatments available.

There are six species of Ebola virus;* the most lethal is the Zaire strain, which was deadly in approximately 60 to 90 per cent of cases. *Zaire ebolavirus* was responsible for the West African epidemic. Initially transmitted from an animal reservoir, probably from non-human primates or bats, into a human host, the disease spreads efficiently from person to person via infected body fluids. The incubation period is thought to last up to twenty-one days. Initial symptoms are general and non-specific: a fever, aching joints, weakness. Similar to other common ailments, such as malaria or influenza, it is easily missed. The virus infects the cells lining our blood vessels, organs and intestines. As our immune system tackles the onslaught, our body becomes the battlefield. Blood leaks from the vessels. Bowels seep fluid. Inflamed organs become painful and dysfunctional. The virus is deadly, but so too is the body's counter-attack, destroying itself in the effort to purge the invader. Over time, the condition develops into more severe vomiting and diarrhoea, which can progress to multiple organ failure and death.

As disease severity worsens, the infected person becomes increasingly contagious. By the time of death, their body is encased in their virus-packed excretions of urine, faeces and sweat. Those caring for the

---

* The six identified species of Ebola virus are each named after the place of their discovery, followed by '*ebolavirus*', the genus name, similar to a first name and family name in people. Four of the species are known to have caused disease in humans. The sixth species was identified in 2018, in Sierra Leone, but it is not known if it causes illness in humans or animals.

sick, offering comfort and washing their bodies, tread a perilous path. The risk of infection for healthcare workers in West Africa was up to thirty-two times greater than it was for the general public.

Her husband is becoming anxious. Why the questions? Why are we not rushing to save his wife and child? He gently places a folded cloth under her head and strokes her face. He brought her to us for help. Her situation is desperate. All he sees are the silhouettes of nurses, midwives and a doctor, conspiratorial and whispering.

With only one capable laboratory in the country, it will take over twenty-four hours for an Ebola test result to be returned. Without treatment for her pregnancy complications, she will die. Inside, there are tight rows of women sleeping under mosquito nets, next to babies bundled in brightly patterned lappa. In the daytime, breast milk, blood, sweat and soiled bed-clothes mix as the women congregate, sharing advice, joy and condolences.

An Ebola epidemic had been declared in March, across the border in Guinea; it had spread to Liberia in April. In Sierra Leone, there had been rumours of suspicious deaths for months, but no confirmed cases. Six weeks earlier, on 24 May, a pregnant woman had been admitted to Kenema Government Hospital's maternity ward because she was having a miscarriage. She was also feverish, with vomiting and diarrhoea. The pregnant woman had left a local health centre to seek further care at the hospital. On that same day in May, a forty-two-year-old mother of two, Mamie Lebbie, sought care at the same local health centre; she was suffering watery diarrhoea. Mamie came from Kailahun, in the south-east, near the Guinean border. She was suspected of having cholera, triggering an alert to be sent to the district surveillance team. On the advice of Sierra Leone's only virologist, Dr Sheik Humarr Khan, an urgent blood sample was sent to his laboratory in Kenema. Another woman, inside the Kenema Government Hospital, was also identified as having symptoms suggestive of Ebola; she too had come from the same local health clinic. The following day, all three women returned positive Ebola blood results. These women became the first confirmed cases of Ebola in the country.

They all had links to the funeral of a highly respected female traditional healer from Kailahun. The healer had been treating unwell people from both sides of the border, ultimately leading to her infection and death on 30 April. The traditional rituals of washing and touching the deceased body followed, so that her death and burial were linked to some 365 Ebola deaths and were key in contributing to the onwards spread, resulting in 14,124 infections and 3,956 subsequent deaths in Sierra Leone. But not Mamie Lebbie or the pregnant woman; among the country's first confirmed patients were their first two confirmed survivors.

In the weeks that passed since those Ebola results there were more confirmed cases, and further spread into the country. Healthcare workers were on alert. Vigilant to ask, could this be Ebola?

A light breeze momentarily breaks the tension. The triage paper used for checking Ebola symptoms has become soft with the rainy season's moisture. Glances pass from one person to another, piercing through the night air. The woman lies unconscious. Should she come inside maternity, or stay outside? Eclampsia or Ebola? If the diagnosis is incorrect, by the time it is realized, the damage will be done.

*

The scene was already set; the actors of a peripheral state government, egotistical international organizations and an impoverished population were in position. The stage had been built on a history of pillage: slavery, colonialism, civil war, corruption, plunder and disenfranchisement. The Ebola epidemic might have begun in December 2013, but the legacy of injustice stretched back centuries. Seeds of mistrust had been planted in a collective memory, with ample time for the roots to take hold.

As the sick attended health facilities and traditional healers for help, their misdiagnoses and the touching, and spreading, of infected body fluids, together with the chronically under-resourced government institutions, provided fertile ground for the amplification of disease. Although ten countries were affected, it was Guinea, Sierra Leone and Liberia that bore the greatest burden of the Ebola epidemic. In total, there were 28,652 cases reported, including 11,325 deaths – although the full extent is certainly higher, and will never be known. It led to the near breakdown of a vulnerable and weak health system. The resulting deaths from the loss and fear of healthcare possibly outstripping those directly from Ebola .

Ebola lifted the curtain on a performance that had been playing out for decades. And the audience could watch, participate or turn away.

2: PRE-DEPARTURE PLANNING

CAMDEN, LONDON

MONDAY, 16 JUNE 2014, 7.30 A.M.

I am on the floor, sitting on top of a bag I have spent weeks deliber-
ating over. I try to squeeze another book inside the rucksack. No
matter how I manoeuvre myself, or the zip, it won't close. My parents look at the room; clothes and belongings are sprawled across the
floor, with me in the middle.

'Have you packed some snacks, for when you arrive?' asks Mum,
trying to sound relaxed.

I glance up from my position on the bulging bag. My face says it all:
Do. Not. Talk. To. Me. They retreat.

My parents had travelled down from their home in Manchester to
bid me farewell. I'm thirty-two years old, a doctor, their youngest child
and only son, pausing my career, and all our lives, to pursue my ambitions
in the humanitarian sector.

Soon, I will begin a journey to Brussels for briefings from MSF's
Operational Centre (OC). From there, I will continue to Sierra Leone.
MSF has hundreds of projects, working in over seventy countries, providing emergency and medical assistance. I had spent days reading their
reports, (self-critical and reflective); and evenings reading the testimonies of their field workers, (emotive and exhilarating). I wanted to be a
part of their independent, humanitarian, medical identity, getting to the
places where aid was needed most.

MSF has a complicated organizational structure. It is split into five
separate sections, each with its own culture and operational priorities;
they are, however, united under a single manifesto and logo. The sections are named after the cities where their headquarters reside: Paris,
Brussels, Amsterdam, Geneva and Barcelona. The Operational Centre

of Brussels, or OCB, had been present in Sierra Leone for many years, and their maternal and child health hospital was a jewel in their crown, both in terms of size and the numbers of patients treated.

The project was called the Gondama Referral Centre, or GRC. It was located close to Bo city, the largest city after the capital, Freetown. I was aware of the project, as it was a well-known destination for obstetricians working with MSF.

I had sat in a stuffy London pub on Great Portland Street with another obstetric doctor, Pip, who had spent two years out in the field with MSF, six months of which were in GRC. 'You'll be fine,' she'd told me, as she recalled massive haemorrhages, tropical infections and near-death experiences.

In the months before I was sent to GRC, a strategic decision had been made at the Brussels headquarters for it to stop providing maternity care. Child healthcare was to continue, and their interest in Lassa fever, an endemic viral haemorrhagic fever in the area, was increasing, but maternity would end in June 2014.

In May, the World Health Organization (WHO) had released an updated report on global trends in maternal mortality. Sierra Leone had the highest ratio of women dying to live births in the world. According to MSF's own calculations, GRC had resulted in an over 60 per cent decrease in women dying from childbirth locally and was providing around a fifth of all caesarean sections in the country. Women from a geographical area spanning over a third of the country travelled there for life-saving interventions and surgery. This project was important. But, at some strategic level, maternal health was not important enough.

Internal organizational pressure led to a swift U-turn and a decision at the eleventh hour to continue obstetric services, though the longer-term future of the facility remained uncertain. Suddenly, a service that had been facing imminent closure had openings for obstetricians which needed filling fast. I was called and asked if I could be there within two weeks.

I had built my ambitions on the stories and experiences of civil wars, earthquakes and refugee migrations. I wondered if I was selling out by going to a stable *development* setting, rather than a fragile *humanitarian* crisis. An awareness was rising up inside me, though there was a lot of talk of ensuring that reproductive health, including access to emergency obstetric care, was available in every humanitarian response, but the reality was very different. Rather than being prioritized, it was often substituted with proxy activities, leaving limited demand for an obstetrician.

Through medical school, I had studied with the intention of becoming an aid worker, considering specialties with this in mind. A decade earlier, I spent several months working with refugees and migrants crossing from Myanmar into Thailand. The maternal health needs were striking. Women came to us with late complications, or needing a safe place to give birth. Sometimes they arrived after delivering in the jungle, with horribly infected babies. Every day, women would attend with complications of backstreet abortions; without access to contraception or legal abortions, they turned to any willing provider. Dire poverty left many with little choice. Sex was an industry, a way to procure goods, to survive, to feed children or keep a job in a saturated labour market. Women, often girls, arrived bleeding, infected and internally damaged. Despite all the harm to the woman, the botched abortion could be distressingly unsuccessful; often the pregnancy continued unaffected. It was here, as a twenty-three-year-old student, that I concluded obstetrics and gynaecology was my path into humanitarian assistance. The needs were vast, and I was drawn to the deeper questions of how to respond beyond medicines and surgery. The specialty offered everything: it was broad enough to keep me well informed on general medicine, while specialized enough to be of value to a population in crisis.

I took further studies and read book after book on how development and aid agencies had entered into situations with good intentions, but poor outcomes. I learnt about the history, evolution and errors of major aid organizations and how their past shaped their work today. Rather than deterring me, this information made me even more curious. How could we keep getting it wrong? Lessons identified were often called 'lessons learnt', but, as I continued to read, this seemed less convincing. My desire to be part of the humanitarian system grew, as my questions of its effectiveness flourished alongside.

Towards the end of March 2014, Ebola virus was confirmed in Guinea.* MSF had assisted in the initial suspicions and identification of the disease.

---

* The alleged index case of the Ebola epidemic has been traced back to December 2013, in Guekedu, Guinea. However, the first confirmatory tests were in late March 2014.

The virus had taken an unusual and concerning course, entering urban areas and crossing international borders – first into Liberia in April, and then Sierra Leone in late May. I had been following the story, but held no desire to be involved in the Ebola response. I was unfamiliar with the disease, and did not see how it could relate to my role.

The week before I was due to leave, I spoke on the phone to Severine, the obstetrics and gynaecology adviser for MSF-OCB. She was out in GRC at the time, and she reassured me that there had been no Ebola cases in the area of the project, the outbreak remaining contained in the east, around the Guinean border. The general consensus was that Lassa fever was of much greater concern, in terms of exposure and risk. I left for Sierra Leone knowing Ebola was there, but without any genuine anticipation that I would encounter it. In retrospect, it seems ridiculous; the epidemic, as we know now, was unprecedented. But, in early June, we had a dragon under our feet only just beginning to awaken; the ferocity and fire were yet to come.

Standing outside the MSF Operational Centre of Brussels, I felt like I was about to enter a special society. Through those doors, huge decisions were made on access to life-saving interventions, often with uncertain consequences. I was about to walk into one of my textbooks, words and thoughts lifting off the page to become people and discussions in meeting rooms. This was the inner sanctum of one of the most recognized non-governmental organizations in the world, a searchlight shining out to me through a haze of humanitarian scepticism.

People rushed around, smiling, chatting, shaking hands. A dynamism filled the air; the energy was a vibrant, and firm: 'Let's get the job done.' In a moment, I had moved from outsider to insider. I wanted to get the job done too.

As the administrative team sorted out my visa applications, a woman around my age came and joined me at the desk. Alice was also heading to Sierra Leone; she was flying out as part of the first MSF Ebola response team in the country. I was impressed by her calmness. There was no shred of fear on her face, just a concern about whether she could fit all the dolls and teddy bears in her bag for the children she would work with. Alice was Danish, a psychologist, and her role was to provide psychosocial support to survivors and families affected by the outbreak.

'I'm an obstetric doctor, heading out to GRC,' I told her.

She squinted her eyes. 'So you're a very important person then.'

I thought it was a strange comment from a woman who was about to head into an Ebola outbreak. I shrugged, 'We're all important people'.

Making my way around the office, each person I met gave me more papers to read, documents to sign and encouragement that I was joining a great project.

Severine, the obstetrics and gynaecology adviser, had travelled into Brussels especially to see me before my departure. We sat together at a long desk, the walls on either side decorated with large maps and magazine-style pictures of refugee camps, MSF operating theatres and striking faces staring into the lens.

Severine spoke modestly, with an air of understated competence. 'You can see the full obstetric textbook in one shift,' she said. 'That's how it is, in the field.' She had worked in many MSF missions, including GRC, before taking the headquarters position. She had the stories and understanding of being a doctor from a high-income country working in a resource restricted setting. 'Obstetrics in the usual MSF settings and obstetrics in the UK are separated not only by geography, but in nature too,' she said.

I already knew I would be dealing with cases and carrying out procedures I had never had to perform before, because the situations leading to the necessity for such procedures were unheard of in London. Gaining another ten years' experience in London would be no guarantee of exposure to such operations.

Severine shared her experience of performing obstetric hysterectomies, repairing ruptured uteruses and the technique of replacing blood directly from a haemorrhaging patient back into the same patient's body during surgery. 'I brought these for you to see.' She pushed a small pile of textbooks towards me. 'These are my bibles in the field. If you're faced with an unfamiliar situation, they can be lifesavers.'

We discussed working alongside local and international colleagues, differences in work ethics and expectations, and ways to manage the inevitable tricky situations arising from the power, economic and cultural dynamics at play.

As we spoke, I was increasingly reassured that I had backup, but I also felt trepidation. I was entering into a mixing pot of more than just complex obstetrics.

'The national staff are still feeling quite sensitive about the decision to close obstetrics at GRC,' Severine said. Her voice changed a notch. 'Some staff had already taken new jobs when MSF reversed the closure. These people, they thought they were losing their jobs till a couple of weeks ago; many are the breadwinners for the family. It has caused quite some loss of morale. It damaged our relationship a bit. The expected closure has also impacted our patient numbers, but I think the news will travel and they will return.'

'So obstetrics will stay?' I asked.

'This decision was last minute. I believe it will be temporary, but maybe we can change their minds.'

I was astonished that ending obstetric activities was still on the table, given the maternal health indicators. I wondered how the Sierra Leonean staff would relate to me while their long-term future remained uncertain.

'You need to know about Lassa fever,' said Severine, moving the briefing forwards. 'It's a major concern for the project, particularly on the obstetric side, where we've had several staff infections.'

I was asked to complete forms in case I caught Lassa fever and medical evacuation became necessary, or if I had symptoms after my mission was over. I signed that I understood the protocols of infection control, and was given more to read about the disease, its symptoms and ways to reduce the risk.

Lassa fever is transmitted to humans in the urine and faeces of the multimammate rat;* strict measures were in place to keep the rodents out of our work and living areas. Once infected, the disease can be passed between humans through direct contact with bodily fluids – hence, a clear risk of exposure during childbirth and major surgery. Lassa fever and Ebola share many similarities, but there were also important differences. Lassa fever was endemic in the region; it had been a part of the differential diagnoses for many years and was particularly recognized as a complicating factor leading to death in pregnancy. The majority of people who contracted Lassa fever displayed no symptoms or complications at all. However, for those who did become unwell, there was a 20

---

* The multimammate rat (which isn't actually a rat) is a reservoir for Lassa fever. The rodent appears similar to a mouse or small rat. Once infected, the rodent excretes the Lassa virus, potentially for all its life. They live close to humans, scavenging leftover food, and breed rampantly.

per cent risk of death. Crucially, there was an antiviral medication, called ribavirin, which, if given early and appropriately, appeared to be effective against the disease.

As my day of briefings drew to an end, I felt ready. The time was now. This large, busy and chaotic office had opened its arms to me and I wanted to be embraced. In a short day, I had met many people, in some cases for just a few minutes, who would cross my path over the years to follow in ways I could not anticipate.

'We are going to watch Belgium play in the World Cup,' said Severine, gesturing to a group of her colleagues. 'Join us?'

We all headed over to an open-air square, where we drank and chatted until the game began, shown on a huge screen. When Belgium scored, the crowd cheered and spontaneous dancing broke out. Beers were thrown up in the air in celebration. A real sense of optimism surrounded me and I breathed it in as much as I could. Summer was in the air and everyone was relaxed.

A woman with a short blond bob haircut sat next to me. 'I'm Liesbeth,' she said. 'I hear you're heading to GRC.'

News travels fast, I thought.

'I spent over a year working there,' she explained. 'You're going to like it; it's a great first mission. Very social, low-security setting and beautiful country.' Liesbeth was looking at me, but I felt her mind was seeing the past.

Her reminiscence was broken as another round of beers arrived at our table.

'Proost!' said Liesbeth, and we clinked our drinks. 'I'll be joining you out there next week. Last time I was there, some of our colleagues caught Lassa fever. There was a lot of stress then.' Liesbeth's voice was gentle, but I sensed a flicker of emotion as she recalled the challenges of trying to get the correct safety measures in place. 'The staff needed to feel they were protected. They were asking for a lot and we really tried, while we could see standards were not being maintained.' It was clear she had had a difficult time, but also, she had come through it with solid achievements and character. 'So, I'll be lending a bit of extra support to the project, just for a few weeks.'

'Great – I'll be waiting for you,' I said, feeling glad there would be a familiar face joining me within my first week.

Drunk, I wobbled my way back to the hostel. I spent the rest of the night trying to download textbooks on tropical medicine, messaging friends and staring at my bag which needed to be totally repacked.

The next day, I met Alice, the psychologist, in the boarding queue for the plane to Freetown. On arrival at Lungi International Airport, about seven hours later. There was little to suggest the threat of Ebola other than a couple of small posters pinned to the wall at immigration. Alice and I spotted a tall bearded guy with an MSF-logo holdall bag. Frederick was an experienced water and sanitation specialist (usually referred to as a 'WatSan') who was also heading to the border with Guinea, where the newest MSF Ebola Treatment Centre was due to open. The three of us continued our journey together.

Lungi airport sits on a peninsula facing the capital, and the quickest way to reach Freetown is by ferry. By the time we arrived at the jetty, the sun was already beginning to set. The warm salty air smelt like holidays, women walked along the beach with baskets balanced on their heads and children pranced around in the sand. It was an idyllic scene.

Frederick and Alice were familiar with the routine of arriving at a new project, but, for me, everything was new. We got to the house where we were to spend our first night in Sierra Leone and were met by an administrator, who gave each of us a mobile telephone and an envelope with instructions and security rules. We left our bags and together headed to a local restaurant, where we ate rice with dried fish as we discussed what the next few weeks might hold for us. They both appeared relaxed, and there was no discussion of Ebola impacting the work I would be doing. After that night, we were heading to two very different realities, or so we thought. That was Wednesday evening, 18 June.

3: GONDAMA

THURSDAY, 19 JUNE 2014

I woke early on Thursday morning, hot and sticky. I pulled myself up and out from under the mosquito net and took a cold shower. I was to be interviewed by a representative from the Ministry of Health to gain my licence to practise medicine in Sierra Leone. I wanted to make a good impression and had packed long khaki trousers, a smart sky-blue shirt and black leather shoes specifically for the interview. It wasn't yet 9 a.m. and I was already sweating. Evidently, I had chosen a poor colour for concealing perspiration. I looked terrible, with sweat patches across my shirt. I focused on my breathing to try to keep calm, fanning myself to keep cool. None of it helped much.

I sat alone in the stuffy waiting room; two secretaries sat opposite me, typing and sweating. Eventually, I was called into the representative's freezing air-conditioned room. The air hit me like an ice wall – at first a relief, though I soon felt hypothermic. The representative was a formally dressed, slight and skinny man. He sat behind a large heavy wooden desk, which, by comparison, made him look even skinnier and smaller. Peering over his glasses, he seemed to size me up and gestured for me to take a seat. He rustled through an application form, which had been completed on my behalf by the MSF in-country team. He looked at me, said nothing, then looked and rustled through my papers again.

'What is the purpose of your time in Sierra Leone?'

'I'm here with MSF; I'll be working at the obstetric referral centre.'

His eyebrows moved together, forming a cross of creases between them. 'I see you have a master's degree in conflict and development. What's that got to do with your time here?'

I paused, feeling the thin ice below me as I uneasily manoeuvred for an answer. I began trying to broaden the conversation, inviting him into subjects such as the long-term impact of conflict on development and sustainable healthcare. This wasn't what I had been expecting.

'Well, I don't see how you can work here.'

My heart pumped hard and my hands became clammy as I felt my stomach open up. I was going to be denied a permit and sent home. I didn't even understand why, except that he was unimpressed by my choice of studies.

'But I'm a doctor. I'm trained in obstetrics and gynaecology; you have a lot of women dying here.'

He looked at me again, then at my papers and back to me.

'You're not a qualified doctor.'

We looked at each other across the large wooden desk. I was confused.

'Can I see those papers?' I asked.

The only qualification listed was my master's degree. Desperation lurched within me. I opened my bag and pulled out my own copies of my medical certificates, explaining each one.

The man's face softened as he leafed his way through the pages. He looked sternly at me again. 'You did not fill this application yourself.'

The atmosphere relaxed and we continued our conversation in a friendlier way. He stamped my papers and signalled our time was up.

I returned to Alice and Frederick in the waiting car, where I threw off the formal gear, returning to the comfort of my shorts, T-shirt and flip-flops. 'Let's go!' I said.

We planned to drive directly to Bo, some three and a half hours away, where I would disembark and Frederick and Alice would continue for another four hours or so to the north-eastern border town of Kailahun. The road out of Freetown wound through green hills, the steep slopes sweeping down to the Atlantic Ocean. We glided along the tarmac, past little clusters of stalls, shacks and small groups of women with children, standing around large wooden mortars, pounding rice with long sticks. I drifted in and out of sleep in the hot car, vaguely aware of the murmuring voices in the front, as Alice and Frederick talked about the project they were heading to. I opened my eyes, registering the towns we were passing through, occasionally catching a blast of West African pop music from outside. Finally, we pulled off the highway into a large walled compound.

Flying overhead was the iconic MSF flag: a sketch of a figure standing, arms and legs apart, drawn from red and white diagonal lines.

A tall Sierra Leonean man approached our car. 'Welcome to Bo Base!' he said, as we all got out. I offered him my hand to introduce myself, but he just looked at it and smiled. 'We don't shake hands here.' He then demonstrated the alternatives – either putting a right hand to the left chest or tapping elbows. At first, I thought perhaps this was a cultural variation to handshaking, but it was my introduction to the *no-touch* policy. We were directed to a Veronica bucket – a large bucket mounted on a wooden stool, with a tap fixed near the base and a bowl underneath. 'Wash your hands with the chlorinated water before entering any buildings, then rinse the tap before turning it off,' the man said.

At first glance, Bo Base looked like a garage: a large tarmac courtyard, filled with white Toyota Land Cruisers. Men stood around, hosing down the Land Cruisers and checking their tyres.

We were directed through a side-door into a large concrete building and up a dark, narrow staircase. We climbed up the steep incline, at the summit it opened up to a large atrium. There were couches arranged in a big horseshoe shape, and scattered around the perimeter were tables, chairs and electric fans. Several offices and smaller meeting rooms surrounded the main gathering space, which was comfortable and welcoming, filled with natural light from the many windows.

The three of us made our way over to a long table where a group of people were eating lunch. Every day, new expats passed in and out of Bo Base, either coming to GRC or on their journey to Kailahun. We joined the group and began investigating the food situation. I felt awkward, uncertain how my vegetarianism would be viewed. I picked at the cold pasta salad, trying to discreetly remove the pieces of pink meat. Gradually, everyone introduced themselves: logisticians, administrators, medics. Two women marched in together, speaking in rapid French. It was evident from their purposeful manner that they were in significant positions. One was tall and statuesque, as if made of alabaster, and she came and joined us at the table, while the other disappeared into a side office.

The woman introduced herself as Kathleen, cocking her head and smiling at the three new people at the table. As she ate her lunch, she told us she had come to GRC in a senior nursing position, but had recently changed her role to 'Ebola focal person', given the uncertain situation in the country.

Alice looked at her for a moment, took a deep breath and announced, 'So, you're a very important person now'.

Kathleen stopped eating. 'What does that mean? When I was a nurse, I was very important.'

I smiled, recalling my own first meeting with Alice.

The other woman came back into the room from the side office. She didn't sit with us, but headed straight to one of the faux-leather couches and pulled out a pack of cigarettes, lit up and took long hard drags. She said nothing, just looked straight into the smoke rising in front of her face, scrying for something. She had a sharp penetrating stare, and her eyes narrowed as she turned to the table.

'Barbara, this is Benjamin, our new gynae,' said Kathleen.

From the couch, Barbara motioned for me to come over and join her. She introduced herself as the project coordinator, or PC, responsible for security and the daily functioning of the project. She reminded me a bit of Dalia, my oldest sister; they had similar long brown curly hair. Her intense mannerisms were similar too, and in this I found comfort. I was on familiar ground.

There was no time for small talk: 'I'm heading to the hospital in fifteen minutes,' she said. 'You can join me. I'll give you your briefing over there.'

I said goodbye to Alice and Frederick, who would be continuing their journey east, and climbed into the back of a Land Cruiser with Barbara and Kathleen. GRC was about six miles from Bo, but the roads were in such a terrible condition that the journey took about thirty minutes. I had arrived at the beginning of the rainy season; these muddy potholed roads would become increasingly waterlogged and, at times, impassable.

I gripped my seat as I was jolted and thrown about, while Barbara continued talking, unaffected. 'You'll be replacing Crys,' she said. 'She's been here for three months. She works with two other gynaes: Marlon, the team leader – he's been in the project a long time; He'll soon be replaced. He –' Barbara hesitated – 'he's very tired. And then there's Mamadou, from Guinea. He's working on his English. You'll have to speak slowly. Mamadou's going to take over the position of team leader when Marlon leaves.' Barbara glanced at me in the rear-view mirror, 'The whole team is tired, you'll see.'

The car crossed over a long narrow bridge, and through the red metal railings I could see the waters of the River Sewa gushing over the large rocks below, crashing into small whirlpools. Crowds of people were vigorously washing their clothes and their bodies on the sloping shores. At the end of the bridge, the metal railings were torn open, twisted like a ribbon and dangling over the side, where a vehicle had hurtled through, dropping into the river below. Not hugely reassuring. We took a sharp left past a small village of resettled Liberian refugees, and continued down a straight mud road, past a primary healthcare centre, which MSF also supported, to the heavy metal gates of the Gondama Referral Centre. A sign was fixed next to the gate; in large painted letters, it declared this a place for *serious problems in pregnancy and delivery*.

I already knew one of the doctors working in GRC. I had met Alessandro back in March, when we spent a week together in Germany on a preparatory course for new MSF volunteers.* He was tall, lanky, the epitome of an extrovert, and he spoke in a thick Italian accent, his long arms moving in time with its rhythm, as if conducting his own orchestra. During the workshops on humanitarianism we had shared opinions. Over meals and drinks in the bar, we had continued the debates, which evolved into lengthy conversations stretching into all reaches of our lives. We confided our ambitions and our fears to each other, what we hoped to gain from our time with MSF and what we were afraid we'd miss out on at home while we were away. Alessandro had already been in Sierra Leone for three months, and when Severine had mentioned my name regarding the availability of an obstetric post, he had told her, 'Take him'. Knowing he would be there among all the unfamiliar faces was some comfort to me.

Barbara had work to do, and I was keen to find the obstetrician, Crys, and see the maternity department for myself. Barbara called Crys on her mobile, but she was scrubbed in theatre for a caesarean section. Hearing this, a wave of anxiety rippled through me. I was actually here, and I really would be performing surgery in this place. Barbara gave me directions, but within a moment I was lost. GRC was made up of separate one-storey buildings and a street map of deep troughs, built to drain the

---

* Although international aid workers are often referred to as volunteers, they are paid for their time working with MSF. The local employees receive a salary.

heavy rainfall away. There was no obvious system or plan and I had no orientation as to where I was. I was a stranger in a strange land.

'Is this the maternity?' I asked a Sierra Leonean nurse standing at the entrance to one of the buildings.

'You need to put scrubs on before you come in here,' she said, dismissing me.

There was no moment of welcome. No formalities at all. This may have all been new to me, but for those working in the department I was just another expat who would come, stay a while and then leave, like the many others before me.

Once I had discovered where to find scrubs, I got changed into the oversized vestments. The large V of the scrub top reached down to my midriff. I yanked it back, hoping to appear less exposed. I put a mob hat and face mask on and cautiously stepped into the operating theatre. Standing on either side of the operating table was the surgeon and an assistant, both completely covered from head to toe, with just a small slit for their eyes, as if they were operating in synthetic burkas. I tiptoed over and let my presence in the theatre be known. Crys was stitching the uterus; I watched as she efficiently brought the two sides together. A knock came from the swinging door connecting the theatre to the delivery room, and a head popped around the side. A tall, broad Kenyan midwife shouted across the theatre, 'Are you almost done? We need to do another.'

Crys shouted back over, 'What's the problem?'

'Fetal heart rate is slow, not coming back up.'

'OK, get her prepared.'

My heart pounded. There were so many questions rushing through my head. In all the literature and discussions before I came out to the field, the indications for a caesarean section were explained to be predominantly for the life of the mother. One fifteen-year-old girl out of every twenty-one in Sierra Leone, at that time, was estimated to die from childbirth complications during her lifetime . Many of the women would go on to have a high number of pregnancies. Performing a caesarean section was a decision to be taken judiciously. Leaving a permanent scar on the uterus would expose the woman to higher-risk pregnancies in the future and additional complications. Fetal distress was hard to judge when only using a handheld fetal heart rate monitor. If the diagnosis was correct, distress due to a lack of oxygen reaching the fetus's brain, then you risked performing a caesarean for a baby with a poor chance of survival, in a place with limited resources for resuscitation or ongoing care. I understood the logic to this, even though it sat a world away from the type of obstetric care in labour I was used to, which was largely fetal-focused, with high rates of intervention and neonatal intensive care units. Working in a maternity ward back home was like being in a constant pressure cooker, the clock always ticking and there was huge stress to ensure interventions happened rapidly. If a midwife on a labour ward in the UK announced that a fetal heart rate was slow and not recovering, the alarms would be ringing. The crash call for emergency teams would have gone out. Within minutes, the woman would be on the operating table and the baby out. Here, this same diagnosis was met with routine normality, no rush. Get her prepared and put her in the queue.

The caesarean section over, Crys de-robed, revealing a confident and forthright person, with a trendy disposition. I could easily imagine her working in any large European or US city.

'Let's get a cup of tea,' she said over her shoulder as she began heading out of the department. It was more like a command than a suggestion. I ran behind, my brain still trying to figure out what was going on. Wasn't an emergency caesarean for fetal distress about to begin?

'Nothing happens quickly here,' Crys said, as if reading my thoughts. 'You'll get used to it.' She turned back to the team. 'Call me when she's in.'

I didn't know where to begin, I had so many questions about working in GRC. What was the daily routine? What were the local nurses and midwives like? Who could I trust and who should I not? Where were the notes written, and who should I call if there was a disaster? What about blood for transfusion? What about HIV? What about Lassa fever?

In the break room Crys made her tea, rearranged a fan so it blew directly on to her and then lay down on a couch. She was already experienced at working in this setting, having spent time in Afghanistan, Pakistan and other MSF projects. There was no messing around; we were straight down to business and she was giving me the proverbial coffee.

'This is not doctors without borders. It's logistics without borders.' She began a monologue of all that was right and wrong with MSF, sharing her frustrations and aspirations for a different way of working. As with many disgruntled humanitarian-sector employees, even as she complained, she was simultaneously thinking out loud about where and when her next mission would be. 'Maybe I'll try Emergency or ICRC, see how they do it.' Crys turned towards me. 'Lassa fever has been a major worry here. You need to question every patient for symptoms before approaching them and keep direct contact to a minimum. Trust no one.' She sat up and sipped her tea. 'I'd be frightened, if I were you. Marlon and I, we're getting out at the right time. This Ebola, it's out of control; if it gets here, you'll be in real trouble.'

I felt my stomach turn over. 'What do you think will happen?'

'I don't know. Maybe you'll all be evacuated. It's hard to say, but they won't let you keep working. It's too dangerous, and they wanted to close the maternity anyway. I'm just glad I'm getting out of here now.'

I walked over to the water dispenser, on the wall above it there was a map of Sierra Leone. Someone had placed little paper butterflies on the map.

'This is pretty,' I said.

'The butterflies?' Crys looked up from the couch. 'They are where the Ebola cases have been reported.'

I studied the flight path. It seemed, sooner or later, a little butterfly could be landing near our clinic.

With Crys I felt secure; she had an air of authority and cool competence. I regretted that I was replacing her; I would have much preferred to be joining her. We headed back over to maternity, where the woman for the next caesarean section was having a spinal anaesthetic placed by the nurse anaesthetist.

'Is it OK if I do this one?' I asked.

I felt, the sooner I got the first operation over with, the better. And to have Crys with me – rather than being alone, in the middle of the night – seemed ideal.

A strict system of infection control was observed in the operating theatre, designed to limit infections to patients (there was a high rate of serious wound infection) and Lassa fever exposure to the staff. Once inside, shoes were changed to wellington boots, all of which were huge on me. The scrubs I was already wearing were exchanged for fresh scrubs and a surgical cap, which would be worn for the surgery only.

In the scrubbing area, I dressed in a heavy apron, which went from my neck down to the floor, a tight 'duck-beak' face mask and a balaclava-like hood that covered all of my head and neck, leaving only a small slit for the eyes. The hood also had a face mask attached, which needed to be torn in the middle so the duck-beak could slip through. Lastly, large goggles, similar to those worn when snorkelling, were placed over the eye slit and the elastic pulled tight, the toggle resting just behind the crown of my head. The goggles were scratched from the repeated washes between surgeries, making everything appear clouded. With the additional layers on, and the adrenaline of uncertainty before my first MSF surgery, I began getting hot and sweaty. I did not yet have the standard surgical gown on.

After washing my hands and arms three times with surgical scrub and then once with alcohol gel, I made my way into the operating theatre, where the patient was having her spinal anaesthetic. The 'runner', who assists in the theatre with non-sterile tasks, helped me with my surgical gown. There were only extra-large sizes, and the gown floated and trailed behind me like a blue wedding dress. The standard was to wear a normal set of surgical gloves, with a second set of gynaecological gauntlets over the top. The gauntlets reached up to the elbow. Unfortunately, these too only came in sizes significantly bigger than my hands and arms, leaving little unfilled stumps of glove at the end of each finger and a loose arm-fitting that risked dropping down during surgery.

The patient was lying flat on the table, with her pregnant belly sloping to one side. I asked for a midwife to check the baby was still alive before I cleaned the woman's abdomen. Through the Doppler machine, we heard the gentle gallop of the fetal heartbeat. Together with Crys, we prepared the area for surgery and placed surgical drapes over the patient's abdomen.

Though the set of surgical instruments were adequate for the operation, there were slight differences from the standard sets I was used to: instruments that usually came solid were hollow, there were fewer clamps and the ratchets were loose. Everything was familiar, but different. I was desperate for my first surgery to be slick, leaving a good impression. Instead, I was clumsy and cack-handed. The oversized gloves meant I couldn't feel the tissues properly and had a poor grasp of the instruments. As I became hotter from the layers covering me, my goggles became increasingly fogged. Sweat and condensation began collecting in the bottom, little puddles making me feel like I was constantly surfacing from a swimming pool. The delivery of the baby was uncomplicated, but using the needle to suture the layers of uterus and abdomen back together was torture, as my fingers ended about a centimetre behind where they appeared to be. I knew I was performing well below my ability. By the time I reached the skin, I was exhausted and deeply disappointed in myself. I could not see through one side of the goggles. I needed to work with my head tilted to stop the collection of sweat from going into my single seeing eye. What should normally take thirty minutes took me close to an hour.

By the time I took off the surgical gown and apron, my scrubs were completely soaked with sweat. My hands looked like I had been in the bath too long from all the sweat accumulated inside the gloves. The face masks were dripping. Embarrassed, I attempted to justify my difficulties to Crys. She smiled and confessed, 'I normally don't wear the goggles at all. I was trying to set a good example'. She looked me in the eyes, 'But you should.'

I changed back into the dry scrubs, sat to write my notes, then thanked the theatre team and headed out to find Barbara for my briefings. GRC was split between two sites: one was the hospital; the other, across a mud road, was for administration and storage. I crossed over and found her in the administration building, sitting diligently at a desk. Barbara grabbed her cigarettes and we headed outside to a concrete cylindrical hut, referred to as a tukul.* Storm clouds were gathering above us, there was a low grumbling of thunder and the air had become heavy. As we sat down, a large crack split the sky and the rain began to pour. Barbara, unfazed by the natural drama unfolding, lit a cigarette, took a long steady drag and held it a moment, before blowing the smoke out and turning to me.

'This is your first mission.'

I wasn't sure if it was a question, statement or judgement. Barbara had years of humanitarian experience behind her; she had worked in some of the most challenging and unstable countries of recent history, both with

---

* A tukul is an East African cone-shaped hut, usually made of mud, with a thatched roof. We used the term more generically at GRC, to refer to any cylindrical gathering place.

MSF and other international organizations. I was full of admiration for her, and simultaneously intimidated. She sat thoughtfully, and a moment of quiet passed as she continued to smoke.

'This will be your best mission, and your worst. The first mission is something special. It's intense. Everyone cries at some point during their first mission, you'll see. And the people you meet, that connection of being on first mission together – so special. I'm a little envious.'

She took another long, thoughtful drag. The rain continued to fall heavily around us. Barbara got her pad out and began working systematically through her list of subjects she needed to brief me on: living arrangements, security, transport, Lassa fever, the team structure and the lines of communication. Who did what and who to call when things went wrong. In the MSF hierarchy, I was a low rung on a tall ladder. The rain stopped, but our conversation continued. We moved from the project to my wider views and personal goals.

'What do you think about the Ebola situation?' I asked.

Barbara lit another cigarette. She explained that they had decided to prepare, in case the outbreak spread to the hospital. 'We think it is unlikely, but it's better we have everything in place.' In her opinion, although it was over a decade since the civil war had ended, the country remained volatile. It was not possible to predict what would happen. This felt like more than a briefing; she was sharing. Barbara's physical similarities to my sister were mirrored in her personality. I looked upon her as a protective sibling from that first day onwards.

I returned to Bo Base, collected my bags and took a car to the house where I would be living. Each house had a name – either a city or an exotic location – and I was in Vienna House, with eight other expats. It was gated, all on one level and spacious, with an outside seating area. Kathleen was also living in Vienna, and she showed me around, explaining the intricate rules for infection control. As with all other buildings, before entering or leaving, I needed to wash my hands with chlorinated water. There were different coloured bins for different waste, buckets of chlorine for used plates and cutlery, and chlorine for soaking vegetables in. There was a supermarket we could buy food from, but we were no longer allowed to go to the main market, as it was crowded and may result in contact with someone who was unwell. Bread could be bought from the roadside kiosks, but it had to be re-cooked in the oven to reduce any risk of illness from a vendor's dirty hands. The many rules were intended to mitigate the risks of all illnesses, and they created an environment where behaviour was dictated by an invisible enemy. Every meeting when hands weren't shaken, every meal where food was reheated and every time chlorine was used, we were reminded that a risk was present.

My bedroom had a large bed with a mosquito net tied above it, and a small wooden desk and chair facing the window, looking out to the entry gate. At the end of the corridor was the bathroom and shower. I unpacked my bag and tried to make the room feel like my own. Whenever I heard the front door open, I would poke my head into the corridor and introduce myself. Each person would exchange pleasantries and then move on to their own business; there was no moment of excitement or extended conversation. In the end, I sat and ate my dinner alone, before retreating back to my room.

I lay on my bed and thought about the last twenty-four hours. I had only just arrived and had already performed my first surgery, but I also felt out of sorts. Crys and the other obstetric doctors seemed more experienced than me and I worried I would not live up to the requirements of the project. The other expats that I had met so far, although nice, were not chatty in the way my friends back home would be. A feeling of aloneness washed over me. As I let my mind run free and thought about the people and problems I had left behind in London, I heard a gentle knock on my door.

'Hi?' I said, scrambling to my feet.

'Hey, I'm Juli.' A young woman with short brown hair stood casually in the doorway. 'I just wanted to say hi. I remember my first night on my first mission in Afghanistan. It's weird, I know. So, if you want or need anything, just come and find me.' She waited for a response, but I was still processing her thick South African accent. 'And don't worry about this house. It's not too sociable. Most people come here and then move somewhere else. I'm moving next week, to the house next door.'

'Thanks,' I said, but I had lost my earlier enthusiasm. I was now feeling withdrawn and wanted to get back to lying on my bed.

'That's my room, over there. Come by any time.' Juli turned her back and, with a spring in her step, headed down the corridor to her room. I stood watching, then returned to my earlier position.

4: SO MANY I STOPPED COUNTING

BO, SIERRA LEONE

FRIDAY, 20 JUNE 2014

The following morning I was collected with a group of other expats by the small convoy of Land Cruisers that came to ferry us along the potholed roads to the hospital every day. I jumped in the back with seven others, and there were another two plus the driver in the front. I introduced myself to those around me, including Marlon, the obstetrics team leader. He was sitting opposite me. He smiled then plugged his headphones in and returned to listening to music and staring out of the window. I felt awkward, with no conversation, uncertain where to look.

When we arrived at GRC, I joined Marlon, Crys and Mamadou in a tukul for the handover and briefing. Crys was finishing her twenty-four-hour shift, and there was frustration in her voice as she tried to get Mamadou to understand her English. During the night, Crys had managed cases of placenta praevia, a ruptured uterus and a hysterectomy. I was impressed by how calmly she recounted the cases: just a standard day's work. These were serious conditions, all beyond my normal independent practice. And, though I knew the theory of how to deal with each, the excitement of being faced with these cases was matched with a sense of daunting dread. When Crys had finished handing over the night's patients, she headed off to get some sleep.

The maternity department was set out systematically. One long building, split according to stage of labour and intensity of nursing needs. The far end had a side entrance where the ambulances and taxis pulled up, and this led directly into the delivery room. At the entrance was a desk and chair, where a nurse would complete a screening questionnaire for signs of Lassa fever. This was a tick-box sheet, intended to highlight any combination of symptoms which may require further consideration by the medical team.

The delivery room had three beds, in varying states of disrepair: rips in the cushioning, parts missing and rust down the sides. These were separated from each other by a curtain or piece of boarding. Women brought to the delivery room often arrived in poor condition, having travelled long distances with an ongoing emergency. It was also a resuscitation room, where women were stabilized and prepared for the operating theatre, which was next door.

Next to the operating theatre and delivery room were two long Nightingale-style wards. Neat rows of hospital beds were lined up against the walls, with a baby cot at the foot of each bed. The first ward, which was closest to the operating theatre and delivery room, was intended for the patients needing higher-level nursing, such as the immediate post-operative patients. There were also four beds reserved for women who had eclampsia, requiring close monitoring. Past the screen shutter doors, the second ward was for women who were on the road to recovery, or antenatal patients being kept in hospital for observation. Next to these wards was a small separate room for patients with wound infections. These were a common problem, some horrendously broken down, filled with pus and extended deep into the abdomen of the patient. There was also an overflow tent outside for when there were no beds left on the wards, which the most stable patients could go to.

Outside the complex, behind the area where ambulances came, was a small building that was locked. This was a standby delivery area, in case there was a patient with Lassa fever (and now Ebola) inside the main maternity block. This backup area could be used for births to avoid risk of contamination from the infected patient, or while decontamination took place. The room had never been used.

I joined Marlon on his ward round, watching as he went from bed to bed. Marlon was Salvadorian and had been in GRC almost nine months. He would be leaving in a couple of weeks and it was evident that, psychologically, his mission was already over. He was worn out, just treading water till he got his ticket home. The nurse followed Marlon with a metal trolley, the wheels making a gentle squeak as we migrated from one bed to the next. There were patient notes piled on the trolley, a box of disposable gloves and a light-blue alcohol gel dispenser. A stethoscope dangled over the edge. The round was simple and monotonous. Marlon asked each patient the same questions, and usually offered the same plan too. The effort to avoid direct patient contact, never touching anyone without gloves, face mask and apron, together with the necessity of using the nurse as a translator, held Marlon at a distance from the patients. Regardless of the admission questionnaire, every patient was viewed through the lens of Lassa fever.

'When on call, you're responsible for all new admissions till the next morning,' Marlon told me. 'You rest the day after, and then return the following morning to see the ward patients and help the next person on call. The day after that, you work twenty-four hours again.'

Once Marlon had completed his briefing with me, I joined the hospital logistician for a tour of the grounds. Alex had long blond hair tied back into a pigtail and wore sporty sunglasses; he came across as confident and in control. This was also his first mission, but he had been around a while already. He knew everyone's name and couldn't take more than a few steps without someone stopping him to ask a question or greet him. Though he wasn't medical, he shared how he found the daily stories of children dying upsetting. 'It's hard to see that every day,' he said, gesturing to a board where the numbers were tallied up for the monthly statistics.

As we strolled around, he showed me the different wards, the hygiene systems and the secure area for Lassa fever patients. His pride, though, was the new Ebola isolation area, just completed. This was a large tent fenced off at the back of the hospital complex. He explained to me how it worked, the flow system that needed to be respected and the different zones, and, while I heard what he was saying, I absorbed almost none of it. There was still a perception that we probably wouldn't need this; it was only there just in case.

Finally Alex led me back to the tukul meeting place, where Mamadou was sitting, slowly reading aloud from a paper in English, sounding out each word with exaggerated intonation. He had a deep voice that rumbled when he laughed, which he did often, and he took his poor English in good humour. We spoke for a while – a bit in English, a little in French. Despite his tall, muscular stature, I found his soft face reassuring. We bumbled our way through a conversation comparing clinical cases and areas of gynaecological interest. Mamadou would become team leader when Marlon left, but first he was going to Guinea for a few days to see his family. I didn't ask, but I wondered if he was leaving because of the Ebola outbreak, and if he would return.

A staff meeting was taking place at the maternity department that afternoon, all the nurses and midwives were sitting in a circle and talking with high animation. I cautiously made my way over and asked if I could join, introducing myself to the group. About twenty Sierra Leonean healthcare workers looked at me, eyeing me up for size and substance. I wanted to give them confidence in me, but also to ask that they go easy on me. This was my first mission with MSF and my first obstetric job in Africa. I knew they were far more familiar with the local obstetric emergencies than I would be. Each midwife and nurse introduced him or herself to me. I tried to chant their names in my head, but it would be impossible to remember them all.

'You know it is important you remember our names,' said Isata, a midwife with a quick voice and sharp eyes, her face framed by her hijab. 'I'll test you when we work together,' she added, without smiling.

One man stood out for being the quiet one in the team, but when he spoke, everyone listened. Suma had a statesmanlike presence. He was self-assured, but not arrogant. A trained anaesthetic nurse, he now managed the department. Whenever the shouting began to crescendo, he would subdue the crowd. A few serene words from him brought a transient tranquillity, till the next outburst.

Sunday would be my first twenty-four-hour shift. I prepared some food to get me through the day and night and I read around the subjects I feared most: ruptured uteruses, hysterectomies and destructive procedures. I had also begun reading more guidelines on Ebola and viral haemorrhagic fevers in general. In the end though, I was resigned to the reality that whatever came through the door I would do my best and I hoped, more than anything, that my first shift would not include any maternal deaths. In all my years in the UK, I had never witnessed, never even worked in a hospital at a time when a woman had died from childbirth.

I arrived early in the morning and made my way over to the maternity department. I still didn't really know anyone. The nurses were congregated around a wooden table at the end of the ward, chatting and laughing. One of them had her phone turned up full blast, playing

West African dance music. The patients lay on their beds, neatly lined up. Most had a relative with them, but many were missing a newborn baby. Of the women who arrived at GRC, around one fifth were carrying babies that had already died . A further group would deliver a live baby, but he or she would be too early, or too exhausted, to make it through those vital first minutes of life.

The nurses helped me get dressed up in a light yellow gown, face mask and mob cap. This was nothing compared to the garb I had worn in the operating theatre, but still, on the humid ward, moving from bed to bed, I could feel the sweat dripping down my back and soaking through my scrubs. With each patient, we asked the same questions: what was she in for, what treatment did she require, and would she like contraception? The importance of providing post-partum family planning options could not be overstated, and the nurses were exceptional in their approach. They would point to their arms, saying, 'Captain Band,' the local slang for a hormone implant. They would raise an eyebrow at the teenage girls and ask, 'You don't want another baby?'. The girls blushed and giggled as they offered out their arms.

As we finished, I sat with the nurses and went back over the notes, the plans for the patients and discharge medications. It was all surprisingly straightforward. There was one woman in labour from the night before. She was on an oxytocin drip as the labour had been slow. The hormone, oxytocin, stimulates the uterus to contract, and the woman's labour was now progressing normally. I expected her to have an uncomplicated birth.

I made my way to the tukul and got comfortable with a book and a strategically placed fan. The day was quiet, and after a couple of hours I was getting bored. I wandered back and forth to the maternity department, to see if anything was happening. The one labouring woman delivered and nothing else was going on. I was beginning to get sleepy in the late-morning heat, when the on-call phone rang.

'There is a patient, Doctor. Come.'

Before I could ask anything, the line went dead.

I arrived to find a woman, called Fofanah, already lying on a bed in the delivery room. The nurses had tried to complete the Lassa screening questionnaire before letting Fofanah in, but it had been impossible; she was semi-conscious and, when she did speak, it was in a language the nurses could not understand.* The information we could gather was scant: Fofanah was forty years old and sixteen weeks pregnant; she had been bleeding heavily for three days. Her heart was racing and her blood pressure was so low it was through the floor. She was working hard to breathe and had a burning temperature. Once I had donned all the protective gear, I quickly examined her. Fofanah was still bleeding, but not too much, and was now mostly passing small clots. She was clearly miscarrying, but the pregnancy remained inside her and was the likely source of infection. I enquired if she'd done or taken anything to abort the pregnancy, but her answers made no sense. We began giving Fofanah oxygen, rapid intravenous fluids and antibiotics. Luckily, there was blood matching her group in the blood bank, so I requested two units for transfusion. I then administered a medication to try to complete the miscarriage, to empty her uterus of the infected tissue, but this required time to work.

A team meeting was being held that afternoon in the hospital, so I left Fofanah in the care of the nurses and I joined the rest of the expatriate staff in the large meeting room. I remained unfamiliar with most of the team, although I was happy to see Liesbeth had arrived from Brussels. I greeted her as if she were an old mate – which, compared to the others, she was.

The meeting was to discuss the ongoing Ebola outbreak, still concentrated in the east. However, there were rumours of the situation upcountry being worse than the official reports. There were growing numbers of stories coming from villages further inside the interior of the country, with clusters of illness and death. Kenema, a city between Bo and Kailahun, was known for high numbers of Lassa fever and had the only government hospital containing isolation facilities. These were intended for Lassa fever, but now the hospital was also receiving Ebola cases.

Kathleen repeated the importance of continued vigilance. Any concerns should be raised to her or her team, which was made up of two doctors. Silje was an energetic Norwegian doctor, with long straight hair and a fair complexion, who had arrived in the project a week earlier than me. Her original mission had been to oversee the health of national staff and their dependants, and to work as the doctor for the Lassa fever isolation. Alessandro, my Italian friend, was the other doctor on their team,

---

* There are over twenty languages spoken in Sierra Leone.

having joined because he had an interest in epidemiology and infectious diseases.

While the conversation continued, the on-call phone rang from my pocket. I didn't want to disturb the group, so, instead of answering, I headed directly over to maternity.

I walked in through the ward and found the midwives standing together inside the entrance, waiting for me. 'Where's the patient?' I asked.

'She's outside,' said Massayo, a midwife assistant, handing me the questionnaire used for screening. Nearly every box was ticked. I looked at the piece of paper: fever, bleeding, headaches, vomiting, diarrhoea – the list went on.

A cachectic woman was leaning against the wall, rolling her head from side to side, while her mother and brother stood anxiously by. Around her was a mist of flies. She had an unevenly shaved scalp, which I had not yet seen on women in Sierra Leone. It was striking because I had recently read that, during the first recorded Ebola outbreak in Zaire, women would shave their heads thinking it might cure the severe tinnitus they suffered. I asked, and she confirmed she had shaved her head because of headaches and tinnitus. It was as if someone had punched me in the stomach.

I gathered myself and looked again over the screening questionnaire. I asked if she had attended a funeral. She looked to her brother and then her mother. There was a rapid flurry of conversation I could not follow.

'No,' she said.

The midwives began shouting at her and the relatives.

'What is going on?' I asked.

'They are changing the story! They are changing what they told us!' said Massayo, standing in the doorway, as if blocking entry to the department. 'Her father died and she prepared his body. They all did the traditional funeral.'

I took a slow, deep breath and walked back inside. I looked at the nurses and midwives. We were all thinking the same, although none of us had said the word yet. 'I'm going to get the others,' I said. 'Just keep them there. Don't touch them – any of them.'

There was no panic. Much like when there's an emergency during childbirth, a sense of directed calm took over. I walked out of maternity still holding the questionnaire. Taking care to wash my hands thoroughly with the chlorinated water, I headed back to the meeting. I didn't want to announce anything. I discreetly looked around the room till I caught Silje's eye, and motioned for her to come.

'You think you have a Lassa case?' she asked, as we walked back over to the maternity.

I showed her the questionnaire and then explained about the funeral. 'I'm not sure; could be worse.'

When we got to the woman, she was sitting on the floor, propping herself against the wall. She claimed to be having a miscarriage, to be bleeding heavily, but there was no sign of that. She had told the nurses the fetus had crawled out of her, and then crawled back inside. It was difficult to know what was really going on. Looking at her, she was obviously unwell – perhaps with AIDS or TB, but we could not rule out the possibility of Ebola.

'Are there any other new patients?' Silje asked.

'Just a woman inside with a miscarriage.'

As I began explaining that the other woman, Fofanah, had also been admitted with bleeding and fever, a midwife informed us of a strange coincidence: both women were from the same village. Silje raised her eyebrows. 'I'm going to get Kathleen,' she said.

Fofanah had responded well to the fluids and treatment. She was sitting up and, now she was coherent. It transpired she spoke very good English, her job being an English teacher. I stood a couple of metres from her and asked again about what had happened. Fofanah denied taking anything to abort the pregnancy, but said she had been bleeding for several days. I began going over the screening questionnaire with her, and this time she was able to give clear and detailed answers.

'Have you been to any funerals recently?' I asked.

'Yes – my good friend. She died.'

'Did you wash her body?'

'We prepared her, and stayed in her home.'

'Did you eat in her house also?'

'Yes.'

'Do you know what she died from?' I asked, hoping she could offer an answer that would alter our conversation's destination.

'She had fever. I don't know what it was.'

'Have other people in the village also died from fever?'

'Yes, Doctor – so many. So many, I have stopped counting.'

I stood still, staring at her. Did she understand what she was saying? My mind ran a thousand miles, but outside I kept a calm façade.

'I see. Thank you,' I said. 'I'll be back shortly.'

In the corridor, Silje, Kathleen and Alessandro were going over the screening questions answered by the woman outside. Kathleen was concerned because the woman had hiccups, which, I soon discovered, was another recognized symptom of Ebola. Kathleen had also noted the brother's bloodshot eyes.

Alessandro looked at me. 'You OK?' he asked softly.

'I'm fine. Just, you know. I'm fine.'

I told them about Fofanah, inside the delivery room. We all looked at each other. It was Kathleen who spoke first, quietly and slowly: 'Benjamin, sitting outside the tukul is Barbara. Go and tell her that I want us to begin preparing the Ebola isolation for two patients'.

The walk was less than a minute from maternity. I stepped out. Washed my hands. Took a slow breath and looked at the sky. The sun had set and the shift to night was fast approaching. I'd felt calm as I left maternity, but with each step something inside me trembled. By the time I reached the tukul, I was shaking uncontrollably.

Barbara and Liesbeth sat smoking and chatting. They both stood as I approached. I tried to speak, but words failed me, and, though my mouth moved, nothing came out.

'Sit down,' said Liesbeth.

My nervous system had kicked in and I shivered as if it were winter. I was embarrassed. I wanted to look in control; instead, I was a wreck.

'Kathleen says . . . She says, open the isolation for two admissions.' I began crying, and apologizing for crying. I felt as if my emotions were working independently of me.

Liesbeth moved closer. 'It's OK,' she said. 'You're having a normal reaction to an abnormal situation.'

I put my hands to my face and wiped the tears away, pushing my head back. 'Pull yourself together, Benjamin,' I whispered to myself. 'Now is not the time to lose it.' I drank the water Liesbeth gave me, stood up and returned to maternity.

Everyone huddled in the small annex between the delivery room and the ambulance ramp. The brother of the woman outside was beginning to get agitated; everything was taking a long time and she was yet to receive any treatment. We had not even confirmed if she was pregnant, and, as this would involve handling bodily fluids, it was now out of the question.

Kathleen, Silje and I went outside, wearing only gloves so we would not appear frightening. Standing a couple of metres back, Kathleen explained what was going to happen. She was careful with her words, first checking if they had heard about Ebola, and then gently describing why we needed to do a test. She explained how we would put the patient in the isolation area and that she need not be frightened. The brother was also offered admission, but declined. He would stay outside the tent. As the woman could walk, she would be able to get herself into the ambulance, which would drive her round to the isolation area. Kathleen described the special suits we would wear, and how we would take a blood test. Watching Kathleen at work that evening was one of the best lessons I would receive during the entire outbreak. The family asked a few questions, but agreed.

I went back inside to talk with Fofanah in the delivery room, explaining the situation in a similar way to how I had observed Kathleen doing it outside, but she cut me off: 'Yes, Doctor – thank you. I had been needing that'.

Although Fofanah had received two bags of blood, she remained weak. I did not think she would be able to walk. Plus, she was still in the process of having a miscarriage, still bleeding what we now considered to be potentially Ebola-positive blood. She would need to be moved to the ambulance in a stretcher. It was agreed Silje, Alessandro and I would do the transfer.

'You should start drinking water now,' Alessandro said as we walked over to the isolation tents.

Although I had seen pictures in textbooks, I had never worn the full personal protective equipment (PPE) associated with high biohazard. At this time, there was no big international response to Ebola, no pre-arrival training, nothing actually preparing any of us for isolation, other than doing it. And here I was, my first shift, and we were isolating the first two suspected Ebola patients in the project.

The three of us went over to the Ebola isolation area, only recently completed. It was made up of several tents, interconnected in a 'flow system', from low to high risk. In the centre were two larger tents for the patients. To prevent the risk of cross-infection, we decided to put one woman in each tent. The area had never been used, and a team of staff from the Lassa fever ward were called in to hurriedly put the final measures in place to get us up and running. In the first tent were unopened boxes containing the protective equipment. I had no idea what to put on, or in what order, relying on my Lassa-experienced colleagues to tell me. The stock was limited to extra-large sizes. The only wellington boots, as before, were huge and heavy for me, but I kept quiet, not wanting to appear unable to cope. We pulled on the waterproof yellow all-in-one suits, a heavy apron over the top, two pairs of gloves, two face masks, tightly fitting goggles and a head-and-face covering. Once fully dressed, everything looked, felt and sounded different. It was an alternate reality, and a much hotter, more humid environment. The night was our greatest gift; had the sun been up, I don't think we would have managed at all.

We walked from the isolation, around the back of the other medical blocks, to maternity. The other benefit of nightfall was that fewer people were around to see us in the iconic 'Ebola suits', which could have led to panic and fear among the other patients. With each step I felt the heat building up, my face mask getting wetter with sweat and my breathing more forceful and laboured. My focus, though, was on my feet; there were drains and pipes all around the grounds of GRC and, given the size of my boots, I was aware I could easily trip over.

I went first into the delivery room. 'I am Dr Benjamin,' I said. 'Remember me, from before? I know I look different and I'm sorry for that, but we are just the same people and you don't need to be frightened.'

And she wasn't. Fofanah was incredibly calm, actually thankful we were isolating and testing her. This worried me deeply; it was as if she had always suspected she had Ebola.

We made sure Fofanah had a clean gown on, leaving the bloodied sheets on the bed, and helped her down to the stretcher. After putting a blanket over her, we lifted the stretcher up from the floor. It was made of solid metal bars with just a flap of orange plastic between them. No wheels or folding legs like we have back home. It could only be carried, and it was heavy. Thankfully, we did not have far to go. We got outside to the ambulance, and Silje, Alessandro and I managed to lift her up in the stretcher and load her into the back. But the metal poles of the stretcher protruded from the end of the ambulance, preventing the doors from shutting. We tried pushing it harder, moving it to an angle, but nothing worked. No one else could assist, as we were the only ones in protective clothing, and she, and all that touched her, were now assumed to be Ebola contaminated.

We were already exhausted. It was our first time in the full biohazard PPE and our bodies were not used to this heat. We had no stamina.

'It doesn't fit,' Alessandro shouted across to those not dressed up.

There was one alternative. The three of us would carry Fofanah on the metal stretcher, round the back of the hospital, to the isolation directly. With much apologizing, we unloaded the stretcher, Fofanah winced placing a hand over her abdomen as the stretcher jolted into movement. The walk was awful, the heat of the physical exertion while wearing full PPE almost intolerable. With every step, I could feel sweat pooling inside my boots and swashing around my limbs. Occasionally one of us would shout, 'Stop!'. We would gently put the stretcher down to the floor, and just breathe. I was terrified that one of us would faint. My head was spinning from the heat and I struggled to get air in and out through the mask. The pressure from the strap on the goggles felt like it was pressing through the crown of my head, straight into my brain.

Finally, we got Fofanah inside and on to a bed, apologizing again for the journey. I then gently examined her to check she was not bleeding too much. We would be able to continue the antibiotics while she was in isolation, but surgery to finish the miscarriage, if it did not pass from the medication, would not be possible.

I made my way to the decontamination area, where the other two were still undressing. I could not understand what was taking so long. Having never worn biohazard PPE, I had no concept of the complex process that followed, and by this time my only thought was focusing on my breathing and not fainting. I stood watching, thinking, I'm just going to pull this shit off. It's too hot. It is *too* hot.

Eventually, I shuffled forward. I was so dizzy and disorientated from dehydration, I struggled to understand what people were saying to me. A man stood opposite me with a tank full of chlorinated water. He wanted me to stand with my arms stretched out, so he could wash me down, but I had no understanding. From the side, someone else was shouting more instructions at me and trying to show me. Why does everyone sound so angry? I felt like I was in trouble, or like I was too stupid to follow simple instructions. I would reach out to touch something and everyone would scream, 'NO!'.

As each layer came off, the relief was immediate. I could see. I could breathe. My scrubs were soaked in so much sweat, they were heavy and dripping. As we were given water and soda to refresh ourselves, the on-call phone rang. An unfamiliar voice told me a new patient had arrived.

It was after 10 p.m., and as I walked to maternity I saw Massayo, the midwife assistant, standing in front of the day shift nurses and midwives. They should have gone home hours ago. The staff minibus had long departed and they needed to find a way home in the dark. Hands-on-hips, Massayo demanded to a passing WatSan that they each get sprayed with chlorine water. Was it safe for their families, if they returned home? What if their hands, shoes or clothes harboured the virus? The anxiety that accompanied suspicions of Ebola was only just beginning to appear. The eventual impact of fear would be one of the most significant aspects of the whole outbreak.

The hygiene team had just finished spraying and decontaminating outside maternity, where the woman with the shaved head had been sitting, when the maternity ambulance pulled up with a new patient. This woman had given birth to her eleventh child that evening, in a clinic near to GRC, but the baby was stillborn and the woman had begun bleeding.

'Has she lost much?' I asked the young nurse who'd arrived with her.

'Yes, a lot.'

Cautiously, I stuck my head in the back of the ambulance, where a thin woman, called Mbalu, was lying under a blanket. Mbalu looked back at me, expressionless with dull eyes. At least a litre of blood was on the floor. As she moved, another gush of blood clots spilled out from between her thighs.

The delivery room remained a no-go area, as it had not yet been decontaminated, but I needed to start resuscitating this patient. Mbalu was having a massive post-partum haemorrhage.

The emergency room behind the maternity block was our only other option. It had never been used and there was confusion over where the key was kept. A new team had arrived for the night shift, and by chance the midwife in charge of the department, Fatmata, was on duty. Fatmata appeared to be in her late-forties, she had a sturdy frame, an unflinching gaze and a matter-of-fact way of speaking. She went in search of the key as I directed the ambulance around the back of the maternity ward, careful to point out the deep and open drains in the dark. When Fatmata returned with the key to the emergency room, we discovered there was barely any stock in there. I ran back to maternity with a nurse and we grabbed supplies of protective clothing, intravenous fluids and drugs for haemorrhage.

Finally, we were able to get Mbalu, the patient, out of the ambulance and on to a bed. Blood flowed out of her as if from an open tap. In the rush, I didn't put on all the correct protective equipment; I just wanted to stop the bleeding. I began massaging Mbalu's uterus, which was soft and floppy, when it should have been firm and contracted. As I stimulated it, I felt it harden under my hand and the bleeding briefly abated. I asked one of the nurses to run and get a urinary catheter. While rubbing her uterus, I asked more about what had happened.

Although this was her eleventh birth, only four of her children were alive. Mbalu kept saying, 'Finish, Doctor. Finish,' and pointing to her belly.

I looked at Fatmata.

'She wants you to sterilize her. No more babies.'

The uterus began to relax again and a large blood clot fell out of her. I asked one of the nurses to take over with the massage, while I examined Mbalu for any birth tears. As blood gushed out of her again, I knew we were in trouble. We placed the urinary catheter and gave her all the drugs we had to make her uterus contract. I put on the long gynaecological gloves and explained I wanted to make sure nothing was left inside the womb, causing the bleeding. Mbalu gestured that she understood. Normally, we would do the procedure with anaesthesia, but I was far from the operating theatre and she was losing a lot of blood. With one hand holding the top of her womb, I gently slid the other in and up through the cervix, into her uterus. It felt as if it was moulded from jelly, wriggling away as I searched the inner walls with my fingertips. It was empty. Using both hands, I squeezed and held the uterus, trying to demand, *You will contract.* As I relaxed, the tap turned back on. Increasingly, the blood on the floor looked watery. This was a worrying sign; Mbalu had lost so much blood, she no longer had the ability to form blood clots. The options were limited. I knew soon, I would either have to remove her womb or she would die.

The nurses were struggling to insert an intravenous line, the veins having collapsed from blood loss. The bleeding was unrelenting. We needed to get Mbalu to the operating theatre, which was back in the maternity block. I ran outside to tell the ambulance driver, but he had driven away. We had no transport. I called Barbara for help, but quickly realized there was no time to wait for it to arrive.

'Let's carry her,' I said to Fatmata and the others. I sent one nurse to get the operating theatre ready, and, together with Fatmata and another nurse, got Mbalu on to a stretcher and carried her out through the night, past the closed, contaminated delivery room and down the short corridor to the operating theatre.

Silje and Liesbeth arrived, having got word from Barbara that I was in distress. They looked at me, horrified. Blood was everywhere. I had red streaks down my arm, like the brushstrokes of some macabre artist.

'She is going to die if we don't go now,' I said.

As I began scrubbing for surgery, thoughts flew through my mind: What can I do to stop the bleeding? Should I place a pressure balloon inside the uterus, or tie a large suture, like a pair of braces, around it? Perhaps these could arrest the bleeding. But by the time we were arriving into theatre it was clear the opportunity for those procedures had gone. Mbalu was bleeding to death. Her heart was beating at the limit of efficiency, and Abu Bakar, the anaesthetic nurse, was struggling to record any blood pressure. Her body would not be able to keep going for much longer. I knew I had to remove the uterus altogether.

In the UK, an emergency hysterectomy for post-partum haemorrhage is a rare and significant event. There are blood and clotting products available, and alternative interventions to avoid such extreme measures. The most senior gynaecologists (usually two) would be called in to perform the surgery, and a consultant anaesthetist too. After surgery, the woman would normally go to an intensive care unit for close monitoring and stabilization. In Sierra Leone, that night, there was me, Jon, who was a theatre nurse, and Abu Bakar, and we had the most basic surgical equipment and a severely limited blood bank.

'Doctor, she doesn't have long. Be fast,' Abu Bakar said as he began sedating her with ketamine.

I could not believe this was my first shift, on my first mission, and only my fourth day in the country. It was the first time the theatre staff would see me operate independently, and I was performing a peripartum hysterectomy on a woman *in extremis*. A finger-prick blood test told us we were beginning the surgery with a haemoglobin level of 3.5 g/dL, so low it was virtually incompatible with life.*

Jon, who was a short guy, like me, smiled reassuringly as we got into the heavy layers of protective clothing. He seemed calm, despite the drama around us. No doubt he had seen it all before. I began sweating instantly.

We gathered around Mbalu like members of a sacred order, in our long gowns and facial coverings. We performed the ritual cleaning of her skin and draped her abdomen with green cloths. I'm not religious, but I whispered a prayer under my breath as I picked up the scalpel and made a midline incision from her navel downwards. I buried my hand into Mbalu's pelvis and brought out her floppy and relaxed uterus.

'Clamp, please,' I said, taking a deep breath. I clamped, cut and tied, thinking I might drown under the pressure, but the theatre staff kept me afloat. If I paused, Jon would gently pass me the next clamp, or suggest, 'Maybe tie here, Doctor'.

I felt for her ureters, the rubbery tubes that carry urine to the bladder. It is possible to accidentally remove these during a hysterectomy. I could feel one, but not the other. There are dyes which can be injected or stents inserted to help identify the ureters, but none were available in our operating theatre. I stopped, looked, felt again. In the end, the haemorrhaging womb just had to come out.

Operating in the full protective gear was exhausting. Pools of sweat had collected in the base of my goggles again, stinging my eyes and blurring my vision. In my darkest moments, I doubted I would be able to get Mbalu through the surgery. Expecting she would die on the table, I questioned the futility of the effort.

I had to have my goggles removed several times to let the pools of sweat out and then have them put back on my face, but my vision was

---

* Haemoglobin is a part of the red blood cell which carries oxygen. A normal level for pregnant women is between 11.5 g/dL and 13.0 g/dL. A level below 10.5 g/dL is considered low.

always clouded. Eventually, I made the decision to complete the surgery without the goggles on: a direct breach of the rules, which I knew could get me in trouble, but I saw no real choice. Not being able to see was slowing me down and increasing the chances of pushing a needle or scalpel into my own hand. I expected the theatre staff to disapprove, but no one said a word.

Once I had amputated the womb from Mbalu's body, I looked down into her pelvis. Every edge of tissue was oozing with watery blood, her natural clotting factors having been consumed during the massive blood loss. I began suturing the edges together, placing direct pressure and rechecking. Eventually the pelvis was dry. I washed it out, checked again and then closed her abdomen.

Towards the end of the surgery, it was clear Mbalu had not produced any urine for a while. Had I stopped her from dying by removing her uterus, only to kill her by removing her ureters? Abu Bakar gave a drug to increase the urine output; it was a great relief to me that it worked.

GRC had no intensive care unit. Mbalu was returned to the general ward and put to rest on a bed. We managed to get two units of blood for her, and, although she was weak and pale, at least she was alive.

Throughout the night I kept vigil on Mbalu. By morning, she was opening her eyes. When I checked on her at 7 a.m., a young woman dressed in a spotless white dress was standing at the end of her bed, silently watching over her. I did not recognize her. She kept her eyes low and her gaze fixed.

'Thank you,' she said, without turning towards me.

'Are you a relative? Her daughter?' I asked.

'I'm a student nurse. You met me in the ambulance with her last night.'

I felt sheepish for not recognizing her, and for not having given any thought to the nurse who had been with Mbalu on arrival.

'Thank you for saving the life of a woman in Sierra Leone,' she added.

There was nothing I could find to say in return.

Normally, I would have been the only international staff member in the hospital overnight, but, having isolated our first two suspected Ebola patients, Silje had also stayed to keep an eye them. The woman with the shaved head was not doing well. The blood samples would be taken and sent to the laboratory later in the morning, though it would take at least twenty-four hours for a result. There were only two laboratories in the country able to process Ebola samples, the nearest being at the government hospital in Kenema; the other was further east in the Kailahun Ebola Treatment Centre.

The arrival of the morning Land Cruisers heralded the end of my shift. I handed over to Crys, and together we returned to the bedside of Mbalu, on whom I had performed the hysterectomy.

'Have you thought about Lassa fever?' Crys asked.

I hadn't. Crys was concerned because the baby had been stillborn and Mbalu had haemorrhaged, both signs of Lassa fever. There had been no time to ponder viral haemorrhagic fevers, but what if I had got it wrong? I'd got her blood and fluids all over myself.

I returned to Vienna House to try to get some rest, my mind saturated. Lying on my bed in the uncomfortable heat and humidity of the day, I could hear the guards' radio blaring the BBC World Service outside my window. I closed my eyes and let my mind drift over the past twenty-four hours. What did this all mean? What would be next? If the isolated women had Ebola, what would happen to us all? At some point, I fell asleep.

5: MEDICAL ROULETTE

BO, SIERRA LEONE

MONDAY, 23 JUNE 2014

I woke several hours later, sweat covering my forehead. I rolled over and checked my phone: no messages. I sent a text message to Marlon to see how Mbalu was doing and went to take a cold shower. When I returned, I saw his reply: *Taking her back to theatre, think she's bleeding internally.* I grabbed my clothes and called for a car to get me back to Gondama.

When I arrived, Barbara was talking to Juli outside the tukul. She shouted for me to come over. She looked irritated.

'Benjamin, why are you here? You shouldn't be back so soon after your shift.' Barbara started explaining the importance of breaks and having time off, but I didn't have time for this right now; my mind was entirely focused on Mbalu and getting back to the operating theatre. I cut her short, apologized, and ran to maternity.

Marlon was already operating when I arrived. I decided to scrub and dress up so I could get a closer look at what was going on. Marlon showed me where Mbalu had been bleeding from: one of the vascular stumps deep in the left pelvis.

'She was dry when I closed,' I said repeatedly, more to myself than any other person. 'We checked several times; I'm sure she was dry.' But I knew this could occur. I had seen it a couple of times before, with consultants in the UK. I felt terrible – totally disheartened that, after struggling through the night, the woman had returned to theatre.

Marlon just patted me on the back and said, 'It happens'. The job comes with risks, and you do the best you can with what you've got.

The results from our isolated patients arrived over a day later. During the interim, the woman with the shaved head had sadly passed away. We never knew if she had been pregnant at all, or if she was just desperately searching for somewhere to gain access to free healthcare. Neither of the women had positive test results. Their symptoms had convincingly mimicked Ebola, but our suspicions had been incorrect. Fofanah, the English teacher, was returned to maternity and we performed a procedure to empty her uterus of the miscarriage. She went back home. We will never know if the other woman would have survived had she not been isolated and tested for Ebola.

Over time, I became increasingly accustomed to the work pattern of a twenty-four-hour shift every three days. Maternity was not as busy as it used to be, partly because of the overturned decision to close the facility. It was assumed the news that we were staying open had not yet spread widely. However, it was also apparent that, as stories of healthcare workers becoming infected and dying from Ebola became more common, people were avoiding health centres.

Every day, news and rumours came in about the ongoing outbreak and the hospitals and clinics where the disease was passed around due to poor infection control and hygiene mechanisms. In our daily medical team meetings, Barbara would update us on the most recent Ebola clusters and their locations. The general trajectory continued to be in our direction. Occasionally, we received stories of abandoned villages, with only dead bodies left behind. Impossible to confirm, these stories were nonetheless frightening to hear, and in time they were picked up by the press, who wrote harrowing reports of ghost towns, biblical in their depiction of the shadow of death passing over. What was happening in the hills around us and beyond was important; these were the villages our patients came from. Barbara struggled to get accurate information, and would plead staff to let her know about any information they had, whether confirmed or hearsay. Ultimately, our safety was her responsibility.

Liesbeth had moved into Bangkok House, opposite me. We regularly had dinner together with Juli and Alessandro, discussing the developing situation. If the stories were to be believed, not only was the outbreak uncontrolled, it was spreading like wildfire around us. Nobody knew what our next move would be in GRC. For now, we just had to keep going and play it as safe as possible. I began searching, downloading and reading as many guidelines, journal papers and reports on Ebola and other viral haemorrhagic fevers as I could find. Maintenance of normal healthcare services during an outbreak was vital, but there was a startling lack of information on how to continue providing care safely. Nearly everything I could find was written from experiences of the outbreaks in Uganda and the Democratic Republic of Congo (formerly Zaire). These had been much smaller outbreaks, and had never got a foothold in large urban areas or crossed international borders. While we were dealing with the same disease, the context was fast turning it into something far more sinister.

Transmission was rising exponentially, with the disease a mysterious baton passed on undetected, and often revealed too late. There were alternative narratives too: disbelief that the disease existed, resistance to infection control measures and an unawareness of germ theory.* An unknown menace decimating whole families slotted into ideas about curses and witchcraft as much as it fitted with the science of an invisible pathogen.

Each week, we received updated epidemiological data, with lists of affected villages. Over time, these became more frequent and detailed. This was supposed to assist us in differentiating between suspected Ebola cases and non-suspects. This had its own problems, though; our patients often came with urgent and life-threatening complications, making a lengthy questioning both impractical and unethical. It was no secret that we were screening for Ebola, and, if someone needed medical treatment they would not want to be viewed as a possible Ebola case, requiring isolation. Patients would sometimes claim they came from a different part of the country, or would not disclose the illness of a family member or their attendance at a funeral.

Termination of pregnancy was largely illegal and difficult to access in Sierra Leone. Regardless, a high proportion of unwanted pregnancies resulted in women seeking unsafe, illegal 'backstreet' abortions. These were estimated to account for over 10 per cent of all maternal deaths in the country – although, as with all clandestine procedures, no one really knew the full extent. Native herbs, or chemicals, might be taken to poison the pregnancy (and often the woman or girl too), or unclean

---

* Germ theory attributes certain diseases to microorganisms, too small to see without magnification, that invade the body.

instruments inserted into the uterus to trigger the abortion. Aside from introducing infection, these sticks and rods could pass through the uterine wall, damaging the bowel or bladder, resulting in terrible complications and requiring major surgery. Even if it seemed obvious a woman had sought an abortion, she would often maintain the charade that it was a miscarriage, perhaps out of fear of the law or other forces. We knew from the writings of previous outbreaks that Ebola infection often caused spontaneous miscarriage, so we were on-guard for any woman presenting with fever and bleeding. This ultimately put all women with an infected abortion as suspected Ebola cases, unless we knew categorically it was self-provoked.

The problem with bending the truth was that it sometimes worked in a patient's favour, and sometimes it didn't. Anyone who ticked boxes on our entry screening form would be further questioned before they could come through the door. The stakes were incredibly high for all of us – patient, healthcare workers and all other people inside the department. Many women arrived so late and in such urgent conditions that any delay in treatment felt deeply wrong, but we also knew allowing anyone with Ebola into the general ward, where infection control was a challenge at best, could lead to widespread infections and deaths among our team and other patients.

One night, a young woman arrived who was in the beginning of the mid-trimester of pregnancy. She was feverish and bleeding; on paper, she should have been isolated and tested for Ebola. This would have taken between twenty-four and forty-eight hours to get a result. She was otherwise well, conscious and articulate. All I needed to know was if she had provoked the abortion, causing the bleeding; if I could explain her symptoms, I could get her inside and begin treatment. But she denied having been to see anyone to terminate the pregnancy. I gave her a rapid diagnostic test for malaria. If it was positive, it might just be enough for me to excuse the fever, but it was negative. This teenage girl stood alone in the dark, her vulnerability stark. She represented so much of why I had chosen this career path, and here I was, able to do something useful for her. But, instead, I was about to prevent her access to treatment. No longer nurses and doctors, the medical staff had become interrogators and judges, dangerously close to squeezing a forced confession. Despite all our reassurances, there was nothing that would convince her it was safe to disclose if she had sought an abortion – or, she was telling the truth. Let her in and treat her? Or isolate her and wait, while she bleeds?

Ultimately, I gave in to my gut, admitted her and began treatment for an assumed septic, botched, backstreet abortion. I was shouldering huge responsibilities and anxiety. Her fever subsided with antibiotics, the abortion was completed and she went home a couple of days later. Roulette, not medicine, became the order of the day.

6: NO ONE LAUGHS AT GOD
IN A HOSPITAL

GONDAMA, SIERRA LEONE

JUNE AND JULY 2014

Among all the hype of Ebola, all the unanswered questions and uncertainties, we remained a centre for obstetric complications. The Sierra Leone Free Health Care Initiative had been launched by the government in 2010, promising access to essential health services for children under five, pregnant and lactating women. Accessible and free of charge, it was widely endorsed and supported within the country and through international collaborators. Our service should not have been required at all; the view from the ground, however, was different. Women continued to make long and hazardous journeys to reach GRC, either because our care was free or their local facilities were not capable of meeting their needs. Time is a luxury we do not have with obstetric complications, and delays in recognizing, reaching and receiving treatment have long been accepted as the underlying reason for high maternal deaths and poor outcomes in low-income countries.

I was becoming accustomed to how blunt and to-the-point the nurses and midwives were when addressing me. The nurse calling the on-call phone would say little more than, 'Doctor come', so as not to waste precious phone credit. As I spent time chatting with those on shift, I gradually built a relationship with the different members of the team. Isata, the midwife I'd met at the first staff meeting with the maternity department, had been true to her word. Any time of day or night, she'd ask me, 'What's my name?' or 'What's her name?'. She was also taking every opportunity to suss me out. 'Which God do you pray to?' she asked one day, as I was pushing a woman to the theatre.

'Whichever one will listen,' I replied, to the approving nods and tuts of two midwife assistants behind her.

The shifts would vary immensely. Sometimes, the only patients to come would have simple problems, needing a course of antibiotics or carefully controlled amounts of oxytocin to help them contract and achieve a vaginal birth. Other times, a disaster would arrive and we would work to pick up the pieces.

Early on a Wednesday evening, late-June, I wandered around the grounds of GRC. The children's emergency room was full. I saw Juli swiftly move from one child to the next, her South African twang rising above the sounds of nebulisers whirring, monitors beeping and the coughing of little lungs. She was direct and sure in her instructions, efficient in procedures and, despite the whimpering children around her, beamed in her element. Her overt competence made me feel proud, though I wasn't sure why.

I settled in the GRC tukul to read one of the textbooks. I positioned the fan as I had watched Crys do on my first day, hoping for a peaceful shift. I took a moment to consider the heavy clouds of the rainy season when the on-call phone rang, 'Come doctor'.

An eighteen-year-old girl lay flat on the examination couch. Her abdomen, distended with a full-term pregnancy, looked like a camel resting on her belly: two humps rose from under the skin. She moaned and made a feeble effort to push. This was her first pregnancy and she had been in labour for two days at home in her village.

After dressing up in the layers of protective clothing, I cautiously ran my gloved hand over her abdomen. The contractions were short and mild, accompanied by her gentle whimpering. I asked if she could bend her knees so I could understand what was happening inside: her cervix was fully dilated, but, instead of a head, the baby's soft buttock was presenting. Lucky to have a working ultrasound scanner, I confirmed the baby was still alive, and could see his head was extended all the way back, as if looking directly up to his young mother's face. Even if she were able to deliver the breech, with the head deflexed, it would likely get stuck – a nightmare complication. I explained this all to the midwives and then to the patient, and we agreed to proceed with a caesarean section.

A caesarean section at full dilatation is not the same as when performed before or earlier in labour. The uterus balloons out, easily tearing. Other organs, such as the bladder, tend to become swollen and stretch up across the lower part of the uterus, risking injury. It was with these complications in mind that I began the operation.

As surgeons go, I'm shorter than average; to be able to reach under the baby's buttocks, I needed the operating table all the way down, plus a box to stand on. I reached down and gently cradled the baby's breech in my hand, lifting it up and out of the incision. The mother had been pushing for so long on the baby's bottom that one cheek was three times the size of the other, with a deep blue swollen bruise.

The baby was completely still.

A vigorous rub with one of the surgical swabs elicited a pathetic mew. 'Good boy,' I muttered, clamping and cutting the cord. I handed the baby over to the midwife, with simple words, 'Rub, rub, rub'.

Soon enough, a healthy, angry cry was heard. I completed the caesarean and the young mother was reunited with her bruised baby boy. After such a long labour, she risked developing an obstetric fistula – a debilitating condition where a connection forms between the vagina and other internal organs, resulting in continuous and uncontrolled leakage of urine, faeces or both. The leaking can cause skin irritation, a terrible smell and ostracism from the family. To prevent this, we would leave the urine catheter in place for at least a week after surgery, allowing the bladder to rest and repair.

The following shift, I felt a sense of *déjà vu*. Fudia was a seventeen-year-old girl, also in her first pregnancy, and she had been fully dilated since the morning of the day before; it was now early evening. In the UK, a woman would not be left fully dilated for more than four or five hours, as the complications to both mother and baby increase rapidly at this stage of labour.

When she arrived at GRC, Fudia was breathing quickly, her pulse was high and she had a fever. She had first tried to give birth at home, high in the hills. When the baby didn't come, she went to the local clinic, where she stayed a full day trying to push the baby out. They then told her to go to the hospital in the city, but her family had no money for transport. Finally, Fudia got to a hospital in a different town, but her family had to buy the operating theatre team sterile gloves and medicines from a pharmacy before Fudia could have a caesarean section. Then there had been a power cut and, when the power resumed, there was no doctor. At this point, the staff decided to send her to GRC, but there was no fuel for the ambulance, and so she waited, contracting, until fuel was found.

A catheter was already in her bladder, showing only a tiny amount of dark brown urine in the bag. Fudia's kidneys were already failing. An ultrasound showed the baby had died, possibly the day before or even earlier. The head was low down and I hoped, with good analgesia and the appropriate tools, I would be able to deliver the baby and avoid a cae-sarean section. Alongside Isata and Massayo, the midwife assistant, we began resuscitating Fudia with fluids and intravenous antibiotics. Her malaria test was also positive, so we began treating that too.

Once in theatre, Fudia was anaesthetized and I examined her again. The smell was unmistakable – the fetus must have been dead for days, and Fudia was badly infected. The fetal head was in an awkward posi-tion (probably part of the reason why it had not delivered in the first place). I grasped the head in my hand and tried to manually turn the baby, so I could apply forceps, but the condition of the baby made this impossible; the decay and maceration was too extensive. I tried to use one forceps blade to push the head round, so I could slip the other in, but the forceps would not lock together. I was wearing full theatre garb, and the physical effort, together with the stressfulness of the situation, had me sweating profusely. I had to get the baby out. I resorted to the ven-touse cup, attaching it to the head, building up the vacuum and pulling. The baby's head came down, turned a bit, came down a bit further and then stopped. It would not deliver. I tried the forceps again to see if the rotation would allow me to get them on, but no, the blades still would not lock. It became clear the baby simply would not fit. It was very large for its mother's small body, and the more I tried to get it out, the more I risked traumatizing the vagina and the girl.

There was a procedure in my mind throughout the pulling, squeez-ing and sweating: a destructive delivery, where a fetus which has died before birth is removed by collapsing the skull, making it small enough to deliver. The method was intended precisely for the situation in front of me. I knew no one in the UK who had performed a destruction, and, though I knew the theory, I wondered if this was the right time, the right person, the right place in which to try. In the days before I had left for the mission, I'd spoken to a retired consultant with decades of experience, who had worked in Sierra Leone, and I remembered his words now:

I would never do a destructive delivery; it's too traumatic. I was hot, confused and defeated, standing in front of a girl who was praying to God for her life as her dead child refused to leave her body and her vagina bled from my unsuccessful efforts.

With a heavy heart, I explained we would proceed to a caesarean section. As with the previous patient, I mentally thought through the fully dilated caesarean technique and complications. When I opened Fudia's abdomen, I saw her bladder was huge, swollen and stretched up across the uterus. Above the bladder were loops and loops of dilated bowel, which were spilling out on to the table. I knew there was no rush; the baby could not die twice. All that mattered was the teenage girl before me. I pushed the bowel back into the abdominal cavity where it belonged, and moved the bladder down, out of my way. The uterus was distended, so I carefully chose the safest place to make my incision.

The head refused to come back up, from the pelvis so I tried to find the feet and deliver it the other way around, but they too were fixed, locked together, refusing to turn. I went back to the head and eventually managed to deliver the baby. The smell was hideous. There was no doubt that what was inside Fudia's womb had begun to rot. I cleaned inside the womb and surrounding area, but there was a problem. After being fully dilated for so long, with the difficult delivery and infected friable tissues, her womb had torn all the way down to the cervix. Prior to going to theatre I had asked Marlon and Mamadou their opinion on Fudia's condition. I called Mamadou again, requesting his help. I closed the caesarean wound and as much of the tear as I could, thankful that Fudia was not bleeding much. Once Mamadou arrived, we examined the uterus. It was in terrible condition from the infection, falling apart as we tried to repair it, the stitches tearing through tissue as if it were butter. Had Fudia not been seventeen years old and childless, we would have proceeded to a hysterectomy. But we tried our best to save her womb. Once the tear was closed and we were satisfied there was no bleeding, we completed the surgery and Fudia was taken to the ward.

Overnight, Fudia continued to show signs of severe infection. By morning, she was conscious enough to talk and move around. We continued aggressively treating the infection with antibiotics and fluids, but her condition worsened. By lunchtime, Fudia had slipped into a state of coma. She died shortly after.

It is hard to explain the feelings that came with Fudia's death: disbelief, sadness, anger. Responsibility. I'm haunted by her and the decisions made that night. In hindsight, had I attempted a destructive delivery, I suspect it would have failed. The fetus was enormous and bloated. Perhaps now I could perform such an operation, but back then, I had neither the experience nor the stomach.

Did saving Fudia's womb end her life? At what price did we consider her future ability to have children? Were our decisions clouded by her age or assumptions on behalf of her community? Would it have made any difference, or was the damage done once the womb's infected contents were released inside of her? When was the point of no return?

A sense of helplessness accompanied my reflections. Fudia was a teenage girl, whose story had already been written before she arrived at GRC, through delay and, perhaps, indifference. What troubled me was that GRC was a safety net, in a country where safe maternity care was promised free of charge. The state, multiple governments and NGOs were supposedly supporting a system to stop women and girls dying horrendous deaths. I believed our presence was justified, but I was increasingly uncomfortable with GRC's function as a parallel service. We were an escape route for when the system did not work. Did our presence relieve those in power of their responsibility to fulfil constitutional obligations? Were we detrimental to progress?

There was a massive shortage of Sierra Leonean healthcare workers – approximately two per ten thousand people; the WHO recommends a *minimum* of twenty-three for basic healthcare. Of these, there was a disproportionate concentration of talent in urban areas, particularly Freetown. The facilities themselves were often not fit for purpose, despite investment and improvements to accompany the Free Health Care Initiative. Not one government clinic or hospital providing emergency obstetric care passed the advised minimum standards. And yet, on arrival at a poorly staffed, substandard facility, often lacking the necessary drugs or equipment, the impoverished patient or relatives would pay from their own shallow pockets to supplement the 'free' healthcare.

I will forever remember Fudia, a young woman negotiating the precarious terrain of her country's health system. Watching her pray in front of me; and my part in failing to answer those prayers.

7: LIGHTNING STRIKES

LONDON

JUNE 2016

Two years later, I was working much as I had before I left for Sierra Leone. The sun shone through the bay windows on the top floor of the North London hospital. I had been back home for several months. Returning had felt natural; everything was familiar, as if it had all been on pause. Then, a thought would appear in my mind, and it was like the plug had been pulled on the treadmill – I would be thrown into a memory, wondering what had happened to colleagues. Sudden feelings of guilt would wash over me, as if I had relinquished responsibility for something. An emotion would surface, like a bubble rising in water, and, the moment I was aware of it, it was gone.

The antenatal clinic was overbooked. Frustrated, heavily pregnant women wandered to and from reception, asking how much longer until they could see the doctor. Towards the end of the clinic, a smartly dressed couple came into the office. I could tell instantly from their body language that they didn't want to be there. They had been sent in by their midwife, who was concerned about the woman's blood pressure. This was her first pregnancy and she had opted for a home birth. There was a detailed birth plan in her notes. She had specified exactly what each person could and could not do, but nowhere was there a contingency plan for if the pregnancy did not follow her instructions. I thumbed my way through the notes. The pregnancy had been normal, and now she was waiting for birth to begin. The estimated due date had been and gone almost two weeks earlier, but still there were no signs of labour starting. Her blood pressure had spiked in the last few days and was now high.

They sat down and I smiled and introduced myself, beginning the waltz of doctor and patient.

'How are you doing? Is the baby moving around plenty?'

The husband answered; the woman wouldn't look at me. This continued for a while. I tried to hide my irritation.

'Mrs Johnson? Can I call you Gemma? Do you know why your midwife asked you to come today?'

Mr Johnson began to respond again, but I cut him off.

'Gemma, I'd really like to hear from you, if that's OK?' I said.

'She said my blood pressure is high, but I checked it again myself and it was not that bad. I'm not coming to hospital. We've rented a birthing pool; it's all set up in the house. Have you read my birth plan?'

At moments like these, I would try to slow the world down. I acknowledged the birthing pool, but insisted we talk about the blood pressure. 'It is quite high, and there's protein in the urine. You have a condition called pre-eclampsia – have you heard of it before?'

Mr Johnson smiled; I was fairly sure I could detect smugness. This was his moment. He took a breath and began: 'We're very well read, Doctor. We have looked online and have some books. We understand all about it and Gemma doesn't think she has it'.

'I see.'

I looked at her blood pressure recordings from the midwife, the repeat recordings from the clinic and her urine test.

'I'm not here to ruin your plans, and I'm certainly not here to try to scare you. I'm sure you're very well informed, but, just so I know I've done my job, I'm going to go back over a few things. You can choose what you would like to do, but I should make sure you're aware of everything.'

The sun was shining in all its afternoon glory through the windows on to my face. The room felt warm, but not uncomfortable, and there was a gentle breeze blowing through. The husband continued to hold a fixed, patronizing smile. Gemma stared at her feet. I wondered why they'd come to the clinic. I was talking, but I was seeing other faces.

Nobody can really explain pre-eclampsia – not fully. What we do know is it is unpredictable and can rapidly develop into a severe and life-threatening event. The condition affects all organs of the body, and cure comes with the end of the pregnancy, though not immediately. The privilege of living in the UK, or another high-income country, is that it is virtually unheard of for anyone to die from the condition. Mostly, pre-eclampsia is detected before escalation to eclampsia.

In the clearest and least threatening manner I could find, I explained what I knew of pre-eclampsia. Frightening people doesn't work – it alienates, and widens the patient–doctor divide. Equally, though, facts are facts, and informed choices can only be informed if information is given. Gemma's blood pressure was high enough to cause her to have a bleed in the brain, which could leave permanent disability or worse. The placenta could separate, leading not only to the death of her baby, but also to significant risk to her own life. The pre-eclampsia could evolve to eclampsia, derived from the Greek word for lightning: sudden and violent convulsions of the pregnant woman. It is a leading cause of maternal death in the world, but not in Mr and Mrs Johnson's world.

Mr Johnson looked at me with pity in his eyes; we both knew my words were wasted. The conclusion of our meeting was decided long before they sat in their chairs, and each person in the room was sure they knew best. Nothing I could offer would be satisfactory. Mrs Johnson would accept no medication to reduce her blood pressure, nor any interventions, pharmacological or other, to stimulate the labour to begin.

I looked at them both, sitting together, united, waiting to start a new life chapter, and I played the personal card.

'Gemma, I understand that this is not what you planned, but here we are. People do die from this. I have seen women die from it.'

The couple appeared unmoved. We shook hands, and they got up to return to their birthing pool and gambling game. The sun had moved down a little, still shining into my eyes, winking at me. Mr and Mrs Johnson went to see a senior midwife, who would no doubt try again to find a compromise. I leant back in my chair and took a slow deep breath. I pushed the images in my head away, the memories of GRC, as another set of notes arrived on my desk.

*

BO/GONDAMA, SIERRA LEONE

JULY 2014

As June turned to July, my life in Bo began to take on its own rhythm, working the three-day rolling shifts and reading as much as I could on

Ebola and the developing epidemic. Watching from the inside looking out, I had a sense of increasing isolation. My evenings were spent having a drink on the veranda of Bangkok House with Juli, Alessandro and Liesbeth. Among the gossip and the chat about who had what films on their hard drive, we tried to make our predictions about how the Ebola situation would play out. Patients, both pregnant women and children, were arriving later and later, as people tried to avoid coming to health centres. The wards, normally overfilled, had empty beds, and this could only mean more deaths in the community.

The maternity patients tended to arrive in little clusters. Hours could pass with no new admissions, then three ambulances would roll in together. I'd sit in the tukul, waiting for the on-call phone to ring, watching the weaver birds fuss over their nests in the trees, listening to their rapid bursts of chatter, and allow my mind wander.

I was imagining, if I had one wish at GRC what would it be? I settled on a secret door that would open on to an intensive care unit like the ones I was familiar with in the UK – the cool dry air conditioning, quiet beeping of machines and the intelligent micromanagement nurse patients back to health. I would be able to discuss cases with the anaesthetist, intensivist or any specialist I needed, get every clinical test I wanted as a priority, and I'd be able to rest knowing the sickest patients had dedicated one-to-one nursing care.

In the UK, I had seen many cases of pre-eclampsia; our antenatal screening picked up most cases early enough to manage with good outcomes. Eclampsia was rarely encountered. The opposite was true in GRC. I assumed the 'pre' went unnoticed till symptoms or seizures began.

One such case involved a woman at full term. Fatou, was transferred midway through labour, having violent convulsions. By the time she arrived, Fatou had been having seizures on and off for several hours. I stood back, encouraging the national staff to manage the situation. Resisting the temptation to get lost in the drama, I held my hands behind my back and gave timely cues on what to do next. The midwives and nurses could manage these emergencies independently. The plan had been for MSF to stop working in maternity altogether just a few weeks earlier; given the uncertain future, it seemed autonomous practice should be nurtured. Fatou stabilized, and a plan was made to deliver the baby and keep the mother on magnesium sulphate treatment for twenty-four hours. The magnesium sulphate does not cure the eclampsia, but it reduces the risk of seizures and gives the body time to readjust. A few days later, Fatou went home with her baby. A happy ending.

Over the following week, there was a flurry of extreme and complicated eclampsia cases. One patient had already been admitted into the department for several days with severe pre-eclampsia. She had been stabilized and had delivered the baby on the same treatment recipe as for eclampsia. She continued to make excellent postnatal progress and, twenty-four hours after delivery, the treatment was stopped. She was walking around and caring for her baby, a proud young mother. A plan was made for a couple more days of observation before discharging her home – another success story. But, around forty-eight hours after delivery she unexpectedly began having seizures – the classic, short-lived but violent convulsions of eclampsia. She was cold and clammy, becoming increasingly confused. Her blood pressure was not high, but she had the tell-tale signs of a headache, seeing flashing lights and swelling down the legs. I came on to the ward to find the nurses scrambling to get an intravenous line inserted. Abu Bakar, the nurse anaesthetist, was priming a bag of fluids, ready to begin a rapid drip. I watched for a while, then cautiously asked what the plan was.

'Fluid and oxygen,' he said.

There is a temptation to throw fluid at all medical emergencies, particularly in obstetrics, where the patients are often bleeding or infected. Eclampsia is different. The fluid leaks out of the circulation into the tissues and spaces between, including the lungs. There is a real risk of drowning a patient.

Abu Bakar was thrown because her blood pressure seemed normal. We discussed her management and agreed to a slow drip, no more than a litre of fluid over twelve hours.

The woman's breathing was rapid, but she had good air entry and her lungs sounded clear. The usual treatment recipe was restarted. She appeared to settle, her vital signs normalized and she had a restful night. As I left the hospital the following morning, she was lying on her bed, talking to her mother, her baby wrapped in brightly coloured lappa in her mother's arms. It looked as if we were back on the road to recovery.

A few hours after I had left GRC, I heard that she had suddenly become breathless. Mamadou had been on call and immediately reviewed her. Her blood pressure remained stable, but she had stopped producing urine. The magnesium sulphate was stopped, as it is cleared by the kidneys and can reach toxic levels if they are not functioning properly, and an antidote was given. But she did not improve. On listening to her lungs, Mamadou could hear they were congested with fluid. High-flow oxygen was started and drugs given to shift the fluid out, but she continued to deteriorate. Over a couple of hours, she drifted into unconsciousness, fighting to breathe above the water in her lungs. She died.

Eclampsia deserves to be respected. It is a serious disease we endeavour to catch early, but it can creep up unexpectedly and present with or without the classical signs. I thought through the girl's management and discussed the case in detail with the other doctors. What did we miss? We had no answer. I wished for my secret door to the ICU.

The staff at GRC saw eclampsia so often they barely raised an eyebrow. One look at the shaking and jerking patient and the magnesium sulphate was already being drawn up. But I feared that familiarity could lead to complacency. Yes, magnesium sulphate treatment is needed, but understanding stabilization and management is also vital and takes more than a reflex reaction. Over and over again, I stood back, watching and commenting . . . 'Airway, breathing, circulation, oxygen, recovery position, control the blood pressure, slow down the fluid, SLOW DOWN THE FLUID.' An emergency should run like a well-oiled machine.

On the following night shift, as I was reviewing a patient in the ward, I heard incoherent screaming coming from outside. An eighteen-year-old was making distressing sounds. She had delivered her baby ten days earlier and had been having seizures since the morning – a long time to be left without treatment. She looked terrible and was completely unresponsive, other than the occasional jerks and her agonizing cries. It had been a couple of days since the other woman with postnatal eclampsia had died – still a raw experience and one none of us wanted to see again. We went through the usual drill, starting the drugs, ruling out other causes.

The girl's eyes were fixed and not moving. She only responded to being rubbed on the chest, and, even then, it was only with screams.

Her oxygen saturation level was dangerously low for a young woman. I feared the worse. I racked my brain to think of what else we could do. We cranked up the oxygen and gave medication to try to offload any retained fluid on her lungs. As I looked upon her, I thought about my secret door. How different things would be . . .

I was called away when two ambulances arrived with patients who urgently needed to go to the operating theatre.

I returned to the woman's bedside after completing the two surgeries. She was transformed – sitting up, trying to feed her baby. She had no recollection of ever seeing me before, she remained well, completed her time on the eclampsia recipe and returned home soon after.

The eclampsia patients continued to come each day, often presenting late, as with all other conditions at GRC. Most responded to the standard treatment and had happy endings, but a few took a stormy clinical journey. It was for them my secret door was needed, and missed, the most.

One morning, towards the end of the first week in July, I was sitting in the Land Cruiser, on my way to meet Mamadou for handover, when Alessandro climbed in the back to join me. 'You look tired,' I said.

'You haven't heard?' asked Alessandro, holding onto his seat as we pulled away.

I shook my head.

'There was another suspected Ebola patient last night, in maternity.'

'What happened?' I asked, grabbing an overhead handle to keep myself steady as we were thrown around.

'A pregnant woman came in, having seizures. She was bleeding from the mouth. We weren't sure what to do; there was a lot of argument. We decided it was better to isolate her.'

'How is she now?'

Alessandro looked out of the window at the swampy road as the Land Cruiser crashed through deep puddles of what looked like molten chocolate. He turned back, his head bowed. 'She died.'

By the time we arrived at GRC, I had enough information to create a picture in my mind. Eclampsia, though a life-threatening condition, *is* treatable. Women displaying the typical seizures, with their whole body violently shaking and spine arched, often bite their lips or tongue, or injure themselves while thrashing around. Between seizures, the women are usually drowsy or confused, occasionally aggressive. It was not uncommon for a woman to arrive both in labour and having eclamptic seizures at the same time. She would be moaning and hysterical from the pain of contractions and the electrical storm in her brain. Once the seizures ceased and her the blood pressure was controlled, definitive treatment would be to deliver the baby. Despite the many cases that we treated, most women and their babies would survive. It troubled me that this woman, still pregnant, was dead.

The full story was no clearer. Adama had arrived after midnight on the back of a motorbike, held upright in a tight sandwich between the driver, in front, and her husband, behind. On arrival, she was unconscious. Her husband told GRC staff that she had begun having seizures in the morning, falling forwards and hitting her face. They had travelled together from a part of the country several hours away. The town was known to have cases of Ebola, and was on our most recent list of locations to be aware of. The husband denied Adama had attended funerals or been caring for sick relatives, but, as the team questioned him he became more anxious. He had travelled for hours along mud roads in the West African rainy season, his wife comatose and fitting, so his impatience was forgivable. No one was sure, though, if his answers were the truth, guesses or plain lies. Trust is everything when decisions have such far-reaching consequences. He said his wife had been unwell for a few days before, but that might have been the prelude to eclampsia.

The concerns from the night team seemed to be around the bleeding from Adama's mouth and nose, but her husband's explanation of her fall explained this, and there are also bleeding disorders related to eclampsia which could cause nose bleeds. This left only her location as a reason to choose isolation. The waiting time for an Ebola blood test result was getting longer. Kenema Government Hospital laboratory had become unreliable and was struggling as increasing numbers of staff became infected with Ebola. All samples were now being sent further away, to Kailahun.

When I spoke with Mamadou, Barbara and Kathleen, they explained that it had taken a long time to get Adama inside the isolation area. Like before, teams had to be called in, the unit set up and the family convinced. Though they had tried to treat her for eclampsia once inside the isolation area, Adama had died as they administered the magnesium sulphate. The blood test had been taken from her corpse. We went over the events again and again, discussing the factors in favour of eclampsia and those for Ebola. It was another impossible call. On balance, I leant towards eclampsia, which left me wondering if Adama's life and that of her child could have been saved, had earlier and different decisions been made.

Over the forty-eight hours it would take to receive the result of the blood test, we went through a verbal post-mortem many times. I questioned what I would have done if I had been on my own in the middle of the night: take her inside the maternity block, or keep her outside and isolate her?

Adama was our first patient with confirmed Ebola. Her case also confirmed how fine a tightrope we were walking. We had been lucky. With every woman that did or did not come inside the department, did or did not end up in the operating theatre, we were taking a chance. We were asking questions and not trusting answers. We knew luck, even ours, had limits.

8: BELOW THE SURFACE

BO/GONDAMA, SIERRA LEONE

JULY 2014

Each day, I would balance my fears of Ebola against my desire to treat the patients coming through our doors with obstetric catastrophes. Our knowledge of how Ebola and pregnancy interacted remained rudimentary. We were basing decisions on a crude questionnaire and gut feelings, none of it robust. Many of the women arriving displayed enough symptoms to meet the isolation criteria, but few of them would survive the time it took to get a result confirming whether or not they had the disease. Ethically, we were in no-man's-land.

Outside, the local community was becoming as obsessed with Ebola as we were. Posters were going up everywhere, some promoting awareness of the disease, some denying its existence, and others advertising Ebola-inspired films and music. Local children, who had called out, 'Hello, how are you? Give me dollar!' whenever they saw us, now shouted, '*Pomwee* (foreign person), you have Ebola over there?'.

The campaign to try to increase the awareness and understanding of the disease was intensifying, though lots of misunderstandings and mistrust remained. Information stalls popped up on street corners and roundabouts, with public health announcements being shouted through megaphones. Small crowds gathered to listen as the symptoms of Ebola were listed, a stick being pointed to a large poster with pictures showing a man holding his stomach vomiting, a woman squatting with diarrhoea, someone bleeding, a dead body and a bat. The orator shouted out hygiene measures – 'Wash your hands! Don't touch dead bodies! Don't eat bush meat!' – and ended with the final statement, 'Ebola is real!'.

There was good reason for all the activity. As July continued, the epidemic marched forth through the country. We heard of terrible news coming from villages in the east, such as Njala and Daru, of communities decimated and abandoned. The official toll had surpassed 400 confirmed cases in Sierra Leone, but more worrying was the number of infected people who remained hidden from the data. Reluctance within society to accept that the disease was real remained a problem. There were cases of patients known to have Ebola leaving hospital isolation areas to seek treatment with traditional healers, private clinics, or simply disappearing.

And why should the population believe the official account? The rural areas were disproportionately affected, and the government in Freetown was distant; rarely had this population reaped benefits from the administration. Now, they were being told a lethal disease was spreading through person-to-person contact and there was no cure available, but one should present to the shoddy health system regardless. Messages to report on suspected family members or neighbours enhanced the atmosphere of mistrust. Communities agonized over how best to accommodate or circumnavigate the changes in caring for their sick or dead loved ones. Traditional burial, which involved washing and preparing the body, was banned: an incomprehensible dishonour for many, perhaps worse than death itself. Tensions between communities, the state, and those associated with the Ebola phenomenon simmered beneath the surface.

Besides, more plausible explanations for the epidemic were available. Stories circulated that the disease was a conspiracy invented by the West: failed military biochemical exercises or a cover-up to steal body organs to trade illegally. People were told not to allow us to take their blood tests, warning that we were actually injecting the disease into our patients. The fear and suspicion became huge.

There was also the hyperactive international paranoia. MSF had been calling for increased international attention to the developing epidemic, yet actions were focused on international isolation rather than cooperation. And within MSF there was another voice rising: ours, in Gondama. As we watched and listened to the escalating situation around us, we began asking more and more about what help we were going to get.

In obstetrics we were increasingly being faced with high-risk decisions, putting not only our own lives in danger, but potentially having far-reaching consequences for the wider situation. MSF stood apart from other organizations; they had responded to many Ebola outbreaks before. And, to date, they had never had a national or international staff member become infected through their work on the front line. We were reminded of this on many occasions, to instil confidence in the infection control measures we were asked to follow. The same mantra was being spoken outside the organization to reassure and encourage others to step up and assist in controlling the epidemic.

'But what if we get infected?' I asked Alessandro and Liesbeth one evening on the veranda. 'Won't that destroy MSF's call-out and their claim to be "infection free"?'

'We just have to hope that won't happen,' said Alessandro.

I gave a short, rueful laugh. 'You've seen the maternity – we have body fluids everywhere. When it's busy, it could be a disaster.' They had both finished their beers, but I had barely got started. 'All it will take is one mistake. One wrong decision and we could have several staff and patient infections.'

'They'd have to close GRC,' Liesbeth said.

'Yes, but what sort of international message would that give? If MSF can't protect their staff from infection, no other organization is going to join us. We have to be invincible, but I think, for obstetrics, it's impossible. It's just a matter of time before we let everyone down. And then no one will come, and the outbreak will keep growing.'

We looked at one another, each of us in contemplation. I wondered if I was over-reacting, or, if the organization was fully aware of what was happening in our little corner of illness, blood and surgery?

I took the discussion to Barbara and Kathleen, who explained the challenges with the powers that be, often sitting in an office in Europe. The response was consistent: 'Keep going'. While we were becoming increasingly anxious about the message our potential infections would give the country and wider world, MSF's head office seemed more worried by the message it would give if we were to stop providing healthcare due to fear of infection. Both were legitimate concerns.

As the dust began to settle after our first confirmed patient, we spent our time on the veranda of Bangkok House trying to predict the likelihood of a surge in new cases over the coming weeks.

'Ebola has a latent period of twenty-one days,' Alessandro said to Liesbeth, Silje and me, 'but for most people, by day eight or ten, the symptoms should appear'. He was convinced more Ebola was on its way. As the rain poured down around us, he counted on his fingers, calculating the different scenarios. 'How many contacts does each confirmed case have? Are they local or did they travel? If they travelled, how many places did they stop at? Did they go to other clinics with vague symptoms, and then move on?' He was becoming increasingly animated, his thick Italian accent jumping up and down with each question. 'Who did they infect before being isolated? What if they refuse to be isolated and remain symptomatic, contagious?'

We stared back at Alessandro, as if pupils in front of a teacher.

'They will begin another web of transmission' said Silje, bringing all our thoughts to the same place.

Sipping cider on the veranda of Bangkok House, we had a clear view; the threat was exponential. Like a movie, the explosion was happening frame by frame, day by day, in slow motion.

We still had no further knowledge or guidance on how our work or lifestyles should change. 'Keep going.' There may have been discussions at higher levels, perhaps contingency plans being made, but these did not filter down to the front line.

The department swung between deathly quiet and intensely busy, depending on the local rumours of where Ebola cases were. The day after Adama died, barely anyone came, but my following shift was the busiest I had had since arriving.

Around mid-morning, as the heat of the day was building up, I got the first call. Two patients had arrived together: one was a seventeen-year-old girl having a late miscarriage and bleeding heavily; the other was an eighteen-year-old girl in labour following a previous caesarean section.

Getting a decent description of symptoms from the patients was often a challenge. There are many dialects in Sierra Leone and, depending where the woman came from, translation would sometimes have to pass through more than one person. I had begun picking up the key words in the two most common languages of the area, Krio and Mende. I could ask about pain, if a baby was moving, and instruct the patient to lie down, push or not push. Over time, I collected more phrases, but I was very much reliant on those around me to explain, translate and reassure.

It was common for patients and their relatives to be reluctant to divulge the information needed to make clinical decisions. I assumed the patient either did not trust us or feared she would be reprimanded or mocked by the team. Respect and sensitivity were, regrettably, not skills innate to all the healthcare workers.

Initially, I focused on the seventeen-year-old. I began resuscitating her and gave medicine to help the miscarriage to complete. I then turned to Musu, the eighteen-year-old. Massayo examined her and found her to be fully dilated. On balance, the safest option for Musu would be to have a vaginal birth. Massayo inserted a catheter into her bladder. No urine drained, just a dribble of dark-red blood.

The scar from a previous caesarean section risks reopening during labour and vaginal birth – a rare but serious complication. One of the difficulties with being a referral centre was that, for many patients, we were their final destination after an arduous journey. I often forgot that the woman who arrived 'fully dilated and pushing', may have been just that for a very long time already.

'Has she been examined by anyone before coming to GRC?' I asked.

Fatmata, the midwife in charge, had now also joined us. She stood with her hands on her hips, next to Massayo. She asked the girl, then turned to me. 'Yes, she's been fully dilated since yesterday.'

Shit.

'And she was in a clinic where she was put on an oxytocin drip to give her more contractions.'

Double shit.

Putting a woman with a caesarean section scar on an oxytocin drip without proper monitoring or access to an operating theatre was inviting trouble, because it forced the womb to contract, stressing the scar. She had been left fully dilated, the baby's head stuck in her pelvis, like a cork in a bottle of fizz, with pressure building, for over twenty-four hours. Sending her to GRC now was like delivering a disaster, cooked, dished and ready to serve.

I began thinking ahead, about how I would repair Musu's ruptured uterus, or perform a hysterectomy if the tear was beyond salvage. The clock on the back wall was ticking loudly, anticipation building with every stroke. I asked to re-examine her myself, getting dressed up and approaching her with caution. The fetal head was low and her pelvis felt as if it had a good amount of space. In a busy London maternity ward, we would perform several assisted vaginal deliveries in a shift; over time, fingers become eyes and an instinct develops; you learn what will come out and what will not.

I was confident she could safely birth the baby vaginally. Massayo and Fatmata looked at me sceptically and tutted their tongues. They had assumed I would take her to theatre and had pre-emptively begun preparing her for surgery. The glances thrown between us spoke volumes. I made my decision: 'Let's get the vacuum extractor equipment assembled.'

Fatmata and Massayo moved with reluctance, slowly collecting the rubber tubing, bicycle pump and ventouse cup.

'Look, you have a choice,' I said to them, feeling impatience stir within me as the heat in my gown built up. 'You can either watch me try to deliver the baby, or you can do it and I will be here to assist you.'

Massayo explained everything to Musu with lyrical intonation, and I gently reinserted my fingers and applied pressure to the back wall of Musu's vagina as the contraction intensified. I felt how the baby's head moved and got a clear idea of the direction it was facing. I gradually pushed my hand inside till I could comfortably hold the head, then I rotated the baby till it was looking directly down to the floor – an easier position for delivery.

I passed Fatmata the ventouse cup, while Massayo used the bicycle pump connected with rubber tubing to create a vacuum on the baby's scalp. Fatmata eased the baby's head down as Musu pushed with all the might she had left. Massayo, the only one of us not fully dressed in PPE for the delivery, had beads of sweat across her forehead as she kept pumping. The bicycle pump squeaked like the springs of an old mattress, as Musu made low heaves, bearing down, urging the birth of her child.

I crouched low down on the floor, watching as Musu's perineum stretched, then supporting it with padded gauze as the head crowned. Together, in goggles, masks and sweat, we delivered a screaming baby boy. Musu began crying, 'Thank you, Jesus!' But the job was not yet over. Once the placenta had delivered, I slipped my hand inside, up to the uterus, and felt along the inner walls for the caesarean section scar. Everything remained intact – no rupture. Musu's urine quickly returned, and washed away the blood till it was a reassuringly golden colour.

The shift continued, with new patients needing to go through the same Ebola triage system, no matter their clinical level of urgency. Safe to enter or better to isolate? Despite this, the department felt under control. But as I was settling in the tukul to eat some noodles for my dinner, I got a call. Binta, the night-shift midwife, was sick.

Opposite the maternity block was a small room where staff would get changed. As I approached, I could hear wailing coming from inside. Night had fallen, and there was only a single lamp burning in the darkness of the room. Binta lay on the floor, and initially I thought she had had a seizure or some cerebral event. She was holding her head, squeezing her temples with her palms and pulling a face of intense pain.

'Doctor, help me, help me!'

Binta was normally so calm – unusually quiet and placid in comparison to her otherwise rowdy colleagues – so it was a shock to see her this way.

'There is too much in my head,' she said, her voice filled with pain and her eyes screaming. Binta then began hitting her head against the wall.

I did not know what to do. Should I touch her? Hold and restrain her? Or let her do what she needed to do? I had no PPE or gloves; the continual fear of touching anyone without precaution meant, even in moments like this, the thought sat in my mind like an electric fence.

I reached out and took her hand. 'Binta, it's OK.'

I didn't know what 'it' was, but I had to say something. She got up and walked out of the room. She wore a vacant look, like that of the heroin addicts I had seen in London. She lay down on the wet ground outside, flat on her back. Looking to the night sky, tears silently streamed down her cheeks. I stood, staring at her, then looked at my colleagues. No one said a word, frightened we might reawaken whatever storm had just passed within her.

I slunk away and, once out of earshot, I asked the others working the shift if they knew anything more. Binta was a relatively new member of the team, so no one had extra information, but they did tell me this had happened once before. That time, she had stopped talking and had intermittently cried. I was lost. Clearly, though, she was in no fit state to work.

Binta remained lying on the ground. I went over and began to talk to her, not knowing if or how this would help. Binta looked directly at me, tears still streaming. I asked if there was any history of illness. She shook her head. I checked her temperature and vital signs, which were all normal. There were some rooms in the hospital reserved for unwell staff, so I took Binta to one of these beds and gave her a sedative, arranging for her to be seen by a counsellor in the morning. My mind ran wild with the violent history of this small country and all the possible pain that could have been in her life.

This meant, for the night, I was left without a midwife.

An ambulance pulled up around 10 p.m. with a twenty-six-year-old woman inside, who had been referred to us from a clinic. Titi was in active labour, with a history of heavy vaginal bleeding and a baby presenting breech. Having been screened negative for Ebola and Lassa symptoms, she was admitted to the labour room. The history was highly suggestive of a placenta praevia, where the placenta has implanted low and grown across the cervix, preventing the fetal head from being able to move into place. The surface of the placenta is the junction between the mother and fetus, a spongy interface of blood vessels; as the cervix begins to open, these can pour out blood in catastrophic amounts. Once again, it was a struggle to understand Titi's clinical history from what she was able to tell us, and it was unclear what exactly had happened prior to her arrival at GRC. We knew she'd had three children before, but only one remained alive. Titi had begun her labour earlier in the day and was now no longer contracting, but in constant pain. As lightly as I could, I examined her abdomen; it was hard and very tender, her face wincing and body twisting away from me. If suspecting a placenta praevia, vaginal examination should be avoided, as poking a placenta with fingers can cause torrential blood loss.

I pulled a condom over the abdominal ultrasound probe – even the scanner had to wear PPE – and put as little pressure on to her sore and painful body as was feasible. The scan result was confusing: the placenta was lying at the bottom of the womb, over Titi's cervix, but it looked as if it was folded and not clearly fixed to the wall of the womb. I slowly moved the ultrasound probe up her tense abdomen. The fetal legs and breech eventually came into view, higher than I would have expected. The baby's heart was not beating and I couldn't see its head. I moved the ultrasound probe further along Titi's abdomen, beyond the normal parameters of pregnancy, trying to find its head. Past the start of Titi's ribcage, almost into her chest, I located the fetal head resting along the upper part of its mother's liver.

Surgery for a stillbirth is a tough call; following my previous experience, I wanted to be sure I was making the right decision if I was to take Titi to theatre. I thought it through and considered the differential diagnoses: the placenta was low, possibly a praevia, in which case a caesarean section would be needed to save her life; the uterus was hard and tender, classic signs of a placental abruption, where the placenta has detached from the uterine wall, so a caesarean could be argued for that reason; the fetus appeared to be outside the womb, which could be a rare abdominal (extra-uterine) pregnancy; but, of all things, and most feared by me, this could be a uterine rupture.

As Titi was prepared for the operating theatre, I requested that her relatives go and begin the blood donation process, then I ran back to the tukul to drink some water. I had already been in PPE a while and knew this operation was likely to be stressful and hot. I needed to maximize my fluids.

Juli, who was on call for paediatrics, was in the tukul, sitting at a computer, inputting data while listening to indie music. Her head bobbed as she sang along.

'You all right?' she asked.

In a flurry, I started flicking through a surgical textbook, knowing I would retain nothing, but blindly trying to confront my hidden panic with facts and instructions.

'I'm going to do a laparotomy. I think this woman's ruptured her uterus. The baby's head is in her liver.'

'Fuck!' Juli's eyes widened. 'You need me to do anything?'

'I don't know. Pray?'

In the operating theatre, I stood on my little step, looking down at Titi's tight belly, only my eyes visible through the hood of my PPE. I slowed my breath and prepared to make a vertical abdominal incision. On the one hand, I hoped she had ruptured, so I could justify having started the surgery; on the other, I hoped she hadn't, because I would need to fix it. With the initial incision through the skin, the answer was immediate. Blood and amniotic fluid began pouring out. Before I got to the uterus, I found the lifeless baby floating completely free in her abdomen. It occurred to me I had never delivered a baby from outside the uterus before. I took the feet and delivered as I would for any other breech. The placenta had also completely detached, but was still in the uterus, resting at the base, as it had appeared in the ultrasound scan.

Once we had mopped up all the blood and fluid, I took a careful look at the uterus. It was torn horizontally, from one side to the other, low down across the front wall. There was also a second, vertical tear, extending laterally to the right, like a horizontal 'Y'. I retrieved all the parts of Titi's uterus and held them together to restore the anatomy as best I could, then I began stitching, making sure the right bits were going back to the right places, like putting together a human jigsaw. Once again, I couldn't see the end of the needle through my goggles, so I dispensed with them mid-operation.

As I encountered more uterine ruptures, I understood I was working partially sighted, even without the scratchy googles. Unregulated oxytocin was widely available in the community. Women were being injected at home, in peripheral clinics or by charlatans to speed up the labour and birth. Not all oxytocin would lead to a ruptured uterus, but there was a significant chance.

After my twenty-four-hour shift was over, I would be too worked up and buzzing to go straight to bed. Bo Base was the only area we had internet access, so I would lie on a couch there and check in with the world, reading over emails, scrolling through the news and Facebook. Life back home was continuing. Tara, a close friend from medical school, had her wedding approaching; it felt strange I would be missing it. We had lived together for several years – six of us in an east London terraced house. We had become a family, discovering our adult selves between studying, partying and sharing our life dilemmas. For over a decade, every date, heartache, success and regret had been shared and dissected. Not being there, I felt as if I were a phantom limb, or a ghost. An observer. The absent participant.

One morning, as I went through my post-shift ritual, a new face appeared in Bo Base. Like a deer stepping through a clearing in the forest, her eyes darted around the room, looking for the familiar and the dangerous.

'Hi!' I called out to her. 'I'm Benjamin. You just arrived?'

She came over and sat next to me. Jenny was a paediatrician from Germany, with freckles on her cheeks, shoulder-length wavy ginger hair and a broad smile. This was her third MSF mission, and she was due to spend a year in the project as the hospital manager.

I explained a bit about my experiences in the project and the challenges we were facing, and Jenny told me about her previous two missions. They had both been hard, intense, exhausting deployments.

'I told human resources I wanted a less volatile mission,' she said. 'They recommended a year here. A long-term, stable project, low security, and I can really get to know the people I'm working with.'

'Right,' I said, thinking back over my last few weeks in the project.

Jenny would join Liesbeth, Alessandro and whoever else happened to be around in the evenings for our long conversations about all that was going on in the world. Nibbling chocolate and sipping beer, we would guess the next move in the global chess game around Ebola. Jenny was an excellent listener, absorbing all of our stories and frustrations from work. She quickly became a close friend, and another mentor to look to, with good insight into the culture of MSF. Her job was to have an overview of the clinical activities in GRC, to help develop the strategy of the project and look towards its future.

I had just finished morning rounds in GRC with Mamadou when Kathleen called. She had heard of plans to transfer a pregnant patient to us from the Kailahun Ebola Treatment Centre (ETC) – a survivor. GRC was five hours by road from Kailahun, so it seemed unusual.

'Do you know why they want to send her all the way here?' I asked.

'All I know is she's not got Ebola anymore and the team think the baby has died. They don't know what to do and want to send her here.'

'They don't need to do anything; they can just let her go into labour naturally.'

Something had ignited in me. I knew I did not want this woman to be sent to us. There was an effort to normalize survivors, reduce the stigma they may face and help them reintegrate into society. Pregnant survivors were less well understood.

'Look, why don't you speak to them?' suggested Kathleen. 'Give some advice over the phone.'

She set up a phone call with one of the medics working in the ETC in Kailahun, who told me that the woman had tested negative for Ebola on the blood sample taken the day before; she was ready to be discharged.

The team were concerned that, because the baby had died, she might get an infection.

'Have her waters broken?' I asked, holding the phone hard against my ear to block out the sounds of GRC surrounding me.

'No, we don't think so.'

'Then she probably won't get an infection. I would leave her alone. She will go into labour spontaneously, or you can induce the labour.'

I could sense their anxiety travelling down the phone line as I explained how to induce a stillbirth. Pregnancy is frightening to those unfamiliar with it, and in normal circumstances I would have relented. I was certain, though, I did not want this woman in GRC. We just didn't know enough.

I had read in the guidelines that semen of surviving men could continue to have the Ebola virus for three months, but they said nothing about the fluids of women or pregnancy. What if the fetus had Ebola? What if she bled heavily? How certain could we be that she was not infectious, when her body fluids would be flowing in the same room as other pregnant women? What would be gained by bringing her all the way from the Guinea border to GRC?

Whatever reason I could think of, I did not want her to come.

There were a few more phone calls, and for a while no one knew what the plan would be. I was pacing around GRC, irrationally on edge. I had induced many women with fetal deaths, so that part was not daunting, but her case specifically was.

Eventually, it was agreed a gynaecologist working in an ETC over the border, inside Guinea, would go to see the woman in Kailahun. I hadn't known about Fernanda – she had been working with MSF, treating infected pregnant women, and her work was groundbreaking. She had been testing the fluids of the pregnant women. Although her number of cases was small, her findings were staggering.

In June, she had been caring for a pregnant woman in Guinea who survived Ebola. The day following her second blood test, confirming she was 'cured', the woman developed a new fever. Fernanda undertook an amniocentesis, removing a sample of amniotic fluid to test it for Ebola. She wanted to know if a negative blood test in a pregnant woman could reliably predict if the pregnancy was also negative.

The fluid returned a highly positive result. Had the test not been taken, the woman may have been discharged to a local hospital or may have delivered at home. However, the findings were not yet widely known, not even by those of us working in the field.

Fernanda went to Kailahun to care for the woman, ensuring she gave birth inside the controlled area of the ETC. The woman was the sole survivor of a large family, all of whom had been infected and had died from Ebola. The success of a pregnant woman surviving was a rare joy for those working in the ETC, and the team was deeply invested in her ongoing care. She delivered the stillborn without complication. But, hours later, she began bleeding heavily, perhaps a lingering result of the haemorrhagic features of Ebola. She died within minutes. It was an unexpected and traumatic blow for the team.

When I heard the news, relief came first. Guilt for feeling relief came next. It settled into fear. A woman survives Ebola, but still carries the disease within her womb. The layers of complexity were mind boggling, and through the fear came intrigue. How were we to overcome the challenges we faced? There were two distinct dilemmas: how to manage the pregnant Ebola survivors, and how to manage the pregnant unknowns – women from the general population. The grey zone of uncertainty for maternal healthcare in the Ebola-affected areas had broadened its range.

9: UNPRECEDENTED

LONDON

MAY 2020

'In room seven is Yolanda, twenty-nine weeks pregnant with pre-term rupture of membranes. She's not contracting. She's had one previous birth, which was also preterm.'

I nodded as Louise, the doctor from the night shift, completed her handover.

Inside the room, Yolanda was sitting up on her bed, legs crossed, with the fetal heart monitor attached. Her chin was pressed against her chest as she looked down at her phone.

'Yolanda, my name is Benjamin. I'm one of the obstetric doctors.'

She did not look up. I heard a *tap tap* coming from her phone.

'I hear your waters have broken, and we are concerned this is quite early in the pregnancy.'

The hard tapping sound continued, punctuating the sound of the fetal heart rate. I bent my neck to try to see what she was doing. Unbelievable, I thought to myself. Yolanda was immersed in an electronic card game.

'Are you . . . ?'

'Yeah, yeah, carry on. I'm listening. I just have to finish this.' She continued tapping the screen with a pale pink acrylic nail.

'The thing is, Yolanda, your heart rate is increasing, and though you haven't had any fever I'm wondering if we need to get the baby out.'

I looked at the midwife, who seemed as puzzled as I was.

'So, we're going to do some blood tests and observe how you both are for a little longer. It's a tricky balance, but we don't want you getting a bad infection,' I said, watching Yolanda's nail hammer down on small playing cards on her mobile screen.

'I won!' Yolanda looked up with a smile. 'Sorry about that, I just really wanted to beat this guy.' She placed the phone on the bedside table. 'Right,' she said, finally back in the room with us. 'I trust you, Doctor. If you tell me we need the baby out, well, that's what we'll do.' Yolanda turned to the midwife. 'I'm starving. Any chance of some breakfast?'

As I took off my face mask, gloves and apron and washed my hands, my mind debated the pros and cons of delivering the baby early. Yolanda was showing signs of infection, but she hadn't had any fever – but waiting till a fever arrives is sometimes waiting too long. And, if we did deliver, should we risk the stress of contractions on such a little baby or go straight for a preterm caesarean section?

'What's your plan?' asked Jane, the midwife, as she passed me in the corridor, carrying a tray of buttered toast and steaming tea.

'I think we'll deliver today, but I'll come back and chat with her again. Just let me know if she's playing cards, so I don't disturb her game again.' We both laughed. 'You know, I like her,' I said. 'We're all too serious around here.'

During the course of the day, I popped in and out of Yolanda's room, her vibrant personality more apparent with each interaction. We discussed the different scenarios and I shared my concerns. Yolanda explained the big picture back to me. She had grasped the details of the dilemma with ease, and had an understanding of balancing risks that doctors take years to achieve.

She gave birth to her little boy, pushing him out in the quiet of night. The neonatal team were prepared and waiting to receive him. A cot in the neonatal unit already reserved for his arrival.

I had shown my cards, and this time, the obstetric gamble paid off.

*

BO/GONDAMA, SIERRA LEONE

JULY 2014

The revolving door of international staff became part of mission life. The flow of expats in and out of GRC was continuous: regular faces left, new faces appeared, and returnees returned.

There were concerns a replacement might not be found for Marlon. The international press coverage of the evolving epidemic was increasingly pessimistic. It was assumed fewer volunteers would be willing to step into such an unpredictable situation. I considered the possibility of Mamadou and I remaining the only obstetricians at GRC, and how sustainable that could be. There would be no room for exhaustion or errors.

On Marlon's last day, he was presented with traditional Sierra Leonean clothing – a shirt made from colourful lappa, adorned with gold and silver embroidery – and then marched around the hospital, with maternity staff banging drums and dancing behind him. I watched from the tukul as our colleagues celebrated Marlon's time at GRC and the care he had provided. A part of me stung with jealousy. Somehow, I knew I would leave in different circumstances. A cloud had already begun to gather, though the storm remained out of sight.

Liesbeth had also departed, her mission only ever intended to be short. Her support had been priceless, and, if for nothing more than our late-night conversations and reflections, she had kept me afloat when I felt like I was drowning. She had spoken to me about normal reactions to abnormal situations; Liesbeth, however, had been remarkable in extraordinary circumstances. I hoped I would be strong enough to carry on without the safety net of her presence to catch me if I went spinning into free fall. Liesbeth had given herself to the project, I suspect she did with every mission. Now she needed to give herself, to herself.

An American obstetrician who had worked in GRC twice before was found at short notice to join us for a couple of months. Collette was in the latter part of her career, and her slight frame was deceptive. She was accustomed to field life and, in her high-pitched squeaky voice, would share stories from the front line that were absolutely not for the fainthearted.

Increasingly we had visitors coming to stay with us in Bo for short periods of time, usually as part of a wider tour around the region. MSF specialists from Europe and emergency team coordinators would come for a weekend break, escaping the unrelenting ethical and emotional hardships of being in Kailahun.

Through my reading, I tried to piece together what we knew, and what we did not know, about Ebola. The maternity questions were often unanswerable. Kathleen and Barbara would listen to my concerns that we were dancing on a razor's edge. I knew Barbara was relaying the dilemmas back up the chain of command, but no solutions were returned. Understandably, anyone linked to the outbreak was overworked, trying to keep their head above water; they didn't have time to contemplate difficult questions from a standard project.

I was still in contact with Fernanda, the gynaecologist in Guinea, but language barriers were against us, and our situations were different. Fernanda was working directly with infected women, whereas GRC was a hospital for the general population that might, or might not, include the infected. Where she worked they knew who had Ebola, whereas we continued to perform surgery blindfolded.

Barbara came to me one morning, excited, with news to share.

'We are going to be visited by Michel, the viral haemorrhagic fever expert of MSF. Finally, you can ask your questions.'

Michel had worked in every major Ebola outbreak since 2000. He had been instrumental in the diagnosis of this unknown and unusual disease which appeared in Guéckédou, Guinea, earlier in the year. He was quick to alert the world that the reach of this outbreak was exceptional. He had warned of how the local traditional practices and overt distrust of the health system and institutions would make containment harder, and yet, despite his expertise, acumen and experience, his warnings had gone unheeded .

Over a hundred local and international GRC staff all gathered together for a special morning meeting, with Barbara, Kathleen and Michel sitting at the front. As usual, the departments gave their statistics and news. Barbara stood and addressed the crowd, shouting above the sound of cockerels crowing and the beeping of passing mopeds. She ran over the week's activities and thanked everyone for their hard work. It was Michel, though, that she focused on, introducing him to the audience and giving him centre stage.

Michel was of average build, balding and unshaven. He wore a light tartan shirt with the top three buttons undone. He spoke in English with a thick French accent, slowing his words down, each one punching the air, carefully chosen and clear. He summarized the situation before us, giving a short introduction to Ebola, but not in clinical terms – he spoke poetically.

'Ebola is a cruel disease. It will take the closest people to you: those who love and hold you; those who care for you in sickness; those who wash your body in death. That is how it procreates. That is how it survives.'

His words circulated round my mind throughout the day. In the evening, I would see him again at Bo Base. There was an international team meeting planned and I would have my opportunity for answers.

'We are just rolling the dice,' I said to Michel. 'We are making decisions and people are dying. What about us, the nurses, midwives and cleaners? Eventually, we will get infected and it will be too late. What should we do?'

I had blurted all my anxieties out in one frustrated mouthful. They lay there on the floor in front of us, both of us looking at them. Michel pulled a cigarillo out of his packet, tapped it in his fingers, lit it and blew the smoke out, then he scratched his stubble and nodded to himself.

I wanted the Holy Grail: the answer. Like a devotee poised for enlightenment, I was ready.

'I am not an obstetrician,' Michel said. 'I cannot tell you about delivering babies or your surgeries. You are the expert for your patients. Everything here is unprecedented. Never before have we seen this. Never before did we have an obstetric project working in an Ebola outbreak. There is no example. There is no precedent.'

I stared at him. My eyes fixed open, red and burning from the smoke.

He took another drag.

'This is the precedent,' he said. 'What you do will become precedent. And, when you say it is not safe, when you say it is too much risk, we stop.' Michel's eyes met mine, 'Then, we stop.'

I bit down on my lips and nodded. I understood: there were no answers.

Everyone in the project was reminded by Barbara at our meetings that we could leave at any time. 'You did not come here for Ebola, and, if you do not want to be here, we will help you to get out,' she would say.

I felt deeply reassured by Barbara and Michel, who represented the higher levels of MSF to me. We were in a whirlpool, and MSF was not only a raft to cling to, but offered ropes to pull us out. The trust Barbara and Michel had in us as individuals instilled reciprocal trust in them, and the organization they represented. It gave me confidence to remain, and I was proud to do so.

One expat doctor had arrived and changed his mind during the car journey to the project, the reality of the current context only hitting home once he experienced it for himself – the checkpoints, posters and constant Ebola discussions.

Talking to him in Bo Base, I reflected on my own arrival at the project. Perhaps the outbreak was becoming business as usual, but I no longer felt weakened by it. There was no doubt I remained anxious, but, in an odd way, I also felt empowered. I hadn't realized it, but I no longer wanted to leave. I had found a purpose – a voice.

'I think you should wait,' I said to him, as we sat on the sofas waiting for a team meeting to begin. 'You've not even seen the hospital yet. Take a couple of shifts and then see how you feel. If it's not right, leave. It might not be what you think.'

But he announced that evening he was going home.

Collette had worked at GRC during previous episodes of Lassa fever infection. She seemed unfazed by the Ebola context. She took an interest in the situation, without stepping into it, like a pedestrian watching a fight on the other side of the road. Collette, Mamadou and I continued working as a team, but we had personalities with different approaches: contrasting, complementing and, occasionally, conflicting.

I began my day like all others, sitting down with Mamadou to get handover from Collette, who had just completed the previous twenty-four hours. I sipped a bitter black coffee as she went over the previous shift's admissions. As usual it was a combined debrief and case discussion rolled into one.

The shift had been busy with cases of eclampsia and a uterine rupture. There was also a thirty-seven-year-old woman, on the antenatal ward, who Collette had struggled to manage overnight. This was Hawanatu's fifth pregnancy; all of her previous four births had been stillborn. Hawanatu had arrived the previous afternoon, feeling generally unwell with headaches, visual disturbances and central abdominal pain. Her blood pressure was 240/160, jaw-droppingly high, and her urine showed maximum amounts of protein. There was no denying she was a pressure cooker of severe pre-eclampsia. The baby was still alive, but it was very premature at around thirty weeks' gestation.

Collette had struggled to bring Hawanatu's blood pressure under relative control. If the pressure drops too quickly or is brought down to 'normal' levels, there is a risk that the placenta will stop functioning effectively, suffocating the baby. Hawanatu was now on three blood pressure medications, including a powerful intravenous infusion being titrated one drop at a time, and still the pressure was creeping up.

We all agreed this pregnancy could not continue, and medication was given to induce labour. Though, we also knew this baby was incredibly precious to Hawanatu. We needed to find a way to give both mother and baby the best chance at life.

Once I had the gown and gloves on, I went to see Hawanatu. She was lying on the bed, with intravenous lines in each arm, and her face was swollen with fluid, which is characteristic of severe pre-eclampsia. Looking into her eyes, I sensed she had come to us with hope. She searched my face for good news.

I took her hand and asked, 'Feeling any tightening? Any contractions?'.

'Nothing.' There was dismay and confusion on her face. She turned to Fatmata, who sat next to her, translating from Mende into English, and said, 'The baby is alive – why are they making it come so early?'

We explained how much we all wanted her to have a baby to take home. I hoped she could hear how genuinely I meant that from the tone of my voice, even if the meaning of my words were lost. The baby was premature and, due to the pre-eclampsia, it would likely be small and unwell. I wanted to be honest: there was a high likelihood the baby would not survive, but there was at least a small chance of life. If we did nothing, eventual fetal death was virtually guaranteed.

She nodded sadly, resigning herself to whatever would be.

After the ward round, I found Mamadou and Collette were still in the hospital. We gathered together and discussed Hawanatu's case again. A further dose of inducing medication had been given, but there was no sign of labour. As a group, we agreed: Hawanatu was due for reassessment at 2 p.m.; if there was still no change then, I would deliver by caesarean section.

The paediatric team was busy with severe cases of malaria, malnutrition and tropical illnesses. I went and spoke to Juli, who looked harassed, struggling to complete her rounds as she was repeatedly pulled away to see sick children in the emergency department or high-dependency bay. I explained Hawanatu's case, and her poor obstetric history. Juli's on-call mobile was ringing; she looked at it – the emergency room again.

'I'll come for the baby, if I can,' she said. 'But no promises. It's manic today and it doesn't sound good for the little one.'

At 2 p.m. Hawanatu's blood pressure was still fighting to get higher and she had had no contractions – but there was also a new problem. Fatmata was pushing the handheld Doppler machine into Hawanatu's belly, and she could not find the baby's heartbeat.

I threw on my PPE and grabbed the ultrasound scanner. I managed to locate the heart and visualize the chambers: it was beating, very slowly. We did not know how long it had been this way. If we were getting this baby out alive, it had to be now.

A 'crash' caesarean section was not something I had seen happen in GRC, but now was the time to try.

'We have to go now – fast, fast, fast,' I said.

I was frantic. I felt the weight of this woman's destiny rested on me. The guilt was already churning inside me.

I explained the situation to Abu Bakar, asking, 'Can you give a quick spinal?'.

He looked concerned; Hawanatu had received a lot of medication to control her blood pressure. A side effect of spinal anaesthesia is that it reduces blood pressure. Combined with the medication, it could danger- ously plummet.

Hawanatu walked into the operating theatre, drip lines dangling from both arms like some odd oversized jewellery.

'I'll get the baby out fast,' I said to Abu Bakar as I turned towards the scrubbing room. 'We can control the blood pressure. The baby is about to die.'

Abu Bakar was on it, but time and circumstance were against us. Abu Bakar also needed to get dressed in PPE to perform the spinal and pre- pare the drugs.

The adrenaline was pumping hard through my veins; each second passing could be a second longer than this baby was able to cope.

I called Juli.

'I'm on my way' she said, I could hear she was walking outside as she spoke, 'and I'm bringing a team.'

I felt reassured hearing Juli's voice, but knew first, we had to get the baby out alive.

Jon and I were scrubbed, dressed and ready before Abu Bakar had completed the spinal. All I could think was, *We cannot give this woman her fifth stillborn child.*

The moment the spinal anaesthesia was completed, we cleaned the skin, pinching Hawanatu to check she could not feel.

'Scalpel,' I said, and in we went.

Within seconds, I was cutting through the thick tissues of her premature womb, avoiding breaking the amniotic membranes. Gently, I peeled the membranes off the inner uterine walls, lifting the delicate head to the bulging sac, which was now presenting through the incision. Premature babies are easily bruised and traumatized; delivering the baby still inside the sac provides a naturally protective cushion. It ruptured as the delivery completed, a gush of fluid splashed out and there lay a very small, wet, motionless baby girl.

I took the cord: clamp, clamp, cut. As gently as possible, I passed the pale, floppy baby to the waiting nurse, who then relayed it to our waiting neonatal team in the room next to the theatre.

I was fairly certain the baby was dead on arrival. I had seen no signs of life in the few seconds before transfer. In total silence, we completed the caesarean section, glancing at each other through our goggles, waiting to hear if a cry would come from next door.

Jon nodded to me in his PPE as a small whimper grew into a howl. The girl weighed little more than a bag of sugar, but she was a warrior, fighting to stay alive. She was transferred across to the neonatal ward to be kept warm and fed. We all knew it would be one day at a time.

The next morning, Hawanatu was already on her feet, insisting she would go and begin caring for her daughter. Her blood pressure immediately became easier to control as she began a vigil of kangaroo care, nursing her precious daughter in the warmth of her bosom.

Every day in GRC we witnessed sad stories, both obstetric and paediatric. The risks were far from over for the baby, but for now we could smile, knowing we had done our best to give her and her mother a fighting chance. The story of the case spread through the team, a brief antidote, a breath of air.*

In Bo Base, after my shift was over, I sat scouring news websites, reading the same stories by different journalists, and opinion pieces posted

---

* Mother and baby remained in GRC for almost two months; they were both eventually discharged in a good and healthy condition.

on Facebook and Twitter. Bad news hammered my computer screen – doomsday headlines about the ongoing epidemic coming from all sides. Outside our bubble, the world was increasingly feeling the Ebola heat.

On 20 July, Patrick Sawyer, a Liberian-American lawyer, flew from Liberia to Nigeria, and collapsed on arrival at the airport in Lagos. He was a known Ebola contact, and later tested positive, dying after several days in hospital. Now, the authorities were searching for anyone who may have had contact with him. It marked a watershed moment in the course of the outbreak. The possibility of Ebola being transported by air had become a reality. If it could happen in Lagos, why not London, Paris or New York? I was reminded of Alessandro's predictions of exponential spread. Lagos was, after all, the largest city in Africa and one of the most densely populated places on earth; it offered the virus a massive opportunity to open its wings and wreak havoc.

The same week brought reports of the first confirmed Ebola case in Freetown, a city of over one million people. The woman, a hairdresser, had been admitted to hospital in the capital. Most concerning was that her family had forced their way into the isolation unit and removed her. Considered 'a risk to all', a search was underway to locate them.

On the veranda of Bangkok House, we argued about whether these events would lead to an international response to halt the epidemic, or further stagnation and posturing. Observing from ground level, it was disappointing. The WHO was not coping, incapable of catching up with lost ground, and international reaction paled in comparison to international reporting. MSF continued sounding the alarm, calling for participation and direct intervention. The response felt inadequate.

In Liberia, another aid group had also stepped up to confront the virus. Samaritan's Purse, an evangelical Christian humanitarian organization, alongside SIM, another global ministry group, were working to treat the infected. There were virtually no other organizations with the experience to manage those infected, but Samaritan's Purse were willing, if done with support from MSF. The evolving Ebola surge in Monrovia, though, was hazardous.

'Did you hear about the Americans?' asked Juli. She was sitting at the end of the table, scrolling through news on her phone. She told me that two of the Samaritan Purse aid workers, an American doctor and nurse, were confirmed to have contracted Ebola.

The panic dial turned up further. 'No one will dare come now,' I said, my head spinning. 'Not if Americans are getting infected.'

MSF was still chanting its mantra that their staff had never been infected in all the previous outbreaks: *If you follow the rules, you'll be safe.* It was an invitation for the world to take action to help stop the spread, but the global headlines were sexier and built a counter-argument that struck at the core of human vulnerability.

Closer to home, we had other problems. Kenema Government Hospital had high rates of internal Ebola transmission. The hospital was overwhelmed and underprepared. Increasing numbers of healthcare workers were getting infected and dying. Approximately 25 per cent of the patients in the Kenema ETC were staff themselves. This was impacting all healthcare and causing absences of traumatized and terrified staff.

The numbers of cases in the community around Kenema were swelling too. Faith in the hospital had dwindled. More and more of the infected chose to remain at home, see the traditional healer or travel to other parts of the country – taking Ebola with them.

Alessandro would update us on news of local sporadic cases: dead bodies left untouched on hospital wards and certain streets where families had been infected. The situation in Bo Government Hospital also worried us. While not in the same league as Kenema, we knew infection control and isolation were not being maintained.

'A lot of the staff at GRC are also working in the government hospital,' said Alessandro. 'We don't know how exposed they might be, or if they pose a transmission risk. Barbara is checking with human resources what the rules are with staff working double contracts. We might be able to make them choose one job or the other.'

'The problem is, it's not only those working at other facilities,' Jenny said. 'Healthcare workers are getting infected at home. They're providing private care to their neighbours – inserting IV lines, giving medications, all sorts of treatments.'

Whether as a business or for altruistic reasons, having sick people arrive at one's doorstep was a hazardous venture. Pressure from MSF to dissuade colleagues from double contracts or providing shadow health services were countered by the need to earn money. Now, more than before, health workers needed to support extended families and assist neighbours in times of sickness.

It was also decided around this time that those of us working in GRC should begin taking turns to work in Kailahun at the Ebola Treatment Centre, to gain experience.

The situation was changing. The healthcare was complex in ordinary times, but now it felt as if there was a python moving slowly around us, advancing surreptitiously, circling and flicking its tongue, determining when the time was right to close in and choke us.

The trajectory of the epidemic did not look good. International reaction appeared to be little more than lip service in response to MSF's siren, while confirmed Ebola cases were spreading like ink on water.

10: KAILAHUN

GONDAMA/KAILAHUN, SIERRA LEONE

JULY 2014

Six years earlier, I had sat in the lecture theatre at the University of London's School of Oriental and African Studies, concentrating as Professor Jonathan Goodhand shouted at us, willing us to believe: 'The capital is not the centre of the country; the border is where decisions are made and the future is written.'

Guéckédou in Guinea, Foya in Liberia, and Kailahun in Sierra Leone: each is a border town where the three countries meet, and each was battling Ebola. Cross-border permeability of both goods and peoples had lent a generous hand to the viral spread.

'If you want to know the destiny of a country, look to the borderlands.' Professor Goodhand's words swam in my mind as I prepared to head east.

I made the journey to Kailahun early on a Friday morning towards the end of July. Alongside the other border towns, this was the epicentre of the Ebola epidemic. MSF had set up emergency projects in each town, battling the outbreak on all fronts. The worrying stories of local populations resisting efforts to contain the disease, on occasion turning violent towards the health workers, had me wondering how the atmosphere further east would be. Kailahun District had been where the spark that ignited the lengthy civil war had first found tinder. It had remained, to some degree, marginalized and neglected.

I was travelling with a driver and Josh, a Sierra Leonean WatSan, and we were taking with us a small package of vital importance: the blood samples of suspected Ebola patients at GRC. Each sample was triple packed, in sealed and chlorinated containers. As we were about to leave,

Josh and I stood together by the Land Cruiser, staring at the box of samples on the back seat.

'Do you want to sit in the front or the back?' I asked.

Josh looked at the box, to me, and back to the box.

'I'll take the front seat,' he said. 'You?'

I eyed the box as if I had X-ray vision, picturing the small tubes of blood inside.

'I think we can travel up front together.'

We strapped the boxes in using seat belts, and squeezed ourselves into the front seats.

As we headed east, we passed through Kenema City. The police were out on the streets and tension could be felt in the air. It had been only days since a former nurse from Kenema Government Hospital had spoken out to a gathered crowd, saying she wanted to let the people know the truth. Ebola and the ETCs were a cover-up, she said, and inside the hospital cannibalistic rituals were happening. The news spread quickly and soon an angry mob had gathered. Thousands marched through the streets demanding the hospital open its gates and release the patients inside, or they would burn it all down. The police shot tear gas to disperse the crowd, but the rumours continued, to the extent that they were discussed on local radio shows, feeding the suspicions about the epidemic narrative.

Shortly after passing through Kenema, the tarmac road ended. The Land Cruiser jerked forwards and backwards over the mud roads. I turned to check our back-seat passenger had not been thrown to the floor, glad not to be too close to the box.

As we reached Kailahun, we were greeted by smiling, waving children, and adults nodding in acknowledgement of who we were, and what our car represented. The ETC was surrounded by lush green forested mountains. It was midday and the sun was beating down. The rains had finished, leaving a clear blue sky overhead. After five hours of being thrown around on uneven roads in the same vehicle as the blood samples from suspected Ebola patients, I was keen to deliver the package. I grabbed some gloves and took the box over to the lab. The sooner the samples were processed, the better for us all.

The Ebola Treatment Centre was made up of tents set on a large area of cleared forest. It was a logistical feat in itself to create a fully functioning complex, with a laboratory, wards and sanitation facilities, in this remote area. Broadly speaking, all ETCs followed a similar structure, being split between 'Low Risk', 'High Risk' and 'Outside' areas. When entering any area, we had to rinse our hands and spray our boots with chlorinated water, and, if going into the High Risk area, we had to dress in the full PPE.

I found the medical team and introduced myself as they were preparing to make a ward round inside the High Risk area. Several new patients had been admitted during the morning. Having already experienced suspected Ebola patients at GRC, and the routine of dressing in PPE, I was asked to assist in the medical activities of the isolation unit.

Movement through the ETC flows in a one-way direction, from lowest to highest risk. This way, the person passing through cannot transfer the disease from a confirmed patient to a possible patient awaiting a test result. Adjacent to the dressing area is patient triage, where individuals suspected of having Ebola are questioned about symptoms and any possible contact with other unwell people. In triage, they are stratified into whether or not they meet the case definition, and to which area of quarantine they should go; if considered to be a 'non-case', they are discharged directly.*

Once I was dressed and goggled up, I walked with Anthony, a tall and lean Nigerian doctor who had worked at GRC previously so we discovered we had several friends in common. He was shocked to hear we were still doing surgery.

'I would feel safer here than at GRC,' he said.

My mind kept returning to this remark as I passed through the multiple orange plastic fences into the High Risk isolation area. There is something totally unreal about walking through an Ebola isolation unit. I had read so much about the disease – it had become like a toxic teenage infatuation, and I had both fallen asleep and woken up thinking about Ebola – I was not expecting to be shocked. But I was.

Not all Ebola patients look sick.

There appeared to be two types of Ebola patient – the well and the unwell. I was ready for the pitiful sight of grown men weakened and dying, people wilted from profuse diarrhoea and external bleeding. While those haunting images I had read about were true, I also found

---

* The 'case definition' is the set of criteria used, based on symptoms or risk factors, to determine if a person should be tested or diagnosed with a disease.

groups of young people sitting around talking and eating together, listening to the radio and playing cards. This was the other face of Ebola: the surviving class.

The unrelenting sun baked through my outer yellow plastic garment, letting all the heat in and none out. It was so hot inside the tent wards that the patients who were able to move tended to sit outside in the mud pathways between the tents. Within minutes, I could feel the sweat dribbling down my body, soaking through my scrubs, which became heavy and sodden. Trying to work in the heat was unbearable, and coupled with the stress of the environment, the stakes of getting everything right and not exposing oneself to the disease, it made for an incredibly intense experience. No one was allowed to enter High Risk alone. You took a 'buddy' and watched over each other – in my case, this was Anthony.

I had spoken to some of the other nurses and doctors at GRC who had been to Kailahun before me, and their reactions had been varied. Some, like Alessandro, wanted to return, convinced this was where we should be: at the front line, containing the outbreak in force. Others were disheartened, and returned frustrated with what they had seen and the level of care available.

The new admissions needed to have their bloods taken, Anthony and I were doing the phlebotomy round. Once inside High Risk we realized some equipment was missing. I walked over, like a turkey wrapped in tinfoil, to the inner perimeter fence and shouted over to the Low Risk area. Nothing comes fast enough when you're cooking in PPE. My goggles were misting over and my head pounded from heat, salt loss and the goggles tight' band. The equipment was thrown over the bright orange fence. Once inside the High Risk area it would never come back out.

Two ambulances had unloaded a group of new patients through a fence at the back of the ETC, directly into the 'confirmed' area. They were all laboratory technicians and healthcare workers from Kenema Government Hospital, and they had all tested positive for Ebola already. They each needed repeat blood tests to determine how high the amount of virus in their body was, and if they had begun making antibodies to fight the disease. The first patient I met had been given a tent to himself; unbeknown to me, he was a national hero.

Dr Sheik Umar Khan was a leading expert on viral haemorrhagic fevers. He had led the research and treatment of Lassa fever in Kenema

and was an author of the WHO guidelines for this West African outbreak. He was also the lead doctor in the Sierra Leonean battle against
Ebola. At some point – allegedly through treating an infected pregnant
woman in Kenema Government Hospital – he too was infected.

'Hello, Doctor,' said Anthony, as we entered the tent. It sounded as
natural as one colleague greeting another in a hospital corridor. But there
was nothing natural about the gravity of the situation. Anthony took his
blood samples, talking of inconsequential things as he punctured the
skin. I sprayed the vials with chlorine and began the biohazard packaging procedure. Dr Khan said little. We wished him well and moved on to
the Kenema laboratory technicians in the next tent.

Eventually, I had to get out of the PPE. My head was spinning, I
could barely see and was feeling faint. Fainting in an Ebola isolation unit
is a very bad idea.

It is on leaving, rather than being in the isolation unit, that the greatest risk of transmission is posed to health workers. I am forever grateful
to the stern Sierra Leonean hygienist who stood before me, instructing
the decontamination process. I circled my finger in the air to show I
was getting dizzy. She ignored it. Breathing rapidly into my double face
mask, I was getting hotter and more aware of the claustrophobia, becoming increasingly frustrated I couldn't just pull the fucking thing off.

'Spread your arms!' she shouted from behind the red line separating
our worlds: the contaminated and the decontaminated. The cool spray
of chlorine washed over me, still in full PPE.

'Turn.'

The relief of feeling the wash was immediately apparent, both physically and psychologically.

'Wash your hands.'

At every step, the hands, still in two pairs of gloves, needed to be
washed in chlorine.

'Remove the gloves, outer pair only.'

There was no emotion. No sympathy that I was melting.

'Wash your hands.'

She shouted her instructions with military precision, her tone clear:
do as you're told.

'Remove the goggles.' Standing side-on to me, she demonstrated, head
tilted, pulling them forward and over the head, with eyes kept closed.

I felt immediate liberation as the air hit my sweaty face. I could see again. I was back in the world. From behind the hygienist, I could see another woman crouching, watching every move, her bright blond hair radiant in the midday sun. She was observing me.

'Wash your hands.'

At last, I was de-robed. With one final spray of my boots, I could cross the red line. I had to wash my hands again in the decontaminated zone, and then I was free to go and rehydrate. I looked like I had just walked through a swimming pool in my drenched scrubs.

Waiting for me was the woman with blond hair. Everything about her was electric and vividly alive.

'You all right, there?' she asked.

The American twang threw me for a moment. The heat was still evaporating off my body, my mouth dry and head banging. I took time to process the words being thrown at me.

'I saw you swaying. Thought you were going to go.'

She led me to a plastic seat, and I flopped, arms, legs and chest spread, breathing deeply – anything to bring my temperature down.

'Here, drink this.'

I took the cold can of soda and pushed it against my neck. It felt good, cooling the blood pumping through my carotid artery.

Mary-Jo didn't need to say that she was a seasoned humanitarian; it was written in her clear eyes and confident kindness. Most people called her MJ. She was a nurse by background and had worked in other Ebola outbreaks before this one. The local staff had a huge respect for her; she had constant energy and a watchful eye to spot anything, even the subtlest of wobbles, that might put them at risk.

Despite the scale of the epidemic and the amount of work to be done, there was a lot of sitting around in the field site. Pre-hydrating, rehydrating, discussing who was going inside when and to do what. Those first days at the ETC were a crash course in Ebola case management. A lot of the skills from working in busy London hospitals were transferable; delegation and coordination with limited resources were nothing new.

With more patients arriving sporadically, often in groups of families or villages, and others leaving, either walking out of the front door or carried to the morgue, there were always jobs to be done. The complication of needing PPE meant work needed to be carefully allocated and thought out in advance.

Occasionally, though, everyone stopped what they were doing – the doctors, nurses, cleaners, everyone – and all attention was directed to the decontamination exit from the High Risk area.

Like a celebrity, the survivor would exit surrounded by an excitable crowd of whooping and clapping. The beaming faces of the crowd were reflected in the broad smile and shining eyes of the survivor. It was always an intensely emotional moment, though often bittersweet. They were sometimes the only survivor from a family, returning to an unpredictable future. Would the community accept them back? Would their belongings and home have been destroyed? Who was still living, and who was not? Despite all the concerns, the sense of optimism and hope was irrepressible.

On discharge, survivors were given new clothes to wear, food supplements, psychological support and assistance from the health promotion teams. Men who survived were given a condom supply to last for three months – a popular debate was just how many condoms that equalled.

Everyone felt a huge sense of achievement during the discharge of a 'cured' patient. But MSF was not curing Ebola; only an individual's own body could win the fight. The medical care was supportive only – through nutrition, hydration and treatment of other infections, such as malaria – though I sensed the emotional and psychological impact on a patient of seeing they were not alone – and of course witnessing the euphoric discharge of others – had an important restorative effect.

Over the course of those few days in Kailahun I got to know the team, working long, hot and hard shifts. The international staff stayed in a guest house, which also hosted other NGOs, press officers and local travellers, and doubled up as the office space for the MSF team. Each evening, everyone would gather to share updates on patient numbers, admissions, discharges and deaths. The epidemiological changes were relayed by Grazia, an Italian doctor with vast outbreak experience. She had been working hard to put together the line lists, mapping out the spread of disease from individuals to their contacts. Grazia was intimidatingly intelligent, an expert in her field, and she had a look of knowing things were going to get worse before they got better.

The conversations would carry on as we all gathered together for dinner, sitting at long tables, while wall-mounted TVs played Nigerian soap operas at full volume. The epidemiologists and health promotors saw the outbreak in much broader terms than those working purely inside the ETC. Emily and Ella were both from the United States, and they had trained a large Sierra Leonean community outreach team numbering over eight hundred staff. Now, as health promotors, they worked together taking vital information out into the villages to dispel myths, educate on disease and explain ways to stay safe. They shared their stories of the holding centres in villages, where the suspected were left alone to wait for an ambulance or fate. At community meetings, they discussed the epidemic and tried to counteract circulating rumours at grass-roots level, and they were building relationships between the Ebola response and respected community leaders – imams, priests, chiefs and healers. Like a sponge, I tried to absorb everything I could.

At the evening meeting, the case of Dr Khan was raised. Nobody had expected such a high-profile patient, but here we were, deep in the rural mountains, and a leading expert was in our care. The WHO was asking questions, the Sierra Leonean government was nervous, and it was rumoured that the President was planning to fly out by helicopter to visit.

The team was locked in a debate of medical ethics and utilitarianism. Should Dr Khan receive special treatment or not while inside an MSF ETC? There was an experimental treatment called ZMapp, which had not yet been used in humans, but had produced promising results in monkeys. The drug was in very limited supply, but, should MSF agree, Dr Khan could have it administered. The discussion was tense and uncomfortable.

There were no human clinical trials of the drug on which to base a decision; it was not clear if there could be unexpected reactions, side effects or toxicity. The question of 'do no harm' came up, but then, what if it worked? What if he would survive without it anyway? What about every other patient not receiving the drug?

If he had the drug and then died, would MSF be blamed for his death? Would this give fuel to the conspiracies about Westerners experimenting on Africans? Then again, if he died without it and it was known the drug had been available, would the same accusations be thrown?

Every argument was convincing and every argument was flawed.

Outside, after the meeting, I had a beer with a South African doctor called Stefan. He was tossing the dilemma around, trying to find some way to reconcile the conflicting and personal issues raised. I'm sure, at some level, we all had the same thought: *What if it was me?*

The team, tired and opinionated, continued debating. I abstained; I felt too new, too much of an outsider, underqualified to play a part.

Over the course of my stay, I became increasingly involved in assisting the medical team. I was working with Morris, a community health officer from the local area, who had already been working in the ETC for several weeks. He was an intelligent man, with a calm nature and a mature outlook, so I was glad to buddy up with him. Each day, before donning the cumbersome PPE, we would check through the patient files together, making a plan of action before entering the High Risk area. This way, we knew which patients we needed to see and any specific tasks to complete, keeping our time inside to a minimum. Preparation and efficiency were key.

Once we had on our PPE, we would check each other to make sure we had not left any small patch unprotected. We were about the same height, which made checking easier. As if staring at one's own mirror image, we meticulously looked around the sides of each other's googles, facial hood and mask. When satisfied that we were safe, we entered the High Risk area.

Our first port of call was the 'suspect' patient area, where patients had been admitted within the last twenty-four hours. They had symptoms, but no obvious history of contact with the disease, and were waiting for blood test results to determine whether they moved through to 'confirmed' or were discharged. Most of the suspect patients looked well; only one man was lying on his bed inside the hot and humid tent. I had seen him on admission the day before, when he walked into the unit himself to declare his concerning symptoms. He had begun having bouts of watery diarrhoea and his appetite had diminished. Today, he was still alert and able to hold a coherent conversation. We talked a bit about basic care when suffering diarrhoea, and a quick assessment showed he was not clinically dehydrated, so I encouraged him on oral intake and made a note: *Not for IV*.

In the tent next door, separated by orange fences and troughs of chlorine solution, were the 'probable' patients. They too were waiting for a blood test and official confirmation, but entered the ETC with a solid contact and symptom history. The day before, six members of one family had come from a village known to have an uncontrolled outbreak; they all tested positive and moved along the conveyer to the 'confirmed' area, filling the beds of recently deceased or discharged patients. The probable patients appeared to be in a worse condition than those who were suspect. Most were lying in the fetal position, one hand resting on their stomachs (a common symptom of Ebola is stomach ache). They looked weak and apathetic.

A small boy was quietly curled up on his bed. He was nine years old and visibly malnourished; he could've easily passed for much younger. He had arrived late in yesterday's shift, in an ambulance with his mother. The roads around Kailahun were in appalling condition, and the journey in the back of the ambulance as it navigated each muddy bump and pothole, when already feeling sick and frightened, must have been awful. When the ambulance doors were opened, the mother was found to have died during transit. Now, recently bereaved and alone in a strange and bleak place, he was faced with strangers dressed head to toe in bright yellow suits, wearing masks and goggles. Terrifying. He was lying in a pool of watery diarrhoea and, though awake, did not show any sign of recognition or make eye contact. He was frozen with fear. We took the small blood test, gently cleaned him and made a note for him to be helped to eat and drink.

We passed through another set of orange plastic gates, which separated the 'suspect' and 'probable' areas from the confirmed Ebola patients, and walked through another chlorine foot-bath. It was not possible to see all patients during the ward round. It was too hot in the PPE and there were too many. Holding a soggy piece of paper with the names of specific patients of concern that Morris and I had identified earlier, we worked our way around them. Although we made notes as we went, we would have to shout our findings to another medic from the inner perimeter fence at the end of the round, who would write it all down again. Whatever we had taken inside could not come back out, including paper and pens.

I began to look for the first patient on our list. Lying in one of the tents, I found a very unwell looking woman. She was not on the list, but clearly she was of concern. Her breathing was rapid and shallow, and her eyes, although open, were glazed over, looking far away and beyond. There was no sense of recognition or interaction. Her arms were tensely flexed and rigid, hands in fists, as if she were ready to begin a boxing match. She was incontinent of urine and faeces. Clearly, she was in the end stages. I made a note, washed my gloves in chlorine and moved on. We would discuss her deterioration in the medical meeting later and decide to place an intravenous line, but when the following team entered the 'confirmed' area they found she had passed away.

The first patient on my list was Ramatu, a middle-aged woman who had been doing reasonably well, but not anymore. She was lying on the floor outside, strong enough to get out of the hot tents, but she looked weak and listless. I knelt down next to her to feel her pulse, check her temperature and count her breathing.

'*Ramatu, aw di bodi?*' I asked, in my poor attempt at Krio.

She looked at me; I was reassured that she could respond to her name. She told Morris and I that she had no complaints, no more diarrhoea, and she was managing to eat. The description she gave was a million miles away from how she looked. Most of Ramatu's family had died, and in recent days her husband had passed away too. Her situation reminded me of what Michel had said about the intimate nature of the disease's transmission: it kills those you love the most, the people you are most likely to care for, or who care for you.

I asked again how she was feeling.

'Sad,' she said. She was emotionally exhausted, giving up her own fight, now, to join those she had loved and lost.

I made my notes and arranged for the psychologist to see her, but despite his best efforts, she would not speak with him.

On my rounds the following morning, I found Ramatu lying in her bed, in the same boxing posture as the other woman, eyes open and body fixed in rigor mortis.

Alongside the ward rounds, I had been given a special maternity assignment. Mariama was a thirty-year-old woman with painfully swollen breasts requiring attention. She had been admitted to the isolation ward with her four-year-old son. Having recently given birth, she was still breastfeeding her baby when people in the village began dying from fever. Mariama's mother was the first in the family to die. Then, one by one, Mariama's children died from the same illness, including her suckling baby. Now, the only one left living was four-year-old Augustine. Mariama was tall and lean, alert and attentive, able to walk about the isolation unit freely and talk normally. Her left breast was large and heavy with milk, as she no longer had a baby to feed. I went over the technique to empty the milk, explaining how the pain would resolve with repeating the procedure. Breast milk, like any bodily fluid, carries the Ebola virus, so she also needed to understand how to safely dispose of it.

Together, we went to see Augustine. He lay on the floor, looking like he had arrived from a famine. Flies buzzed around his head, his eyes were sunken and dull, and his skin was loose with signs of severe dehydration. His gums were bleeding, leaving dried scabs over his lips and tongue. His liver felt enlarged, and he grimaced when moved. During the examination he only made an occasional whimper, otherwise remaining floppy, working hard to get air into his young lungs. Mariama confirmed Augustine had profuse diarrhoea. He desperately needed hydrating. As a team, we discussed little Augustine, and where we were going with his treatment. What was a reasonable measure between assisting him and unduly distressing him? We decided to insert an intravenous line, to try to replace his lost fluids.

The following day, I reviewed Augustine. His veins had been too thin and too wilted to accommodate an intravenous line, but Stefan, the South African doctor, had managed to pass a line into Augustine's bone marrow instead: intraosseous rehydration. While he was still very sick, there was a significant improvement. His skin had regained turgor, and he was more aware of what was happening, even fighting off my examination a little. We were cautiously optimistic. Another lengthy team discussion followed, as we debated attempts to build up his nutrition. Decisions that would normally be easy became contentious in the Ebola context; the line of what to treat and how was ethically and emotionally challenging. Together, we decided his improvement was a sign to give him extra support, and we agreed on placing a nasogastric tube to feed him nutritional supplements. Later that day, however, we found little Augustine lying still, next to Mariama; her last remaining child had been lost to this pointless epidemic.

It is hard to convey humanity in an Ebola isolation unit. As a health worker, I am used to reaching out and touching my patients, letting them know they are not alone. In the ETC, any contact was through double gloves and triple-layered protective clothing. My eyes were the only part of me visible, behind their misted goggles and the small slit in my head dress. The distance created by the PPE was compounded by the linguistic and cultural differences, and the lack of understanding about Ebola. I have never felt so far removed from and, at the same time, so intimately close to a stranger as when I rested my gloved hand on Mariama's, and, with only my eyes and the subtle movement of my head, conveyed my deepest sympathies.

Regretfully, I learnt to develop this communication, repeating it several times during those few days in Kailahun.

Despite the unfortunate and frightening circumstances, a community had developed among the patients in the isolation unit. They would sit together outside the tents around the 'confirmed' area, listening to a radio or chatting in small circles. A group of children, who were doing surprisingly well inside the ETC, had come together to create a pseudo-family, the older kids caring loyally for the younger ones, offering a stark sign of hope during difficult times.

The night before I was due to return to GRC, I sat in a small meeting with some of the doctors and nurses. MJ stood next to a whiteboard, energy emanating from her. 'We need to get ready; numbers are going up. You guys have ideas? How are we going to organize this place?' she said.

Stefan opened a can of beer and leant back, the sun setting behind him. Geraldine, a Swiss nurse with a thick accent, big intelligent brown eyes and long brown hair, began explaining how she thought the ETC should be organized. She was clear and precise. I watched her and knew she was part of the answer.

'You need a coordinator,' I said.

As usual, I had returned to my comfort zone for inspiration: the London labour ward. At home, it was standard to have a senior midwife (or nurse, in the emergency department) coordinating activity – not getting directly involved in patient care, but seeing it all from above, knowing what's been done, what needs doing and who needs a break.

The next morning, we all went to the ETC and cleaned the large notice board; we were trying to devise a more efficient system to follow patient progress, test results and outstanding tasks. We also left space for the name of the shift coordinator. Geraldine was taking first duty.

I gathered the empty boxes used for transporting blood samples and bid farewell to Morris and the rest of the team. I took a last look at the tents lined up against the dark green of the surrounding forest. Professor Jonathan Goodhand was right: this remote land of mountains and burnt buildings – this was the centre.

Stefan texted me the following morning, 29 July. Dr Khan had died, ravaged by the beast he was meant to conquer. He was thirty-nine years old. He never received ZMapp, nor had he ever known it was available. The nation was devastated; he had been their hope, and now hope was gone. The shock of his death forced many to acknowledge Ebola was real, and, if it could take Dr Khan, it could come for you too. In particular, the President appeared more shaken than ever before.

As the rainy season advanced, the daily thunderstorms attacked the parched red earth, beating it into submission and flooding what had once been dust. The large droplets bashing the corrugated iron roofs created a deafening cacophony, like thousands of steel drums being struck by an angry mob. Everyone and everything stopped for the downpour. The rain came with such fury it took my breath away.

Back on the veranda of Bangkok House, I stared straight into the sheer rage of the storm. Like the rains, the epidemic was sweeping across the country, permeating through the different layers of society. The resistance to believe in the dangers of the virus was evolving into a national disaster. Some of the loudest and longest storms felt like they would never end, but eventually they always did. The same was true of an Ebola epidemic. The spread of the disease leads to violent outbursts of illness. However, in a time with no vaccine and no cure, it will ultimately burn itself out. What remained to be seen was how far this storm would spread, who would be left standing and what would be washed away.

Not so far away, in Monrovia, the Liberian capital, a course of ZMapp was shared between the American nurse and doctor who had contracted Ebola while working for Samaritan's Purse. It was two days after the death of Dr Khan, and exactly the same treatment declined on his behalf, without his knowledge. The team treating the Samaritan's Purse patients grappled with many of the same dilemmas as the team in Kailahun. The doctor and nurse were later airlifted to an intensive care unit in Atlanta,

USA, where life-supporting care was available. They both survived, but it could not be confirmed whether this was due to the ZMapp. They were the first humans to ever receive it.

In epidemiological terms, the sun was yet to begin its descent on the outbreak. For all the political rhetoric of the last few months, it appeared that the world was only now beginning to sit up and take notice of the unfolding disaster. I may not have been qualified to give an opinion on why the moment had finally come at that point, and not with MSF's warnings several months earlier, but it was hard not to notice its arrival had coincided with air-travel transmission and the infection of Westerners.

In West Africa, the epidemic continued to slowly burn, but until sufficient international coordination got under way to release the necessary resources to extinguish the fire, we knew the needlessly sad stories we were witnessing would continue.

11: STATE OF EMERGENCY

RWANDAN BORDER WITH THE DEMOCRATIC REPUBLIC OF CONGO

JULY/AUGUST 2019

Bursts of colour ripped through the grey metal fence. The crowds pushed forward and backward over the Rwandan–Congolese borderline. The disorganized queue of shouting women moved as a single chaotic swirl towards the checkpoint. Like cattle waiting to enter the slaughterhouse, they were shoved and slapped by border guards holding twisted metal rods with sharp pointed ends.

Small yellow and brown bananas piled on their heads, sacks full of dusty clothes, flip-flops or flour strapped to their backs, the throng of women moved to make money at the Gisenyi border market. On the other side, the sprawl of Goma city and the troubled Kivu regions simmered with militia groups, massacres and a prolonged Ebola epidemic. Each day, over 40,000 people crossed the barbed wired no-man's-land between these economically interlocked neighbours, carrying goods, contraband and, perhaps, disease.

The nurses charged with monitoring the surge of people for signs of disease dispersed through the crowded queue. They stood out like stone pillars among the colour and noise in their long, dirty lab coats. The smell of sweat filled the air. The atmosphere was humid and pungent as the travellers shouted and shoved. Each nurse was armed with a thermo-scanner, trying to detect any person with a fever, but the crowd moved with unrelenting purpose; slowing it down only built the pressure, like water against a dam. Business is king, time is money, and the border is for unstoppable trade.

I stood at the border, watching the flow of humans and the exchange of goods. It had been a week since the WHO announced a Public Health Emergency of International Concern in the Democratic Republic of

Congo. Rwanda, like David to Goliath, held a slingshot, not quite sure where to aim. Over a million people live across the borderline separating the two cities, sharing history, language and culture. Gisenyi and Goma are inseparable for all matters, including life and death.

'So, a woman arrives at the hospital in labour. Are you worried?' I asked the fifty Rwandan doctors and nurses sitting in neat rows on wooden benches. The fresh air was gently blowing through the open meeting space of the Gisenyi Government Hospital.

'There's no outbreak over here, right?' I went on. 'It's in Goma, over the border, but you get patients from both sides, you get the travellers and traders. So, should we be checking? Asking where they've been? Checking if they have a fever? If anyone they know has been sick or died recently?'

The men and women sat up, nodding in agreement. Their eyes followed me as I paced, attentive to my movement.

'But currently, you're not checking. By the time you realize – *if* you realize – they will be in the hospital with all the other women and babies. They will have been inside the operating theatre and feeling unwell on the ward for days. You, your patients and their visitors will have been exposed.

'What if this woman says she's come from Congo and has a fever? What if she is obviously unwell? What will you do? Where will you tell her to wait? What if she is literally about to give birth?'

The eyes looking at me have no answers, only a realization that they are not yet ready for this, but they need to be, because it is already happening less than hour away from where we are talking. I'm looking into my crystal ball and I'm seeing GRC.

'Preparation,' I say, handing the task over to the team. 'Let's talk about how to get ahead of Ebola, before Ebola is here.'

*

GONDAMA, SIERRA LEONE

JULY/AUGUST 2014

On Wednesday, 30 July 2014, a state of emergency was declared across Sierra Leone. We were going into lockdown: schools and markets would be closed, military troops drafted in and Ebola-affected communities put into quarantine.

Thursday was declared a National Day of Reflection by the President of Sierra Leone, Ernest Bai Koroma. The population was requested to stay at home and consider the implications of the epidemic. For myself and the staff of GRC, however, it was business as usual.

I began my shift optimistically. With the restrictions I could relax a bit and chat with colleagues. There were not many inpatients; there had been a further decline in numbers due to the fear of catching Ebola in healthcare centres. We took the opportunity to a run a refresher on PPE. There was a mix of overuse and persistent lapses in maintaining a safe standard for infection control. After lunch, I got comfortable outside the tukul, pulled out a book to read and positioned the electric fan. Through the fence, I watched men and women walking to the river banks with large round sieves balanced on their heads and carrying heavy-looking spades. They were searching for the minerals and wealth buried in the muddy waters.

The on-call phone rang: 'Doctor. Patient. Come.'

On the bed in the delivery room was a woman making the deep vigorous noises of someone with the uncontrollable urge to push a baby out. Massayo passed me the triage sheet, so I could see the woman was not a Lassa or Ebola suspect, and began reading off her notes on the maternity assessment form.

'This is her third birth,' she told me. 'The two before were both normal deliveries. She's been in labour for over a day and pushing since early morning.'

I noticed that the patient's abdomen had the tell-tale signs of an imminent uterine rupture – dipping deep in the middle, where the uterine muscles were pulling in. The urinary catheter had only a small dribble of blood inside it.

'Before coming to GRC, they gave oxytocin to make the contractions stronger,' Massayo added, following my stare.

The baby's heart rate dropped slowly down with each contraction, making a difficult ascent back to normal between the forceful pushes of its mother. It was stuck in the wrong position and too high to assist a vaginal delivery. All the signs of obstructed labour were there. If not relieved, the uterus would split, emptying its contents.

In the operating theatre, the caesarean proceeded smoothly. The baby came out, startled and limp, but the heartbeat was present, and a midwife whisked him away to be resuscitated. As I was closing the final layers of the patient's abdomen, Jenny stuck her head around the operating theatre door. As hospital manager, she had begun taking daily walks around GRC to see what was happening and speak with staff.

'Do you need me to call a second gynaecologist?' she asked.

I looked at her through my goggles. I could make out the freckles on her face, but was not quite able to read her expression.

'No,' I said. 'I think we're done, here. Why?'

While I'd been operating, two new patients had arrived. Jenny told me they both looked serious.

I left Jon to put the final stitches into the skin and made my way next door, to the delivery room, where I was faced with pandemonium.

The two women were lying flat on adjacent delivery beds. The first to grab my attention was a twenty-year-old having her third child. Her last delivery had been by caesarean section. She was making a lot of noise, screaming and wailing, but, to my ears, it was the sound of progress. I turned to the woman in the bed next to her. Tennah was a nineteen-year-old who had delivered the first of her twins at home in the morning. Now, she was here, with the second twin's purple arm hanging out between her legs. She was not screaming. She lay still, only making an occasional grunt.

I went to the quiet one first.

Tenneh acknowledged my presence with a flicker of her wide-open eyes. A stunned look of terror covered her face. I turned to the midwife, Isata, to find out the vital signs.

'No blood pressure, Doctor,' Isata said, holding Tenneh's arm in her gloved hands, feeling for a vein. 'Her heart rate is 150. Breathing rate, forty-five a minute. She has a high fever and her haemoglobin is four.'

The situation was grave. Around me, the nurses and midwives were fluttering in disorganization. I took a deep breath. Order and control were needed. Direct commands began to leave my mouth, not because I was being rude, but because there was no time to be polite.

'You —' I looked at Isata, 'take the IV fluid and squeeze it into her as hard as you can.' I turned to the gathered nurses. 'You, get oxygen now and put it on the highest flow. You, get a second IV line in and then take a manual blood pressure. You, get antibiotics. Massayo, go to the patient in the other bed and don't leave her. Whatever is happening here, you stay with her.'

I turned to Jenny, who had been watching the scene unfold. 'Can you run to the blood bank? Beg them to give us any compatible stock they've got.'

I donned all the personal protective gear and felt Tenneh's abdomen. It was scorching hot to touch, tight and tense, with a deep ridge in the middle where the uterus doubled in on itself. A quick ultrasound scan showed a dead, trapped twin. The baby was lying in an awkward position, making vaginal delivery impossible. The head was buried into its mother's upper left abdominal corner, neck and body wrapped in an almost perfect circle, with the legs and feet high up at the top of the uterus. And one arm hanging down through the vagina.

There were two options for getting the baby out: reach inside, grasp a foot then try to bring the legs down and deliver the baby breech first, or do a caesarean. But, before I could do either, Tenneh lost consciousness.

Her pulse suddenly dropped from racing at 150, to a steady, slow 60, and there was still no recordable blood pressure, even with two IV lines and fluid being forced down them as fast as possible. Her breathing was now nothing but an occasional gasp. Tenneh was dying in front of us.

I hesitated, my mind searching for a solution. I felt responsible and helpless.

Jenny returned with one unit of blood. Immediately, we started the transfusion and inserted a third intravenous line. Tenneh's condition was beyond critical.

I began speaking my thought process out loud, to anyone willing to listen: 'Airway: it's open and clear. Breathing: she's breathing, but slowly and we've got oxygen going. Circulation: pulse is slow, no blood pressure, fluid going in, blood going in, no urine coming out. Uterus displaced.* Antibiotics given. Fetus still in. What are we missing? OK, let's start from the top again.'

While we continued resuscitating her, I tried to get the baby out. Tenneh was unconscious, not stable enough for theatre, but maybe, if

---

* Moving the uterus to the side helps relieve pressure on the woman's heart and circulatory system.

I could remove the baby, it would help treat the infection and make resuscitation efforts easier.

I put long, gynaecological gloves on, and asked two of the nurses to support Tenneh's legs. I reached through her vagina, past the prolapsed arm. All the amniotic fluid had drained out and the baby was tightly fixed inside. Like a contortionist, I twisted my arm and got my hand round the head and chest. I found the other arm and kept going. The feet were all the way up past the tight constriction ring where the uterus was contracting, folding in upon itself. Squeezing my fingers together into a pincer grip, I pushed, urging them to find a way, but it was impossible. The feet were beyond my reach.*

Straightening up, I repeated my resuscitation monologue. 'Is there anything else we can do to help?' I asked the nurses and midwife looking upon Tenneh.

'No, Doctor,' said Isata, squeezing a bag of saline, rushing it down the drip.

Though I had looked after women who had subsequently died, I had never seen a woman's heart stop beating on my watch. I turned to Jenny, and mouthed, 'She's going to die'. I was out of ideas. I began preparing mentally and practically for the oncoming cardiac arrest.

The fourth time I went through the vital signs, we finally found a blood pressure: 60/40 – bad, but better than nothing. Slowly but surely, Tenneh's pulse began rising, her breathing became stronger and her blood pressure started to increase. Our efforts were kicking in, not a second too soon.

Massayo shouted from the cubicle next door, 'Doctor, come here, please'. I did not want to leave Tenneh. 'What's wrong?' I shouted back.

'She's fully dilated, Doctor, but the baby's not coming.'

Before I could respond that it hadn't been too long, Massayo added, 'I've tried the vacuum cup, but the baby don't come. It's still in the same place'.

A failed assisted delivery is considered an obstetric emergency, especially in a woman who's had a previous caesarean section. But so is a

---

* Turning the body of an entrapped baby inside the womb requires a firm grasp, hence needing to reach for a foot. It is not possible to hold onto the round fetal head as it will slip out of the assistant's hand.

teenage girl trying not to die. I looked down at Tenneh and told the team to keep doing what they were doing. I pulled off my protective clothing, replaced it with a new set and attended to the patient next door.

The baby was alive. Its head was still quite high in the pelvis, but deliverable. Unfortunately, it was looking upwards. I desperately wanted the operating theatre to stay free for Tenneh, once she was stable. This baby needed to be born vaginally.

Massayo explained to the woman what was happening as I reapplied the vacuum cup far back on the baby's head. As the contraction built up, I shouted in Mende for the patient to push: '*Too-kpey! TOO-KPEY!*'

Nothing moved.

Sweat poured down the sides of my face and round my goggles as I crouched low on the floor, poised with one hand stabilizing the suction cup and the other in position for applying traction. All other noises were muted; I was completely focused.

'*TOO-KPEY.*'

I felt the head descend as she pushed down, and it rotated under my hand to look downwards. As the head crowned, it became clear this was a big baby. I slowly eased the head and body out. As the newborn baby cried, I passed him to Massayo with the cord still attached. I pulled off the gown, gloves and googles, and made my way back to Tenneh.

Her eyes were open and her breathing normal. Unbelievably, she was talking to Isata. I had sent all her relatives to donate blood, in anticipation, and now we transfused another unit and prepared her for the operating theatre.

Trepidation tiptoed through me as I cleaned Tenneh's bulging abdomen with the dark-brown iodine disinfectant. A caesarean for a baby lying transverse, after the amniotic fluid had gone, can be tricky. I cut a large incision from her umbilicus down. I wanted all the space I could get.

Once I entered, I saw litres of blood pooled either side of the uterus: it had ruptured. The thin translucent outermost layer of uterine tissue had not torn, creating a congealed mass of blood which extended across the front of the womb, completely obliterating the usual place for a caesarean section. I picked-up the skin of the uterus, cutting into it like opening cellophane packaging and released the trapped blood. The baby's feet fell through the incision, holding them I delivered the deceased second twin, now with ease. The rupture was small but had ripped through the arteries to the uterus on one side. In late pregnancy, these carry over half a litre of blood every minute. Goggles off, I ligated the torn artery and repaired the uterus. By the time I finished her haemoglobin was 2.4 g/dL – desperately low. I begged for blood and got another unit.

Afterwards, I sat outside the theatre, writing my notes and reflecting on the situation. Alessandro knocked on the door. 'I heard from Jenny; she said you're having some tough cases. Is there anything I can do?'

He sat with me as I wrote instructions for the ward nurses on the post-operative plan.

'The cases coming here – it's like a different specialty from what we have back home,' I said, pondering my competence. 'And this PPE really doesn't help.'

From the theatre, we heard shouting: 'Dr Benjamin!'.

I dropped my notes and ran back to Tenneh, who was bleeding from everywhere.

Not blood, really – a watery pink. Her uterus was relaxed and the blood was pumping out from her vagina. It poured from the edges of the wound, as if her body were crying tears of blood. After losing so much blood and receiving large amounts of fluid, and with severe infection, her body had no clotting left. We gave drugs to contract the uterus and tilted her body, head down. I got Jon to press on the bleeding wound and I asked Alessandro to call Mamadou. I clenched my fists and pushed them deep into Tenneh's abdomen, compressing her aorta, a major blood vessel, to reduce blood flow to the uterus and buy time until help arrived. I did not want to operate again, but knew it was a possibility, and, if it had to happen, I wanted company.

Together, Mamadou and I assessed the situation. Tenneh could be bleeding internally from the surgery, or it could be the lack of clotting and her relaxed uterus causing vaginal bleeding. We decided to reopen the stitches and check inside. The same watery blood was there, but no active bleeding. The surgery was clean and dry – a huge relief. Mamadou thought we should proceed to a hysterectomy, but I was unconvinced. With no clotting, we risked causing more bleeding by operating again. On the other hand, if we left the uterus in she could bleed vaginally. Either way, she could not afford to lose any more blood. We looked at each other across the operating table, the girl's open abdomen before us. These were impossible decisions, in extreme circumstances. Neither of us wanted to back down, but I was the first to concede, and we performed the hysterectomy.

Once Tenneh's abdomen was closed, we begged to get another unit of blood for her. Blood was more precious than gold in GRC. The laboratory technician came to complain, but soon realized the drastic situation we were in. Throughout the night, Tenneh's blood pressure remained low or unrecordable. I kept pushing the fluid. Hour by hour, we checked for a change. As the sun began to rise, so did her blood pressure, and at 7 a.m. something very special happened: urine. Everything was starting to go in the right direction. I left in the morning, shattered, but sure Tenneh had turned the corner to recovery.

I woke in the early afternoon. I absorbed my surroundings, looked up at the mosquito net, listened to the crow of cockerels and the rumble of the generator outside. After replaying the previous shift in my mind, I texted Mamadou. It was 3 p.m. and I had one question only: *How is she?*

At 2.50 p.m., Tenneh, a young mother, her life before her, had become another participant in the sad statistics of global maternal health. Each death is a tragic story of poverty and motherless children, and a reflection of sociopolitical attitudes, priorities and understanding. Tenneh's death had nothing to do with Ebola. The world was awakening to the Ebola epidemic, but we were also witnessing another emergency: a protracted health crisis.

Over the following days, I was caught between recollecting Tenneh's journey and fixating on the developing Ebola response. I felt the best line of defence would have been for the international community to spur into action, tackle the epidemic's source and join us. Instead, it seemed paranoia had won again. Emirates Airline banned all flights to Conakry, the capital of Guinea, on 3 August. Two days later, British Airways announced it was suspending its flights between London, Freetown and Monrovia. Further international airlines followed suit, either reducing or cancelling flights. High-income countries had prioritized isolating the region, rather than ending transmission. This was not a solution; in fact, it would become a hindrance, reinforcing geopolitical stigmatization and diminishing the accessibility of the worst-affected places – the places where access was needed most.

12. INVISIBLE INSURGENTS

GONDAMA, SIERRA LEONE

AUGUST 2014

The week after Tenneh died, I arrived at GRC on a Thursday morning for my long shift and headed over to the tukul to get handover from Collette, a cup of strong instant coffee in my hand. Collette had just finished her own twenty-four hours, and was sitting at the table completing her notes. The story of her shift began like any other: the eclamptic teenager, obstructed labours and caesarean sections. I was beginning to think about how I'd manage each case, when she started telling me that an ambulance had arrived from the hospital in Kenema.

'They had been trying to induce this woman's labour for days,' she said, 'but it wasn't working. Her membranes are ruptured and she has a fever. Her blood pressure's also on the high side, so I've started magnesium'.

My eyes widened. Everything around me stopped.

'Collette, is she inside the maternity department? Was she a patient *inside* Kenema Government Hospital?'

Jenny, who had been sitting at the next table, going over some papers, looked up and caught the expression on my face. Instinctively, she moved in a little closer.

'Then, you wouldn't believe it,' Collette continued, 'another ambulance came from Kenema. This time, with a woman in her ninth pregnancy – they also couldn't get her into labour. The baby's dead. They said she's been in the hospital for two weeks already, but is not doing anything.'

I could feel my pulse rising, my heart pumping in my throat.

'Did they have IV lines already in?' I asked.

'Yes.'

Kenema Government Hospital was an infection control disaster. Local colleagues knew many of the healthcare workers who had died there, in particular related to maternity. In the weeks to come, we would refer to that time as the 'Kenema Massacre': during July and August, over forty healthcare workers from Kenema were infected with Ebola, with at least twenty-two hospital staff dying. The place was a disease amplifier.

Jenny and I were like deer staring into the headlights of an oncoming truck. The crash we had all been trying to avoid – was this it?

The women were inside the maternity department, one on each ward. They each had features of suspicion – fever and intrauterine fetal death – but most concerning was they had been inpatients inside the overwhelmed Ebola-riddled Kenema Government Hospital. We had heard Ebola patients were able to walk freely in and out of isolation. Staff, patients and visitors were getting cross-infected. The women had had invasive procedures performed inside the hospital – IV lines, blood tests, vaginal examinations – and there was no way of knowing what level of precaution, if any, might have been taken.

I went straight to maternity. I needed to get an idea of what we could be dealing with. I wanted to speak to the women, but first I needed PPE. I wasn't taking any chances.

I went to the ward – there was no PPE there. I went to the delivery room – it was all finished. The night team had been working without PPE. I looked at them, dumbfounded. What had we been talking about all this time – stressing about? I asked the nurse to collect some more PPE from the warehouse, so there would be enough for the shift. Another nurse walked out of the delivery room, wearing gloves, and into the general ward, picking up charts and touching door handles. I was watching and wondering, *Where have those gloves just been?*

Once the PPE arrived, I gowned, gloved, face-masked and head-capped up. We used a 'light' form of PPE on the wards, though even this *too* was unbearably hot. The world was immediately more distant, separated in humidity, haziness and discomfort.

I went first to the woman in her ninth pregnancy, Yabom. I wanted to understand what had happened while she had been inside Kenema Government Hospital for two weeks. I asked if there had been anyone dead on her ward.

'Yes,' she said. Her thin, twig-like arms rested over her prominent belly, a pink intravenous cannula was fixed to the back of her
hand with white tape, peeling up at the side and smudged with rust-
coloured dirt.

'She was in the bed next to me. She just died – I don't know from
what. And they left her body there for a long, long time. I covered her.'

I sucked in air through my damp face mask, pulling my thoughts
together.

'Do you remember, was the woman bleeding?'

'Yes, she was.'

But, in a maternity ward, bleeding can mean anything.

We went back over the history of Yabom's admission. The baby had
stopped moving and she had been feeling unwell. The hospital knew
the baby had died, which meant she had been carrying it for over two
weeks post-mortem. They had tried to induce the labour with tablets,
but nothing was working and now she was having fevers. That's when
they decided to send her to GRC.

I took the ultrasound probe and glided it across Yabom's abdomen,
methodically building an image in my mind as I scanned up and outwards. I could clearly see there was no fetal heartbeat, but the rest of
the findings were strange. The placenta wasn't attached to anything; it
was hovering under the baby. It didn't look like a placenta praevia; it
was freely floating. Nothing made sense. The placenta could have completely detached from the uterus, but Yabom's belly was soft. Normally,
if the placenta detaches, it causes heavy internal bleeding and the uterus
becomes hard and painful. She was at ease, calm and patiently waiting
for her stillborn child to pass.

As I continued to think about Yabom's predicament, I stripped off the
PPE, washed my hands and arms thoroughly in the chlorine water and
went across to investigate the other woman. Kadie was young and in her
first pregnancy. Her waters had broken, but the labour hadn't followed.
After a week of waiting in Kenema Government Hospital, with other
patients walking in and out of the ward, she had developed fevers and
was sent to GRC. Kadie too had had several internal examinations and
IV lines inserted.

I went outside to think. Neither woman was obviously unwell enough
to consider an outright suspected case, but they both had a high risk of

exposure. What if they were in the early stages of disease? What would be the risk, if they delivered and we had body fluid contact? There would be no point testing them; even if the test was negative, it could be a false negative – we had seen this in the treatment centres when it was taken too early. What if they had already had Ebola and survived? Would the pregnancy still pose an infection risk? So many questions, each with high stakes, and no answers.

As I was pondering all this, I heard a commotion, shouting and angry voices coming from maternity. I went back in and saw An, a visiting expert in infection prevention and control, standing red faced, with her hands in the air. A nurse had just delivered a baby with no gloves or protective clothing on. An was livid. She turned to me and I uttered the words no one had yet dared say: 'We need to close'.

Later, those of us on duty huddled together in the tukul and began heatedly discussing what all the morning's activities meant for the safe continuation of services.

'We have no idea what risk the two patients from Kenema pose to the others,' I said, 'and some staff are still not taking precautions. It is too dangerous. The risk is too much and we will lose this game sooner or later. Luck is all we have had till now, and it will run out'.

Jenny reminded us that headquarters in Europe still expected us to keep going. No matter what, we weren't to stop activities. But we all agreed that this message felt increasingly distant.

'They're out of touch with our reality,' Alessandro said.

'If we get infected that's it; no one will come to help,' I said, pulling my knees into my chest. 'The world is terrified and looking to MSF to lead the way. If we have a disaster here – internal transmission – they will say "if MSF can't do this, then we won't".'

The concerns that MSF stopping would send a bad message were countered by the risk of us becoming infected. Surely, the damage of the latter would surpass the former? We had witnessed the catastrophe of Kenema, and heard increasingly worrying stories of healthcare-associated infections across the region.

'The lives of the staff have to come first,' Silje said. 'They are the future of the health service.'

We all nodded in agreement. Without the staff, the long-term impact for maternal health seemed even bleaker.

Those of us who had been up to Kailahun pointed out that working in the ETC felt safer and more secure than working in general health-care. The patients there either had Ebola or they didn't. The set-up was specific and infection control tight. At GRC we were working in a grey zone: our patients might have Ebola, or might not, or might go on to develop symptoms after admission. There was nothing to tell us how to stratify the risk. Our knowledge, at that time, was rudimentary.

'If a person isn't symptomatic, that means they aren't contagious, right?' I asked. 'But what if you perform a caesarean section and have a scalpel or needle injury, and then the patient develops symptoms after-wards? What about the fluids of pregnancy? How do they correlate?'

No one knew.

I explained that both women would need to have their labours induced. 'Will it be safe to have other patients in the delivery room when they give birth?'

An was shaking her head. 'Infection control practices are evidently still not in place,' she said. 'We need to minimize collateral risk to others.'

We called Hilde, an MSF doctor experienced in viral haemorrhagic fevers, who was working in Kenema, trying to help the hospital get its isolation unit in order. She heard our concerns, but had no answers either.

'We have to stop taking admissions,' I said. 'The wards have one patient each from Kenema, and there's a good chance they will both need surgery. We have no way to guarantee the safety of patients coming in.'

'If you do surgery, you'll need to fully decontaminate the theatre afterwards,' An said.

Jenny ran a hand through her red hair. 'Perhaps it would be better for patients to go to the Bo Government Hospital till we have this sorted,' she said.

This seemed like a good idea to me. 'We need proper infection con-trol and patient flow,' I said. 'We need to protect our staff, our patients, ourselves. This is more than a health issue – it's our security too.'

The discussion flowed between us: the known and the unknown, the ethical quandaries. In the end, we all came to the same conclusion: we needed to stop, before our luck did.

Jenny called Barbara and told her. There was no resistance. Barbara was already on her way to a meeting and would relay the message to key stakeholders, ensuring the radio announced that GRC was not taking maternity referrals.

I went back to maternity to complete the ward round, but soon heard there was a taxi with a patient at the front gate. Jenny and I went out together to explain that they needed to go to Bo Government Hospital.

Lying in the back seat of the taxi was a woman at full term. Her head rested on the lap of a man, his eyes bulging and intense.

'The baby is here. The baby is here,' he was saying, pointing to between her legs.

I looked at him, at her, at the taxi driver. 'What do you mean? Is she delivering?'

'The head, it has been here since yesterday.'

'You have to go to the government hospital,' I said. 'We're closed. It's not safe to come in.'

'Please, help us,' the man pleaded. 'Help us.'

'You need to go; we can't help you right now,' I said.

We walked away, the woman staring, never having spoken a word, and the man calling out from the open door. The taxi didn't move.

Inside GRC, I could see through the fence that the taxi was still waiting. What was I doing? Were we right? Were we wrong? There were no answers. All I could come back to was that we needed to make our house safe for all before we took any new patients. But, for those who had made the journey to us, that meant shutting the gate and denying care.

An ambulance pulled up on the opposite side of the road to the taxi and began honking the horn. A guard ran out and explained the same situation to the driver.

A woman opened a small window in the back of the ambulance and began calling over to us. 'Help us! Help my sister! Help us!'

I stood, staring, horrified. What were we doing? We no longer knew anything. I no longer trusted what was in the back of ambulances from far away. Ebola had spread like wildfire and people lied about their symptoms. We were blindfolded at the end of the plank.

We needed to explain to our colleagues what was happening. Jenny called a meeting for 2 p.m., the time for changeover of shifts from early to late, so we could speak to both groups at once. As everyone congregated, my mind and body felt lost, wandering in a wilderness of guilt, anguish and confusion.

Jenny stood up to speak.

She described the situation in maternity, the country's changing context, and finally the decision to stop taking admissions. It was clear that, to the majority, this was the beginning of the end. I felt eyes burning into me. Would they lose their jobs? Is that what I had done – taken away their livelihoods? After Jenny had finished speaking, I stayed back and spoke to those who needed to know more. The message was simple: we needed to do what was safest for us, for staff, and that meant stopping admissions so we could figure out the next move. We also needed to get ourselves prepared for the delivery of the two women transferred from Kenema.

Isata stood directly opposite me, her face impossible to read. Firm and fixed, she stared hard at me. She was a colleague I had come to feel close to; I didn't want to be frozen out.

'What do you think?' I asked.

She said nothing. I felt the world falling apart around us; I was desperate for some sign of hope that we were together on this.

There were very few people left from the meeting, now, and, as the last of them drifted away, Isata stood, slowly and with purpose, she began to move. 'Come,' she said, walking towards the metal wire fence separating GRC from the dirt road and world outside. We stood looking through the wires. The ambulance and taxi had gone. I wondered about their passengers and what would happen to them now.

'I know those people in Kenema,' she said, looking past me, towards the road. 'We all do. They are our sisters and brothers. We have all worked together. I know of five who died already in the hospital.' She paused, took a breath. 'In the war, we knew when the rebels were coming. We would run into the bush. Those were terrible times. But, this Ebola – you don't see it, you don't hear it. It is worse than a rebel.'

'What should we do?' I asked.

Neither of us had answers to offer.

Inside maternity, our priority was to try to ensure safety for everyone: healthcare workers, patients and the two women from Kenema. We rearranged the wards, moving Yabom and Kadie into the area we tended to keep for post-operative patients. I left the beds next to them empty, as a buffer for any theoretical risk should either begin to display symptoms of haemorrhagic fever. I needed to demonstrate restraint between keeping infection control procedures appropriate and not lending myself to overt paranoia or stigmatization. I'm not sure the balance was ever going to be achievable.

The three labouring women I had inherited in the morning from Collette had each given birth, although not without incident. The adherence to infection control had been poor. I was normally sympathetic to this – we all found it a hassle – but, in the current circumstances, my leniency was spent. The delivery room was cleaned and we made sure there was a solid supply of PPE. Once the first patient from Kenema was inside, I didn't want any other patient or unnecessary staff member to be involved.

The drugs I had given Kadie to begin the labour were kicking in. We moved her to the delivery room and I got dressed up into the PPE for the examination. Kadie was not a small woman and it took time to get her on the bed and in position. She moaned and moved with each contraction and, as the time passed, the heat and humidity under the protective clothing deepened. When I was finally able to examine her, I found her cervix was only one centimetre open and still felt thick. I could also feel another layer of membranes – possibly the reason why Kenema Hospital's induction efforts had failed. I took a long sterile hook and carefully passed it through the neck of the womb to rupture the membranes. A small stream of light green fluid flowed out. Kadie found the examination difficult and was screaming and swearing to Jesus as I removed my fingers. She was sweating, I was drenched, and we both still had a long shift ahead of us.

I asked Isata to begin the oxytocin hormone drip and to monitor the baby's heartbeat. Isata and the others present wanted me to deliver by caesarean section, but I wanted to avoid surgery as much as possible. However, while the labour continued, I spoke with the WatSan and explained that there remained a significant chance Kadie would eventually need a caesarean. If required, it would be during the night. We discussed the logistics of making sure we had WatSan support and what level of PPE would be safe, but also suitably comfortable.

As the day drew on, the rest of the international team began to go home. I met the night shift of nurses and midwives, updating them on the events since morning, the decisions that had been made and the plan for the two patients. It was a difficult concept to understand; the patients didn't show signs of Ebola, but they might have been exposed and we didn't know what that meant. Like me, the night shift staff had many questions. I had no easy answers and no easy solutions.

Kadie continued contracting; I knew we should let the labour progress, but, after hours of the hormone drip, there was no change. We were all exhausted, Kadie cried in pain to 'make operation'. At 2 a.m. I called in the backup WatSan support, and together we performed a caesarean section of unknown hazard. There was silence throughout the surgery, all of us engaged in working quickly, smoothly and safely. The baby came out screaming, and soon the surgery was completed. Each of us in the operating theatre undressed, using chlorine water to decontaminate ourselves. Again, we planned to have Kadie transferred to a bed away from the main ward. The invisible enemy and the fear had not gone away with the birth of her baby.

By morning, we had cleaned the delivery room and moved Yabom, the other woman from Kenema, in. As I handed over to Mamadou, we discussed the possible reasons for Yabom's odd presentation, and the ultrasound scan which made little sense. His feeling was to take her for a caesarean; I was more in favour of a trial of labour. His judgement was correct. Yabom had a rare case of abdominal pregnancy, the baby, placenta and sac having grown outside the womb.

I left GRC and headed to Bo Base. I was too tense to sleep. It was Friday, 8 August. I connected to the internet and looked at my phone. There was nothing I could say about the last twenty-four hours that I felt anyone back home would understand. Pete, a tall Australian logistician with short blond hair, had been sending me text messages overnight for updates, and he joined me now for a chat. His light-hearted manner was a relief after the heaviness I had been immersed in. But when he returned to his office, I returned to my phone, and the news and continued discussions of the mounting global threat Ebola posed weighed on me again.

The WHO had declared the Ebola epidemic to be a Public Health Emergency of International Concern, over four months after accusing MSF of being 'alarmist' for calling the outbreak unprecedented. There were now four affected countries and over one thousand people had died from the disease. The declaration enabled the unlocking of emergency funds and resources for global coordination and action. Perhaps now, a sizable, forceful and appropriate response would materialize.

Barbara saw me and walked over. She looked tired. Our eyes met and I wondered whether I was going to be in trouble for having disobeyed the instructions from headquarters to 'keep going'.

'I am so sorry.' These were her words, not mine. 'I am so sorry we let it get this far.'

She explained that a new emergency project coordinator had arrived last night to begin establishing an ETC near Bo. An MSF legend, she was known to everyone by her initials – MTV – and had decades of humanitarian field experience. Her love of adventure was as well-known as her eccentric tendencies and passion for whisky and cigarettes. Apparently, she also had strong feelings on the activities of GRC.

I walked from Bo Base back to the houses. I was in a suspended state; nothing seemed real or unreal, just numb. I had no appetite and I couldn't sleep, though I tried, lying on the bed, listening to the buzz of the guard's radio and letting the stream of questions, thoughts and images run freely through my mind.

That evening, the international team gathered in Bo Base. I had gone early to check through emails, and I was writing reports about our predicament in maternity when I saw a flash of colour from the corner of my eye. I looked up to see a woman wobbling her way out of the bathroom, cigarette dangling from her mouth and tumbler glass in hand, wearing a bright bandana over her head. This had to be the infamous MTV.

As more people gathered, we moved all the sofas and chairs into a 'U' shape, with Barbara, Kathleen and MTV positioned at the front. Barbara began the meeting by updating us all on the week's events – the rise in cases, the struggle for international action, and the challenges in other health centres – and then MTV was presented to the group. Her credentials were impressive: a tour of humanitarian headlines going back decades.

There was a pause as we all waited for her to speak. She took a drag of her cigarette, though there was little more than the butt left, then she theatrically removed it, stubbed it into the ashtray and immediately lit up another, taking a long, smooth drag. She raised her glass of whisky, as if making a toast to the room. MTV had arrived.

Her voice had the sound of a thousand missions, someone who had seen the best and worst of humanity. Though small in stature, MTV filled the room with personality, and, like a professional actress on a stage, she owned the space around her. Everyone was spellbound.

'MSF is bad,' she began. 'MSF is very, very bad. But –'MTV held her glass up high – 'we are the best.'

Her monologue continued through a history of MSF, her aspirations for GRC and for the project she had been sent to begin. She talked about the drama of the world around us, MSF's role and the part we would all play. She moved between singing the words and spitting them at us. And repeatedly she returned back to her mantra on the bad and the best of MSF. By the time MTV had finished, we were all somewhere between stunned and lost.

After the meeting, as I sat chatting with Pete, Juli and Alessandro, I saw Barbara from across the atrium, motioning to me. We were to have a side meeting with MTV, who wanted to speak about the maternity services.

I had already written a report for headquarters on the challenges we were facing inside maternity. Mamadou, Collette and An had all contributed. This included recommendations on how the department could be reorganized to reopen and support ongoing services during the Ebola epidemic. I ran over to Pete's office and printed several copies of it. There was no point discussing maternity if those discussing it didn't have the context.

Barbara, Kathleen, Jenny, Mamadou, Collette, MTV and I gathered around a large table in the meeting room. Everyone sat for a while, reading the report, anticipation building as pages turned. MTV had been in the project for little over a day. Her understanding of the last three months for maternity could not have been more than basic, and she seemed caught off guard by the information in the report. I heard her pencil scratch along the paper as she underlined a few sentences, then she put the report face down on the table. The floor was hers.

'I wanted this meeting so we could understand each other,' she said, making eye contact around the table. 'You must keep maternity open. This –' she gestured to the report – 'doesn't matter. You *must* keep it open. I am a nurse; I know what it is to look after patients. You cannot abandon them now. In Switzerland, my country, we have mountains – this is like climbing the mountains. I would never, never let a team go to a mountain that was not safe. I would cut the ropes to stop them if there was a danger. I understand you feel frightened, but you must continue. If you stop, then you send the women of Sierra Leone to hell. You send them to hell.'

Everyone at the table stared at one another. The room felt smaller than when we had walked in. Perhaps it was because I hadn't slept; space and time were distorted. I should have felt hazy, but somehow my mind was focused. It was my time to speak.

'MTV, I don't know you. I'm Benjamin. I apologize – I haven't slept or eaten much in two days – but I'll do my best to help you understand.' The words moved slowly through my mouth like syrup, but they each fell with intention. 'You don't come and sit here and tell us about sending women to hell. We are the ones who have seen what is happening here. We are the ones who have stayed up through the night, operating and fighting to save lives, not knowing if we should treat or isolate. Do you think this decision to close was easy? You think it hasn't been thought about carefully? We have been tearing ourselves to pieces.' I touched the report on the table in front of her. 'Read what we have written in that report. If you can find answers, if you can tell us how to do this and be safe, please do. We have proposed improvements, changes to make the department and our work safer, but these will take time and resources.'

I took a breath, the others around the table looked on, but none appeared ready to join the discussion. I turned back towards MTV.

'You say you're a nurse and you understand mountain climbing? Then you must know the first rule in any emergency is to assess the danger before approaching. If it is not safe, you do not go. You would not send your team up that mountain if the avalanche was still falling. Obstetric care right now, with what we have, is not safe. You will be sending us back into the path of the avalanche.'

This wasn't the conversation MTV had been expecting. Her face twisted with a look of indigestion, as she tried to appreciate the issues and swallow the magnitude of the situation. Despite coming from opposing positions, I had a fondness for her. She reminded me of a great-aunt; her words, while harsh, were from a place of wanting good.

'No,' she said, finally. 'You have to reopen, immediately. No waiting.'

Barbara and Kathleen both tried to reason with her, but MTV had walked into the room with her mind made up. We tried again. Explained again. But she wanted us to reopen, without accepting the risks.

Jenny spoke up, her face red with angry tears: 'How dare you come here and attack them? You have no right to talk like this. No right.' She got up and left the room.

'I think that's probably a good place to end the meeting,' said Barbara, and the rest of us began to move from our chairs.

Before leaving, I turned to MTV and spoke to her, one-to-one. She smelt of tobacco and whisky. I wanted her to understand that no one here wanted to stop activities, but we had to take action before disaster hit. The irony was we all wanted the same outcome – safe maternal healthcare – but our chosen paths to get to that destination were radically different. If she could help us find a way to make obstetrics safe in *this* context, mitigating for the gaps in our knowledge and designing safe systems to deliver care, we would provide it. I knew, below her thorny exterior, she wanted what we wanted. But, without adaptations, we stood in a building on fire, and we would be burnt.

In the following days, we continued discussions of how to reopen maternity. Jenny and I planned what would be needed to make the department as safe as possible: the human resources required, a one-way flow of patients, and modified hygiene facilities. As we put this all down on paper, we knew it was unlikely we would be given the people and resources we were asking for. The organization was already struggling to meet the huge demand for the Ebola response, and the wider world was not keen on entering the danger zone.

Each day, I would return to GRC, see the remaining inpatients and discuss with the local staff the broader state of affairs. I shared my experiences in Kailahun, the proposed modifications to GRC and the expanding Ebola response. They looked at me uncertainly, afraid of what it would mean for them. I encouraged them to apply for jobs in the new ETC near Bo, the one MTV had come to build.

I was spending more time with those dealing directly with the Ebola response, collecting my own thoughts on the way forward. I agreed with Alessandro that the most immediate concern was stemming the epidemic. Without breaking transmission, without a solid response, the ability to provide safe and comprehensive obstetric care would remain elusive.

Each night, I debated the future and shared dilemmas with my international colleagues – Alessandro, Jenny, Juli, Silje, or whoever was around

– and I also began spending more time talking with MTV. Despite our prickly introduction, we got along well. Her experiences from humanitarian missions across the world were as captivating as her theatrical presentations. Her task now was to find a plot of land that could be rented and converted into a large ETC. Bo was in a prime position for taking cases: a central location, with highway access to most other major cities.

I began pushing to be sent back to Kailahun. Their caseload was increasing and medical volunteers were in short supply. There were also frequent stories of pregnant women being admitted. I received calls from the team to discuss their management, but the mortality rate remained astonishingly high. There was very little knowledge on how to look after a pregnant woman with Ebola, or on how to deliver her baby. The only documented reports were from previous outbreaks in the Democratic Republic of Congo (formerly Zaire), where 93 per cent and 89 per cent of women had died, respectively. There was no published case of any newborn to an infected mother surviving.

The agreement was made: I would return to Kailahun indefinitely. MTV had one other request: she wanted me to come back and join her at the new Bo ETC, once it was near completion.

13: TWO YOUNG BROTHERS

BO/KAILAHUN, SIERRA LEONE

MID-AUGUST 2014

Early on Sunday morning, I got a call from Pete, the Australian logistician. I was to travel to Kailahun at lunchtime. I began throwing belongings into my rucksack. I had learnt from my previous stay that I would need more socks. Wearing wellington boots all day, especially with the heat and humidity, left our feet blistered and in a terrible condition. I rushed down to the local shop and bought half a dozen pairs.

I hadn't cut my hair in months and it was an unruly mop. I was mentally preparing myself for time back in full PPE and wanted to make every effort to be comfortable, so I borrowed some hair clippers and cropped the lot off. I felt nervous and invigorated, putting myself exactly where I said I never would: the Ebola front line.

I met with MSF doctor, Hilde, at Bo Base. We would be taking a lot of equipment with us, as well as a former patient from GRC who had been treated for a ruptured uterus and torn bladder. She could finally go home, travelling with us through the checkpoints to her home village. When the Land Cruiser was fully packed, Hilde and I squeezed together in the front with the driver, Mohamed, while the former patient, her baby and her mother, who had been with her at GRC, sat in the back.

It had been raining almost constantly for three days, which made the inside of the Land Cruiser uncomfortably humid. I tried to find a balance between having the window open for ventilation and not getting a constant shower of rain and mud. It was good to be up front with Hilde, and the long journey gave us plenty of time to discuss what had been happening around the country. Hilde had trained in Belgium as a general doctor, but had a fascination with viral haemorrhagic fevers. In recent years, she had worked with MSF, responding to outbreaks, and had spent a long stint in GRC to focus on their Lassa fever treatment centre. She had been working with two other experts to help Kenema Government Hospital get its infection control procedures in place. These were stressful times, but Hilde was in her element – a rising star in her area of expertise. As she described the horrendous tasks performed to clean up Kenema, her voice changed to the blunt tone of dissociation, punctuated by bursts of motivation. This work was her passion and, while exhausted, she radiated vigour. Hilde had been engaged in the response from the start; she would see it through to the end.

We dropped the new mother who had travelled with us at her village. She was smiling as she left us, but I could not help but feel anxious for her returning to the area. She and her baby had survived what many would not, and now they walked back to an uncertain future, with the dual threat of high infant mortality and a spiralling Ebola epidemic. I watched her walk away with her mother and baby, feelings of pride and trepidation mingling inside me.

Hilde was keen to stop at Kenema Government Hospital to see the team there and check in with them, but, before we went inside, she warned me not to touch anything. They had done a lot of work to clean things up, but, for her, the whole place was still contaminated. Armed with alcohol gel and gloves, we began walking through the deserted wards to the area being used for Ebola isolation. There was no one in sight in the main hospital, just the constant sound of rain hitting the corrugated metal roof, but the isolation unit was a hive of activity, with the Red Cross, WHO, MSF and local teams working together. Hilde was happy with what she saw. She explained to me how it had been when they first arrived, with little separation between those who had Ebola and the rest of the hospital.

Hilde got dressed in PPE, slipping into the suit as if into a second skin, and went into the High Risk area. I waited by a small office next to the isolation entrance, where some staff sat chatting. On the floor was a large cardboard box with a toddler inside.

'Who's this?' I asked one of the nurses, as she dipped a biscuit into her tea.

The nurse was dressed in a pristine white uniform, with a matching fascinator pinned to her hair. She looked down at the box and smiled at him. 'His mother is inside the ETC; she tested positive. He's got no symptoms; we are looking after him.'

No symptoms of Ebola, no testing required. They nursed him here, fed him, played with him. I had not considered what happened to unaccompanied children. Where could they go? But he was also a high-risk contact, much like the pregnant women we'd had in GRC.

I heard, a few days later, that the toddler had developed symptoms and tested positive. I imagined being those nurses who had been caring for and playing with him, drinking tea in their office with him at their feet. Their conflict of sadness for him against the fear for themselves and their own families.

We continued our journey east, and I began to recognize the names of the villages we passed through, infamous from the weekly epidemic updates. They told a sad story of how the disease had travelled from the border regions of Guinea and Liberia.

The journey from Bo to Kailahun normally took around five hours, however the rains had made the roads difficult and as we moved further east they changed from concrete to shale to mud. The journey was broken up with a 'kiss': those travelling from Kailahun back to Bo would meet us along the way and we would swap vehicles; this way, each driver would return home with passengers. Juli had been in Kailahun for a few days, and the South African doctor, Stefan, was heading home with his mission completed. We met on the roadside and, as they came out of the car. I got a sense of the roads ahead. Stefan was covered from his waist down, as if dipped into chocolate, having had to push the Land Cruiser out of the pools of mud. We exchanged details on life in Bo and Kailahun, and Stefan updated me on the pregnant women they had in the ETC.

Hilde and I squashed up front again, continuing our unending conversation as the rain became increasingly heavy. The daylight was beginning to fade and by the time we hit the really bad roads it was night. We were travelling through lush jungle on narrow dirt tracks that rolled steeply up and down and were peppered with pot holes. The area was in quarantine; movement of people was restricted and there were efforts to get food and living supplies to the villagers lying behind the checkpoints. Large trucks, intended to deliver aid, were marooned along the roadsides, lopsided in the mud soup. For the most part, Abu, our driver for this part of the journey, skilfully navigated his way between these trucks and the edge of the road, but the Land Cruiser would occasionally skid. At other times, the wheels on one side would lift up, throwing us all to the side. We would all lean against the tilt, trying to weigh the vehicle back down to the road. I found myself praying under my breath for us to survive the journey.

We came to a stretch of track with trucks deeply embedded in the mud on both sides. The road appeared impassable. Abu stopped and got out of the vehicle. He chatted with the drivers and villagers who were standing around, assessing the situation. Hilde and I began to consider the possibility that we would need to sleep in the Land Cruiser or attempt the journey back to Kenema – though, in the dark, this seemed a risky strategy.

Abu got back in and started the engine, his eyes focused on the swampy path ahead. The corners of his mouth twitched, flickering the muscles of his face.

'Are you sure?' asked Hilde.

'We'll see,' he said, tilting his head to the side, as if it were a spirit level measuring the angles of the mud track. 'If we don't get through, we reassess.'

There was no radio or mobile reception, so we hadn't been able to communicate with the base to let them know the situation, and the rain was now hammering down. With the windows open and engine revving, Abu went for it with full force. He pulled the wheel one way, then, as we began skidding, quickly turned hard the other way. The engine cracked beneath us, letting out a groan. Steam rose from the bonnet, but Abu, undeterred, powered on.

'You can do it!' Hilde shouted, and together we began chanting, as if at a football match.

The vehicle lurched and hit solid ground.

'Go, Abu!'

He smiled and shook his head. In the dark of night, we continued down the mud roads, heading east to the border.

We arrived late at the Kailahun guest house. The team was in the restaurant, eating their dinner of chicken and rice. I recognized some familiar faces, including the health promoters Ella and Emily, and as we sat around chatting I was introduced to the newer members of the team. Gabriel was the archetypal Irishman, with fair skin and burning ginger hair. He was sitting with Vincente, a Spanish man with light freckles, short brown hair and a strong jawline. They were both epidemiologists, and were discussing local chains of transmission and projections of where the outbreak was heading. They had continued working on the line lists Grazia had created before their arrival. These showed how certain villages had been struck by the disease, and how it spread from family to family, sometimes leaving no relative untouched. The lack of ETC beds in the country meant those suspected of being infected were left untreated, in unsanitary conditions, increasing transmission risk. Between the epidemiologists and the stories the heath promoters brought back from the villages, the overall picture was increasingly grim.

After eating a small amount in the restaurant, I headed to the administration office to find out which room had been allocated to me. Hilde was already tapping away on her computer, the fluorescent light from the screen illuminating the concentration on her face. She carried such an overwhelming weight of responsibility I don't know how she slept. I suspected she didn't.

Each day I tried to see the same patients, to review their progress and offer continuity in their care. I met Jeneba the day after my arrival in Kailahun. She was one of the pregnant patients Stefan had told me about, and I took an instant liking to her. She had the same name as the premature baby we had delivered to Hawanatu, the woman with severe pre-eclampsia in GRC, which made me smile.

Jeneba's village had been badly affected by the epidemic; she was one of eleven members from the same family to be infected, most of whom had died, including her youngest child. She was about six months pregnant with her fifth child, but it was evident from our first meeting that the fetus had died. Jeneba hadn't felt any movement for days, and though, in herself, she seemed quite well – no pain and no bleeding, and she was able to walk around, talk and eat – she had a fever and a bit of diarrhoea.

She was sharing a tent with two young brothers, a nine-year-old and an eight-year-old, also from her village, but they looked less promising. The younger of the two was lying in his bed, weak and lethargic. He managed to sit up and drink oral rehydration solution, but he preferred to sleep. His older brother was comatose and bleeding from his mouth and nose. The boys' parents had both died already. They were here alone, except for the care and attention they received from the staff of the unit.

The second day I saw Jeneba, she had improved enough to come and sit outside. She moved herself with the typical slowness of the infected, yet still held her head in elegant posture. We talked over the isolation fence, with the help of a counsellor from the Sierra Leonean psycho-social team. I asked if she knew why the baby wasn't moving?

'Because it has died, and I'd like it to come out now,' she told the counsellor.

I explained how that could be done, but I also explained my reservations, as, with Ebola she could bleed heavily. Together, we agreed that she should first focus on improving, getting stronger and building herself up with vitamins and nutrition.

'When you're better,' I said, because I believed it, 'we'll induce the birth'.

A couple of days later I took the early-morning ward round with Morris, the community health officer I had buddied with during my previous Kailahun stint. It felt reassuring to be with familiar colleagues; consistency created confidence. Morris and I went through the usual ritual of dressing and examining each other for any gaps of skin showing. We made our way through the 'suspect' and 'probable' areas of the ETC, stopping at the patients on our list. I would crouch down next to each patient, my oversized yellow plastic bodysuit puffing out as I did so. Despite the layers of PPE, I made a point to put my gloved hand on the wrist of each patient. I did this partly to feel their pulse, which told me much more than their heart rate – it also spoke to me of force: strong, feeble, bounding or thready. But I also wanted to reach from one human to another, to touch those deemed untouchable. Morris would talk with the patients and explain to me their complaints and progress. He was methodical and exact. When time was critical, as the heat of working in full PPE intensified, his precision was a relief. Our suits crinkled with every movement. Morris and I communicated with our eyes and body language, as if we were divers in the ocean, because verbal communication was reduced to muffled barking.

Inside the 'confirmed' area, I found Jeneba curled on her bed. She was struggling to breathe, gagging with vomit and nausea, gasping for air between the retches. I looked down at her, stunned for a moment at her unexpected and rapid deterioration. I yelled for Morris, who was behind me checking on another patient. I crouched down, taking her wrist in my hand. Her pulse felt like a butterfly trapped under her skin, frantically flapping its flimsy paper-thin wings for freedom. When I looked up at Morris, his eyes showed he had seen this too many times before. We gathered cloths, disinfectant solution and large absorbable pads to clean and dry her. Jeneba's eyes rolled back and round, her eyelids fluttering. The skin over her pregnant belly wrinkled as I wiped off the mess. *She needs more fluid*, I thought, planning ahead, trying to be efficient. Morris drew up anti-sickness medication into a syringe, passed it to me, and I injected it into her vein. I stroked her arm in some pathetic hope it would encourage the medication to take effect, and said, 'It's OK; you'll feel better now,' hoping the sound of the words might soothe her. Morris put his hand on to my shoulder, I looked up to see he had returned with the IV fluids, but he did not open them. He looked only at Jeneba's still chest. I closed her eyes.

There were patients we knew would die. We accepted there were dire limits to what we could achieve in the field hospital, the camp. I probably should not have been shocked. But as we lay her body straight, it was shock which trembled my double-gloved hands.

The epidemic was out of control. Every day, we were receiving more patients. They were arriving from increasingly far away, meaning longer journeys squeezed in the back of ambulances, bouncing along those terrible roads. By the time the ambulances arrived, we would find patients who had died en route, and patients lying, dazed, next to them, disorientated and dehydrated.

We took turns to run around to the ambulance bay, assessing the condition of the people in the back of the vehicles. Standing a couple of metres away, we would shout to the passengers inside, 'Open the window! How many of you are there?'.

We tiptoed to see through the crack of the ambulance window. Trying to count patients and see if anyone was on the floor. Conferring with one another what our next step should be.

The ambulance drivers often did not know themselves what or who they were bringing. They were unsung heros, providing a vital service. Transporting infected people was a hazardous job. I do not know how many of those drivers became infected; I do remember those dark days when we would isolate familiar faces: soldiers from the front line. Incredibly, there were drivers who, having survived Ebola and witnessed all that death inside the ETC, went back to continue their essential work, showing a strength that does not exist in many people. Those drivers saved uncountable lives.

Looking back now, I realize I did not appreciate the drivers and the work they did. They all wore some form of PPE – terrified, I assume, of getting infected and taking the disease home to their families. They would be drenched in sweat, having driven in the impermeable suits. We would give them bottles of water to rehydrate and, once the patients (alive and dead) were unloaded, the ambulance would be sprayed inside and out with chlorine to decontaminate it. On instruction, and quite sensibly, we would not touch anything from the ambulance. The referral papers for patients coming from other hospitals would be held only in gloves and read out to someone else to copy the information down. The driver, their ambulance and all that was in it represented an Ebola twilight zone. They were neither infected nor free of the risk of onwards transmission, and yet they were fundamental to the fight.

Those final weeks of August are a time I see like a film. I'm not there, I'm watching it all play out on screen. The ETC had been expanded twice to meet the needs of increasing patient numbers, and still we were struggling. There were now eighty beds, and it was not enough.

I would often go in the early hours of the morning to collect blood samples and insert IV lines. During those morning rounds, we also took note of which patients had not survived the night. There were so many patients coming in and out, we relied on their numbers to identify them and to know where in the ETC they were located. They represented bed spaces we could empty for the next round of sad and confused souls to arrive.

We were witnessing death on a scale no person or people should ever experience. The young, the old, those in the prime of life, stronger and fitter than I will ever be, bent and bleeding, begging for help, while lying curled in their own uncontrolled vomit and excrement. Often, a person would die with their back painfully arched and limbs upright and flexed – the typical position of a person who has died from their brain swelling. Rigor mortis would freeze them, like a statue from a Greek tragedy. Their twisted form caused great difficulty when laying them to rest in the body bag. Death became so familiar it was a passing comment, a matter of fact. 'Thirty-one, thirty-five and forty are dead; we'll need one child and two adult body bags.' I am chilled to think how those words rolled so easily off my tongue. It was just work. We had to get the dead out to get more living in, and so the wheel turned.

The UK has a strong tradition of providing palliative care. In previous medical jobs, I had been accustomed to ensuring patients with terminal illness or intolerable symptoms were kept comfortable. Now, on the days when demand far outstripped supply, I took a palliative approach to caring for those inside. There were three distinct groups of patients: those who were well enough to look after themselves; those who needed extra support with nutrition, hygiene and hydration; and those who were dying. There was a point at which we could do no more than make sure there was no pain, and provide comfort, cleanliness and dignity. To provide a human touch to say, 'You are not forgotten and you are not alone'.

There were daily discussions and debates about IV lines – who would get one and how many we could handle. We could have put IV lines in every patient, but we could not have managed to give them all fluids and medication. We could not stay sweltering in PPE while the drips ran, and would not be there if, in confusion, a patient pulled their line out and bled. It was essential, with so many patients and shifts of around five expat and fifteen Sierra Leonean healthcare workers, to ration our care to be as efficient and safe as possible. These were always heartfelt discussions, and I don't know that we ever got it right.

I would often sit inside the ETC, staring at the orange fence that separated the High Risk from the Low Risk area, or watch the corridor where the patients entered, where we sorted them. Some – very few – were free to go, as they did not fit the Ebola case definition, but all the others were led into the camp. Here, patients had vacant sunken eyes and slow exhausted movements, and many were emaciated and lying on the floor, staring into a nothingness. The long tents they stayed in, with rows of beds on each side, were often unbearably hot. The patients with enough strength would stay outside, leaving the weakest inside to do what they needed to do. The frequent visits from the WatSan team, with body bags in hand, made no secret of what went on in here. The morgue sat just behind one of the tents. As I sat in my heavy wellington boots, watching all that went on either side of the orange fence, I wondered how the world that had abandoned us would judge us. Sitting there, on the line between life and misery, I felt myself transported to another time and place – a different kind of camp, where people walked in and were carried out.

I stopped remembering patients as they became numbers, aware that this was happening and the reasons for it, both practical and psychological. I decided to memorize the two young brothers, their faces and their story. They symbolized the heartbreaking reality of what was around us – children alone in a place where no child should be. There was no one left to know if they were alive or dead, and no one to remember them when they were gone. On the same day Jeneba died, I'd found the younger brother's corpse. Before I closed his young eyes, I whispered that I would not forget him. The brothers had died within a day of one another. Now, years since that day, I see their faces. They represent the many other faces I have forgotten, those who lived, died or were lost.

Sitting in the epicentre of the largest ever recorded Ebola epidemic was unnerving. Family and friends were asking every day, 'When are you coming home?'. In all honesty, I was asking myself the same question. It was frightening to be there.

What made being in Kailahun unique at that moment was our direct proximity to the infection all the time. In the treatment centre there were the High and Low Risk areas, but the fact remained, that outside the centre, Ebola was among us and it touched every action. In my mind, I was constantly living, eating, breathing Ebola.

In order to be secure, there needed to be a consensus of trust between me and every other person I worked or interacted with, national and international. That's a big ask in one of the world's poorest countries. Everyone entrusted their life to everybody else. If I felt sick, or had an accident, I had to share that information. I trusted those around me to do the same.

I was not staying because I was a doctor – the medical side of the response remained basic. I wanted to be present because I was *human*. I wanted to show unity, to witness the events before me. I also knew, however, that my time to leave was coming closer. Like everyone else, I had my limits.

Michel's speech in GRC continued to circulate in my mind: *Ebola is a cruel disease. It will take the closest people to you: those who love and hold you; those who care for you in sickness* . . . I would often hear these words when families were admitted into the treatment centre, all infected from having cared for a sick relative or attended their funeral. Of the patients inside the treatment centre, some would live and some would not, but I tried to focus on the people who would live *because* their relatives were in the treatment centre. Ebola is a disease of contact; remove the contact, break the chain, and you reduce the risk. This became a mantra I kept in mind, giving another sense of purpose to the work, because, while we couldn't save the lives of all those inside, in collaboration with the community outreach teams, we were helping protect their loved ones outside.

14: TRANSMISSION

'I'll wear what I want,' said Lauren, through her tight-fitting FFP3 respirator face mask. She stood with the full-length blue surgical gown wrapped tightly around her compact body, a plastic apron over her front and another over her back. The tight bands of the FFP3 mask blanched the skin of her cheeks and restricted the natural movement of her jaw as she tried to talk.

'You know we won't have any left for when we actually need them,' I said, leaning back against the wall of the delivery suite. 'I heard they are sharing masks in intensive care because of shortages.' I was tired; we'd been having the same PPE conversations every day for weeks.

Lauren was the midwife allocated to look after a woman in room two. The woman was in labour and also had COVID-19, coughing and occasionally dropping her oxygen levels. Increasingly, midwives had been refusing to care for COVID-infected women. Naively, I had not anticipated that stigmatization would show its face in a central London hospital.

'Look, we've been told there's no difference in protection between that and a surgical face mask,' I continued, making a point of putting a standard surgical mask on my own face, bending the wire over the bridge of my nose and pulling the lower part to fit snugly under my chin. 'Unless the patient is having a general anaesthetic, there's no reason for the FFP3 mask.'

'Well, I need to protect myself,' Lauren said.

'Have you read the guidance?' I tied the single-use plastic apron round my back. 'It's pretty clear. Of course, it could change, but that's true of everything we do.'

'I don't care what it says. I'll wear what I want.'

'You know a midwife fainted last week in this room? She got too hot wearing all this gear. Surely you can see that's dangerous?'

My mind wandered back to GRC, trying to repair uterine ruptures through clouded goggles and handling a scalpel in oversized gloves. I still remembered the fear.

Lauren's eyes looked at me, deadpan. In these conversations, I was always the bad guy. I couldn't care very much about health worker safety if I didn't want them piling on all the PPE in the world.

I rolled my eyes. 'Let's see her.'

Lauren introduced me to Hannah as we entered the room, gesturing towards me with her double-gloved hand.

Hannah lay on the bed, her large belly covered with a patterned NHS hospital gown. Two cords connected her to the fetal heart rate machine, and her finger was attached to an oxygen monitoring probe, the levels reassuringly normal.

'How's the epidural working?' I asked, as I discreetly counted her breaths.

'It's good, thanks,' she said, and began a round of dry chesty coughs. I watched the numbers on the oxygen probe dip down and come back up to normal as she caught her breath again.

'Where are the notes?' I asked Lauren, looking around the room.

'I've left them outside, in the office.'

'Can we ask someone to bring them over, and keep them in here? All our women keep their maternity notes at home; they've been in the their hands and coughed on; they're contaminated'

I listened to Hannah's chest; there was little movement of air in and out at the base of her lungs, on both sides, but the rest sounded better than I had expected.

'Hannah, when it's time to push, I want to put you on a little bit of oxygen, OK? If there are any problems at all, I'll be just outside and Lauren can call me.' I turned to Lauren. 'Let me know when you're about to begin; I'll make sure I'm around.'

Lauren nodded; it was unclear what she was really thinking, as all facial expressions were hidden. When the notes reappeared, I scribbled a plan and bid everyone good luck, then I removed my gloves and apron, and washed my hands.

As I left the room, I was overcome by a sense of impotence. Weeks of training and working hard to improve infection control had born few results. Behaviour change had been dictated by social media and false information. The newspapers and television were blasting out distressing stories of NHS workers not having the correct protective equipment, and it was true. But this, right here, was also part of the problem, because those same stories perpetuated the fear that fed wastage.

I watched from the corridor as Hannah gave birth, midwives entering and leaving the room, each one donning a fresh surgical gown and FFP3 mask, taking an occasional selfie for Instagram. Our supply was running low and there was no delivery of stock planned for another five days. No rational discussion could be had. Emotions were high. There was no trust. I was worried tensions would pass snapping point, and we couldn't afford anyone else snapping.

'Is she OK?' I asked Lauren, as she sat at a computer in our communal delivery suite office, red marks etched around her nose and cheeks from the tight-fitting FFP3 mask – the stigmata that have come to be associated with COVID-19 care.

'She had another temperature after the birth,' said Lauren, blowing gently on a cup of tea.

'Who's looking after her now?'

'Oh, she's with her sister.' Lauren turned back to the computer, leafing through the yellow patient notes from the room.

I looked at her ungloved hands running over the pages, the communal desk the notes sat on, the shared computer keyboard Lauren tapped at. She took a biscuit and dipped it into her cup of tea.

'Those notes are still dirty, you know,' I said to her.

She looked back at me, her face like a stripy red candy cane. She looked at the notes, then at the biscuit in her hand. 'Well, I've started eating it, now', she said, and carried on.

*

KAILAHUN, SIERRA LEONE

AUGUST 2014

I had been doing the afternoon ward round with Morris. The ETC was nearly full in the 'confirmed' area and we were still expecting five more admissions, but by the time the Sierra Leonean staff changed over from the late shift to the night shift the expected patients still hadn't arrived. We were not supposed to take any new admissions after 7 p.m. as it was not safe to move patients inside the High Risk area in the dark, but the roads were so bad patients often arrived late, even if they had begun their journey to the ETC early in the morning.

I sat with the others on shift – Geraldine, the Swiss nurse and our first ETC coordinator, and Tina, a doctor from Belgium. There was also Allan and Dennis, both clinical officers from Uganda who had experienced Ebola outbreaks before, although not on this scale. There was a huge comfort in knowing we had them and their experience on board. We sat and chatted about places we had been to and shared our views on the current situation. As the time drew on, the temperature dropped from the burning hot of daytime to a cool breeze. Thankfully, the afternoon downpour was also over. We called the base to update them that we were still waiting for the patients to arrive. An important meeting was planned and the project coordinators had wanted all international staff to be present.

In the distance, we heard the honking and whirring sounds of an ambulance. Driving down those roads in the dark cannot have been easy. When it finally arrived, the driver told us how they had been on the road for almost ten hours; some of the dirt tracks were impassable. Before we had unloaded the first ambulance, we heard the sound of another vehicle, and soon a second ambulance pulled up. Both were full of patients. It was after 10.30 p.m. and we now had ten patients who would each need assessing in triage and admitting.

The patients all looked absolutely exhausted, and one could not walk at all. There were five who were all from one family, three generations. I pushed any sentimental thoughts deep down and carried on with the job. There was a saying, you could *smell* Ebola. There was no odour to the illness, but after seeing enough cases a sense developed in recognizing the dull look in patient's eyes and their inability to coordinate normal movement. We could *smell Ebola* in them all.

We transferred them in groups of three or four into the 'suspect' area and gave them food, blankets and the first doses of symptomatic treatment. Though working at night was considered higher risk, it was infinitely more comfortable. I didn't break a sweat at all, and was able to work calmly, without the pounding of blood at my temples. Eventually, we had seen and transferred all of the new patients, and, together, tired and hungry, we made our way back to the base.

On arrival, we saw the coordination team smoking in the courtyard. They had saved dinner for us, but also wanted to update us on the meeting we had missed.

The MSF shield was gone. In Liberia and Guinea there had been infections of MSF staff. Investigations were being carried out in both countries to determine how the staff had got infected, whether it was work related and if changes needed to be made in protocol. It was bad news, not just for those people and their projects, but for the wider global perception of risk in responding to the outbreak. I took a beer and sat with the group outside to discuss how this new development might change the response, but I was losing the battle to keep my eyes open and soon headed for bed. I would be on the late shift again tomorrow and hoped for a lie-in.

I had breakfast after most of the team had headed off for the ETC. The housekeeper was cleaning my room when I returned. She was a pleasant lady, singing and humming to herself as she worked. I asked her for a fresh towel and took a shower, feeling the sticky layers of sweat peel off my body, then I sat in the courtyard, catching up on emails.

I wrote to Tara, back home, whose wedding looked like it had been sensational. My old house mates had sent me a running commentary, with photos, over WhatsApp. But it was the stream of pictures from a novelty photo booth I had looked at most: all five of them, squeezed together, in ridiculous costumes, drunk grins and arms wrapped around one another. I was missing from the pictures, but I was exactly where I felt I should be. I'd always known pursuing humanitarian work would come with these added costs.

On my way back to the ETC to begin another shift, I stared out of the window of the Land Cruiser while the others made small talk. The mountains around Kailahun were so green, the buildings still had the scars of war but from between them ran excited children screaming and squealing, waving at us as we passed by. As we pulled into the ETC, I saw a large crowd gathered around the eating area. This was unusual, as we generally avoided any gatherings. We got out of the vehicle and were told to go straight back to the guest house. Nobody knew what was going on, but all expats were to leave immediately for a meeting. An ambulance was expected, so, after some hurried discussion, two expats chose to remain at the ETC and the rest of us returned to base. On the journey we were all silent, unwilling to speak our fears out loud.

In our short time away something significant had changed. The gate was opened slowly. I felt like we were entering a compound rather than a shared guest house. Though we always washed our hands and sprayed our feet on entering, this time the staff started shouting orders at us to do so. With military discipline, we lined up to follow instructions and went straight to the meeting room. Hilde had returned to Bo to meet a new member of the coordination team, so it was up to the medical team leader, Livia, to speak to us all.

Livia was an Italian infectious diseases doctor, who usually spoke quickly and decisively. This time, however, she began slowly: 'I have bad news to share. A doctor living with us in the guest house is unwell. He's working with one of the other organizations. He was tested this morning for Ebola. The test is positive.' Livia paused for a moment, she looked around the room, 'He got tested secretly and won't admit to being sick. It was the lab technician who told us the result. The doctor is still in his bedroom in the guest house. He hasn't agreed to be isolated yet. Geraldine is talking with him.'

No one in the room moved as we absorbed the information, considering what it meant for us as individuals.

'How long has he been feeling unwell?' Gabriel asked.

'Six days.'

There was a unified gasp. Emily, normally composed and cool-headed, stared intensely at the table. I watched as her face began to crease, her head shake and tears rolled from her eyes. 'Six days? Are you fucking kidding me? Six days?' she said with disbelief.

Once a person becomes symptomatic, they are contagious. We were all contacts now.

Like many people, this doctor had at first assumed he had malaria and began taking antimalarial tablets. As he became increasingly unwell, he went into denial.

The anger in the room was rapidly rising as realization set in.

I had spent many nights thinking of this exact scenario in my head – only, in my imagination, I was the one who had symptoms. After working inside the ETC would I admit to being unwell? Would I want to be in those tents, surrounded by death and waiting for my own fate? It was easy to judge others, but what would I have done in his situation?

Gabriel spoke up, wanting to clarify exactly who it was.

People began describing the doctor. He was friendly, would socialize with the MSF team and eat with us.

'The guy with a lisp? Spits when he speaks?' said Gabriel.

Fuck.

Around the room people began sharing stories of when he had accidentally spat at them during conversation.

'What if he spat on the food?'

'What if it went in my eye and I didn't realize?'

The panic in the room was escalating.

'What do we do now?'

Livia took back control of the situation. She confirmed the fears in the room. They were logical, but we had to do our best to stay calm. It was a Saturday and they needed to get hold of whoever was on call for emergencies at headquarters to discuss the situation. There was no doubt this was a serious safety breach. The guest house was to be secured. Livia had already spoken with the owners. Only MSF personnel or those approved by MSF were to enter, and all areas where the doctor was thought to have been would be decontaminated.

Gabriel and Vincente began interviewing everyone in the guest house, to ensure there was nobody else unwell who should be considered with suspicion of infection. Those of us due to be on the late shift were to return to the ETC, but not to discuss what was happening at the guest house till more information was available.

Once the meeting was over, people were dazed. Livia asked everyone to hold back on discussing the situation outside of the group, to avoid media interest or panic before there was a plan in place. I walked back over to the Land Cruisers and made my way to the ETC once again. The same journey, but totally different.

At the ETC we updated the two expats that had stayed behind, reviewed the board of patients and took handover. The day had to continue, work had to be done – the usual admissions, checking in on patients and deciding who would get what treatment. We had just exited the High Risk area at around 4 p.m. when Livia called on the mobile phone. The doctor had agreed to be admitted, providing he would have a tent to himself. They were transferring him from the guest house immediately. Tina and I went over to the board to assess how we could rearrange the patients so a tent could be emptied. We could move some beds so the larger tents had an extra couple of patients. It wasn't ideal, but it would do. We dressed in PPE and re-entered High Risk to help move patients and relocate their beds. Just as we were finishing, the ambulance pulled up. There was no need to question or triage him; we already knew he had Ebola. He was brought into the 'confirmed' area through the back entrance, the same way the healthcare workers from Kenema Government Hospital would arrive.

Despite all the anger I had seen in the meeting, when I met him inside, I felt a great weight of pity. In his eyes, I saw the fear and uncertainty that lay before him. We walked together to the tent which would be his place to stay the night. I went through the usual admission procedures with him. He barely raised his head, his answers monosyllabic and subdued.

After tending to a couple of other patients, I headed out and completed the decontamination ritual, now a ceremony so familiar, I glided through it like a choreographed dance.

I sat in front of the medical team's tent, drinking a can of Sprite and contemplating the world beyond the green mountains – a world reporting on the epidemic every day. *Why is it so quiet here?* I asked myself. *Where is everyone?*

In the back of the tent I heard the mobile ringing again. Tina answered and there was a low, muffled conversation. She came out and sat next to me. 'There's two more,' she said.

I looked at her. There was no panic, just matter-of-fact information.

'A daily worker from the kitchen and the housekeeper. They're putting them in the ambulance now.'

'OK,' I said, nodding slowly. 'We'd better get the admission packs together.'

We switched into work mode, as if any other ambulance was coming. But we all knew this was more than any other ambulance.

As the sun was setting and the air cooled, the ambulance pulled up, honking its horn. We ran out with our clipboards and gloves, ready to begin the questioning. The back door swung open and there, facing me, was the housekeeper, just as she had been that morning, in my room.

'Doctor, I'm here!' she called to me from the ambulance steps, and then she began singing at the top of her voice to sweet Jesus, tears streaming down her face.

'Yes, sister, I see you,' I replied, directing her across to the other side of the orange fence to begin the triage process.

She had been feeling unwell for two weeks – nothing too serious, a bit of diarrhoea and nausea, general lethargy and fevers. The history was not very convincing, but it was worrying; she had enough symptoms to meet the case definition and would need to be isolated and tested. If she did have Ebola, it would mean, for two weeks, she had been coming in and out of our rooms, cleaning and washing, all the while contagious.

The daily worker also met the case definition with similarly vague symptoms. We admitted them both into the 'suspect' area of the ETC. Their blood tests would be taken in the morning, as it was already evening.

We returned to the base for another team meeting. The area was now cordoned off with tape, like a crime scene. *MSF Only*, read the sign.

As I went to sit in the office, my phone automatically logged on to the Wi-Fi and began buzzing and beeping like it was on speed. I hadn't been in contact with any friends or family since the doctor got infected, for fear of saying the wrong thing and giving too much information away. I did not want them to worry any more than they already were.

I looked at the messages appearing in all the different social media:
Are you OK?
You're being evacuated? We saw it on the news?
We are all praying for you!
Message after message. I looked at them, flummoxed. How did they know? I hadn't said anything. I switched over to the news and saw the headlines: *British Medic in Sierra Leone gets Ebola: to be evacuated by RAF*.

The only details given were that it was a British man, who was a medic in Sierra Leone. My friends and family had assumed it was me. The timing was impeccable, the effect exactly what I needed. Responding to all my friends and family – affirming I was OK, I was not sick and I was not being evacuated – reminded me that, though times were tough, they were bearable.

William Pooley, a British nurse who had pitched up to volunteer at Kenema Government Hospital, had been infected. It was all over the news. I struggled to empathize; it was too close to home. I wondered what the fallout of Pooley's infection would mean for the international response. No doubt the UK's level of paranoia would be raised from high to hyper. The country's tabloids would have a field day terrifying everyone about the pending plague. I worried this would only mean bad things for those most affected in West Africa – less assistance and further barriers.

At the evening meeting tensions were running high. Hilde and the new coordinator were still travelling back from Bo but were due to arrive soon. Everyone had questions and no one had answers. If the daily worker was infected, was there a risk our food had been contaminated? The housekeeper had been in all our rooms, so were they safe?

Late into the night, Hilde and the coordinator arrived. The team met and discussed all the events of the last day. Some people just stared blankly, while others were visibly angry, wanting – needing – answers that didn't exist. It seemed headquarters in Brussels had been caught off guard too. This situation hadn't been anticipated – like the spiralling outbreak, it was beyond anyone's experience.

I felt bad for the new coordinator. We were not an easy audience. All of us were physically tired and emotionally burnt. He had never been in an Ebola outbreak before, but was experienced in other insecure environments, so tried to draw parallels. When it came to the safety of the guest house and level of possible contamination, he suggested that if we thought it was unsafe we could all sleep in the office.

There was a hushed chatter between people at the tables, contemplating this offer.

'We've been sleeping in these rooms for weeks,' I said. 'If there was a risk, it's been and gone. We probably have more chance of catching something if we all squeeze in here overnight than we do in our own space. I'll sleep in my room.'

People muttered and nodded their heads in agreement. An offer was made for anyone who wanted to leave. If the situation was too much, going home was always on the table. The reality, however, was there were barely any commercial carriers still flying in or out of the country. We could leave the project, but we might not be able to leave Sierra Leone.

A psychologist had also arrived with Hilde. She spoke to us about mental wellbeing and how to support one another. She offered to see people privately if they were struggling. I liked her; she had a clear and analytic way of talking. It was comforting to listen to her.

We all stayed up chatting in the courtyard outside, where the number of people smoking seemed to have significantly increased. There was so much to talk about, but little to say. Geraldine and I wanted to get to the ETC before the sun was up, to take the blood tests of the suspected patients, and those we thought may have survived and become negative. I headed off to bed, arranging to meet her at around 5.30 a.m.

I got to my room, desperate to wash the day off me. I looked at the towel the housekeeper had given me that morning – the same woman I had now isolated in the ETC – and contemplated for a moment whether it was safe to use. I picked it up and got myself under the cold water. The logical part of me found its way through the cloak of tiredness: Ebola is not transmitted on a clean towel.

I had no meaningful sleep. I lay under the mosquito net, listening to the subtle sounds outside my bedroom door. I wondered about the doctor lying on his own inside his tent, contemplating life; the housekeeper and the daily worker awaiting their blood tests in the 'suspect' tent. I could not shake the image of the housekeeper standing on the ambulance steps and calling out to me, the sound of her singing and the resignation in her eyes. Every now and then, I would lay my palm on my forehead. What if I got a fever? What would I do? Would I go to the ETC, or would the Royal Air Force fly me out? I saw the many corpses we had become so accustomed to, the expressions on their faces and the posture of their limbs. The body bagging and disposal. My poor family, my mother and father. It all sat on my chest as I lay there, waiting for, but not really wanting, sleep.

Soon enough I was released from my thoughts by the sound of my alarm. It was still night outside and there was a cold dampness to the air. I wrapped up in a hoodie and cagoule and headed out to the office to see which vehicle we would be taking.

I liked being on the early-morning shift; it was nice to arrive when the day was fresh and just starting, to check in with the night team and get the bloods taken before the sun rose and the PPE became intolerable. The method for taking blood samples was an operation in itself, and there was a certain ritual in getting all the apparatus together to make it as efficient and safe as possible, ensuring everything was correctly labelled before entering, as the samples could not be touched once taken. Blood samples and people were virtually the only items to come back out of the High Risk area.

Geraldine and I split the list of patients for sampling between us and headed inside, each of us with a buddy to assist with packaging and decontamination of the blood samples. The needles had to be handled and disposed of with impeccable care. There was no room for error. We moved methodically from tent to tent, working our way round the patient flow, from 'suspect' into 'confirmed'. I took the doctor's blood sample. He looked more settled than the day before. It was rumoured an international evacuation was being planned.

The last sample I took was from a child who had been with us for a couple of weeks. At ten years old, he had a cheeky personality and mischievous smile. He was fondly referred to as The President because of the way he strutted and danced around the 'confirmed' area. He had a radio he played booming tunes on, and he would encourage the younger and weaker patients to eat or get up. I was anxious to see if he would be negative. I had already taken blood tests from several children that morning. I always found it more stressful, concerned I would miss their little veins or that they would move. It must have been terrifying to have us bending over them in our yellow and white PPE, pointing a needle at their arm. Even as I was taking the President's blood, he had his radio turned on, and he continued to swing his little body around in a constant state of excitement. Finally, the samples were all done. I checked in with Geraldine and made a note of the deceased patients' numbers, for body bagging. Then we headed out to get undressed and hand the blood samples across to the laboratory.

As I was being sprayed down with chlorine in the decontamination area, I could see the rest of the morning team arriving, which meant breakfast would be arriving too. Geraldine and I had left the guest house before the kitchen opened, but the others had brought bread, omelettes and coffee with them. There was an eating area across the mud road from the ETC, and Geraldine and I headed over to get some nourishment. A small pink plastic basket was waiting for us. We sat quietly, drinking our coffee, letting the caffeine kick in. Then Geraldine returned to the ETC to begin sorting the jobs of the day, while I stayed back to clear up.

As I began walking back towards the road, I heard someone call out my name. I turned and saw Morris.

'Dr Benjamin!' he called out again, and I waved to him.

As he got closer, I thought he looked different. Was he drunk? His walking was unstable. His eyes were heavily bloodshot.

'Dr Benjamin, I need to speak with you.' He came up close, stumbling, almost falling on to me.

Instinctively, I took a step back and asked him if he was OK.

'I've not been feeling too well.'

15: EXODUS

We stood opposite each other, looking at one another for an extended moment. We were out in the open. I didn't want to panic Morris and I didn't want to panic anyone around us. We spoke for a while calmly, like normal, with no protection.

Morris told me he'd been feeling unwell for about four days. Initially a fever and then headaches, now he felt very tired and had diarrhoea. He'd treated himself for malaria, but it had made him feel worse.

I didn't want to say anything, not yet. Not while it was just the two of us outside. I had no gloves and didn't know what his reaction would be. We continued chatting a while longer. There was nobody else around. I asked him to wait while I ran into the ETC to grab a few things, like a thermometer. I instructed him very specifically: 'Wait here; I'll be quick. Don't come into the ETC'.

I entered our administrative area, a place we considered Ebola free, trying to look as unaffected as possible. I washed my hands with chlorine and went to find Geraldine.

'I think Morris has Ebola,' I said.

Her wide brown eyes searched my face. We discussed what had happened outside and what to do next, without causing alarm. He had been coming to work during the time he was unwell, which would mean everyone who had worked those shifts would be a contact. As we spoke in rapid hushed tones, I caught Morris out of the corner of my eye, entering the Low Risk area. I watched as he touched the gate, as he touched the fence. I saw my colleagues touching them after him.

We walked over to him. 'Hey, Morris, what happened?' I asked.

'The guard said I wasn't allowed to stay there, told me I had to come in.'

'OK, well, let's just go chat over there,' Geraldine said, gesturing to one of the storage tents, away from the groups of staff.

Together, we went back over the story. We passed him a thermometer to take his own temperature, which was borderline – just below the cut-off we were using for fever. I gave him a can of Coke and our fingers briefly touched. I looked at my hand. I looked at him.

Outside the tent, Geraldine and I discussed the situation. She didn't think it was convincing, suggesting he should go home to rest.

'Look at him,' I said. 'Look at how he walks. He *looks* like he's got it.'

We called Livia, the medical team leader, to ask her opinion. She was the voice of reason. Her answer was simple: 'Test him'.

'I'm sure it will be negative,' Geraldine stressed to Morris, 'but it's better we check'.

Morris knew the ETC better than most of us. He let himself into the 'suspect' area. We wanted his admission to be as inconspicuous as possible. Geraldine got dressed into PPE immediately to take his bloods. There was still time to get it processed with the batch we had taken earlier for testing. I went to speak with the rest of the nurses and CHOs on shift, pre-empting the inevitable rumours and concern.

I gathered everyone around the board and explained Morris wasn't well, and we were going to test him. They all stared at me. There were no questions and no comments. I requested their discretion; we had to respect his privacy – it was only a test, not a diagnosis. But, before the meeting was over, the news was already out. Text messages were being received alleging we had a staff member infected.

The shift continued in a muted mood as we waited for the laboratory results. At 2 p.m., when both the morning shift and afternoon shift were present, they finally came in. Geraldine had the book in her hand and brought it straight to me.

'All positive.' She paused. 'But, look.' She pointed to the list of seventeen samples. Against each identification number, there was a result showing the viral load. One of them was very high. There was a theory that, the higher the viral load, the lower the likelihood of survival. 'That's Morris,' she said, pointing to it. 'I'm going to go tell him, before anyone sees these.'

We agreed that while Geraldine spoke to Morris I would speak with the staff from the two shifts. We also needed to arrange for the Low Risk area to be decontaminated. It was now High Risk too.

I went to the whiteboard and called everyone to gather round. I had not prepared an announcement and had no time to even consider how to break the news. Morris was our colleague, a friend to many, and now he was our patient. He may also have unknowingly exposed us all to infection.

I took a breath before speaking, knowing we were on the cusp between ignorance and knowledge, between numbers on a piece of paper and a personalized, shattering reality. Thirty colleagues in green scrubs turned their eyes to me as the midday heat beat down upon us.

'As many of you know, we tested Morris this morning,' I began. 'I'm afraid it is not good news. He's being told now, and will be moved across to the "confirmed" area.'

I spoke a few words of reassurance, but had little to offer. After I had finished, there were many questions about what would happen next and how we could know what was and what was not safe. I explained that Gabriel and Vincente would need to speak to each member of staff to determine if anyone had had high-risk contact, or had developed symptoms of illness.

The positive test result of the doctor from the guest house was now confirmed, and both the daily worker and housekeeper were positive too, but with much lower viral loads. This reopened a conversation a few of us had been having for a while: how did we know if everyone with Ebola would be sick enough to be admitted to the ETC? What if there were people who never became unwell, just mildly symptomatic? The housekeeper had already got over the worst of her symptoms and was almost back to normal. Even at her sickest, she had managed to come to work every day. Had we not been contact tracing, she might never have been suspected and tested. And, if that was the case for her, how many others? However, in keeping with the belief that low symptoms were due to a low amount of virus in the body, it also followed that these people should pose a lower transmission risk. In the end, though, all we had were theories and what ifs.

I returned to the base later in the afternoon, drained from the day's events. Tina was sitting in the leafy courtyard, smoking and drinking a beer with a nurse. It was their day off. I went over and said hi, sat down and pulled my knees into my chest. The rain had just finished and the air was fresh. I had assumed events from the ETC would have filtered back to the base, but they hadn't heard anything. As I told them, they both began crying. Their tears took me by surprise. I had been so busy, I had failed to be human. All I could do was apologize for being the one with bad news. I also wanted to say sorry I wasn't crying. Sorry I didn't appear upset. Sorry how I spoke like I was ordering dinner, blunt and to the point.

I sent a text message home, asking my dad to call. I hadn't spoken to my family for a while and I knew the circus around Pooley's evacuation and transfer to London would have them worried. He was calling from home, where he was with my mother, sister and her family. I asked him to make an excuse and go to another room; I couldn't handle an audience.

All the way through, my parents had never once asked me to come home. They respected my decisions and the work I was doing, agreeing only I could judge when enough was enough. Hearing his voice was that moment. I had no words and he thought perhaps it was a poor line, but I couldn't speak for fear that my voice would crack and give me away. I coughed loudly and managed to say, 'I think it's time I came home'.

My father has travelled the world and lived through many of recent history's pivotal moments first hand. He is not a man of many words, but his reflections and thoughts are always full of wisdom.

'If you think it's time to leave, then it probably is.'

It was all I needed to hear. The call was brief; it wasn't good for me to hear all their voices. I had too much in my head, too many images of their faces if I were to become infected. Though not a big drinker, he later told me that, after the call, he returned to the room with the rest of the family, sat quietly and poured himself a large whisky. Whatever his thoughts and anxieties as a parent, his composure and insight not to burden me with them was a show of selflessness.

That night we had another fraught team meeting. The results were now known by everyone and the unanswerable questions were endless. We were waiting for instructions from headquarters to come, but the final decision would be ours. As a group there was calm tension. Most of us were short on sleep and raw nerves were easily exposed. Three options were proposed. We could stage a mass evacuation – it was even proposed we leave that night and travel to a place deemed safe. Alternatively, we could organize a partial evacuation of those who had been potentially exposed to the disease and anyone who felt they needed to leave, maintaining a skeleton team till replacements could be found. Finally, we could continue as we were.

We struggled to get our heads around the implications of each option. I felt we were incredibly isolated – a small boat bobbing in an ocean of Ebola. There was no obvious answer for us as individuals or as a group. Each of us would need to grapple with our own conscience and limits.

An outright evacuation seemed incomprehensible; we had around a hundred patients relying on us, and we knew there were many more out there needing to be brought in. Abandoning our local colleagues was also inconceivable; we had a responsibility to them too. Our departure would give a terrible message to the wider community and do unknown harm to the response if we just disappeared. However, our security was in doubt. We needed to find a balance. Leaving at night made no sense – the risks of driving down those mud roads in the dark probably outweighed those of one more night in the guest house.

The debate continued to wax and wane, a couple of people bursting with frustration at the lack of definitive direction from higher up. I valued our inclusion in the decision-making process, the trust MSF had in us – the affected – to take joint control in the search for a resolution. This was the second time in the space of a month that I had faced the dilemma of closing or leaving a project. These were impossible decisions, in impossible circumstances, and I still felt guilty for stopping activities in GRC, revisiting and questioning every detail.

After much discussion, we took a vote. The overwhelming consensus was for a partial evacuation. Each of us had to decide for ourselves whether to stay, leave, or go for a few days' rest in Bo. We dispersed for dinner with the plan to return in the morning, having each made our decision.

A few of us sat out in the courtyard, smoking and talking. The decision for many was clear: they were either staying or leaving. Geraldine was going to go; she was tired and close to burning out. Tina was staying – she had only been in the project a couple of weeks and could not bear the idea of leaving the patients behind. I sat on the fence, one moment sure I would leave, the next feeling a compelling responsibility to stay.

My thoughts were elsewhere, though, and my conversation with Morris replayed again and again in my mind. How close had he been standing? Did we touch hands? Had he been sick when we were doing the ward round together the other day? Did I put the pen he had been holding in my mouth? Did I wash my hands before touching my face? And, though

I reassured myself, knowing transmission is through bodily fluids and the risk to me was probably negligible, anxiety repeatedly won over reason.

I went to bed, still pondering my next move. I was deeply exhausted, but I also felt leaving was desertion. In the end, I fell asleep, hand on my forehead, checking for a fever.

The sun was not yet up when I went out to make a coffee. No one was going to the ETC early today; we were all meeting again at 7 a.m. to put the final plan together. As I spoke to the others, my own decision formulated.

We decided about half the team would leave for Bo; some were going for a period of respite before returning to Kailahun, and some would continue their journey home. The other half would remain in Kailahun and continue caring for the patients and managing the ETC. The team had been living and working together in a time of incredible intensity, so, whether staying or leaving, emotions were complex and high.

Those heading to Bo would leave in an hour. We had to move quickly. I ran back to my room, put some music on through my phone and started bundling everything into my rucksack. Music and packing distracted me sufficiently from thinking.

Outside the base there was a pile of bags belonging to those of us who were leaving. I chucked mine on top and sat with my friends. The atmosphere was both tranquil and hectic, all at once. Everyone knew that half a team leaving mid-project in the greatest Ebola outbreak ever known was a pivotal moment.

It was only then that my mind was empty enough to let thoughts in. I looked at my friends and colleagues, those I was leaving behind. We couldn't touch – no hugs, no handshakes – but our eyes communicated all to each other. My body felt as if it was being torn open. As I got in the Land Cruiser and looked at my friends on the outside – those who would have to return to the ETC, not knowing what the next few days would bring – it was as if it was all happening in slow motion. My mind pounded with images of the patients and colleagues I was leaving behind. The living and the dying, the children I had watched breathe their last, and those waiting for their tests to confirm if they had survived. I was overwhelmed with the sense that I was abandoning them. Had I made the wrong decision? I knew, as the Land Cruiser pulled away, surrounded by the murmurs and tears of my colleagues, that I would return. This wasn't the end, but merely a pause.

We travelled in a convoy of three Land Cruisers. I sat in the back and, for a long time, we were all silent, each lost in our thoughts. The small villages we passed through, the children shrieking and waving – it all filled me with guilt. We smiled and waved back, but I felt like a traitor.

We arrived in Bo about six hours later, and Pete, the Australian logistician, was there to coordinate and explain what would happen. About ten of us were leaving, continuing on to Freetown. It was a long journey and we passed many road blocks and checkpoints, particularly as we were crossing from the east of the country. There were long traffic jams at the checkpoints, where colourful impromptu markets had sprung up. At each one we would all get out of the Land Cruiser and pass through on foot, having our temperatures checked and washing our hands with chlorine. Before getting back into the vehicle, we would all wash our hands again with our own alcohol or chlorine wash. With every thermometer check, my heart would pound; it was twenty-four hours since Morris had been isolated and a week since the doctor had become symptomatic.

Night fell as we began climbing the bendy road up to Freetown. I was past exhaustion, running on empty as we arrived at the base. Arrangements had been made for us to stay in a nearby hotel, as there were no seats on flights out of the country. Nearly all airlines had suspended their flights, so we were all on standby.

After checking into the hotel, we found Barbara, Kathleen and MJ sitting at a table outside. They had finished their missions and were returning to Brussels, once they could secure seats on a flight. We joined them and ordered beers, glad of the opportunity to catch up.

When Geraldine's mobile rang, she got up and took a few steps away from us to answer it. She spoke in lowered tones and nodded her head. After finishing the call, she paused a moment, then returned to the table.

'That was Livia, in Kailahun,' she said, slowly exhaling. 'It's Morris. I'm sorry.'

When we saw his viral load, we knew he was unlikely to survive. Morris knew it, too. But his death had come faster than anyone had dared anticipate.

It was awful to think of him being a patient in that place, where he had cared for so many others and seen for himself so much death. I tried to imagine how it must have been for those working in the ETC, for the staff to communicate his death, bag his body and continue with work. Impossible.

The resilience of the local staff was astounding; they returned day after day, then went home to their communities, not knowing if disease would knock at their door, or if they themselves would bring this invisible enemy into their household. Many worked for months without a decent break. Never had they known Ebola to visit their world before, yet they walked on with determination. As the outside world, with all its resources and capability, held back in fear and self-protectionism, these individuals stood firm, and in no small way played a part in saving us all.

In the hotel Gabriel continued in his role as epidemiologist, risk assessing each of us. I sat with him on the terrace, the hot sun on my face. We had become close over the last weeks and talking with him was easy. Together, we went over our recent experiences, and what they might mean for the future. As I talked through what had happened in the ETC with Morris, I felt myself drifting off into a place somewhat distant. Gabriel stopped me mid-sentence and asked a simple, but telling question: 'Are you counting days since contact?'.

I was.

After several days, we got news that Brussels Airlines was restarting commercial flights. Their hiatus had been forced upon them due to Senegal's refusal to allow flights from the most affected countries to land, preventing crew changes. MSF had secured us seats on the first flight out. Brussels Airlines' decision, alongside Royal Air Maroc, to maintain flights to the region provided a humanitarian corridor – a lifeline to the commodities and support outside Sierra Leone. The flights they scheduled shame those other airlines who crept away at a time of immeasurable need.

Part 2

16: LIFE IN LIMBO

BRUSSELS

SEPTEMBER 2014

The flight landed in Brussels in the dark morning hours. Europe was autumnal, placid and cold. Throughout the journey the flight attendants had looked highly strung and nervous; now, they appeared proud – and rightly so. We shuffled off the plane. I had been unable to sleep and was running on the last drips of adrenaline. The airport seemed unusually quiet. As we entered the terminal we were met by women in white lab coats, holding thermometers and clipboards. I was on day four, around the time when fever and symptoms would normally appear, if infected. All ten of us passed through without issue. None of us knew what the plan after arrival was. It was too early to call the head office, so instead we sat in the airport, drinking espressos, waiting for the working day to begin.

We arrived at the office as the doors were opening and together made our way in. It was a strange feeling of homecoming. Even though I had visited the Brussels headquarters for the first time only the day before I left for Sierra Leone, it felt comfortably familiar.

The administrative staff had been caught off guard by our return, and needed time to sort out accommodation and onward travel for each of us. While we were sitting together in one of the corridors, Michel, the viral haemorrhagic fevers expert, came over to us. He made a point of giving each of us a big, warm, consuming hug, with a kiss on each cheek. I'm not sure if it was my English sensibilities or because I had not touched another human without PPE for months, but the gesture made me acutely uncomfortable. All the same, Michel represented so much of the Ebola story that his presence filled me with energy. He looked at us with a grin on his face and said, 'You're not in Ebola anymore'. It was an incredible realization.

It was standard MSF practice for all those returning from the field to talk with a psychologist. When it was my turn, I found the office to be exactly as I had expected, with a couple of comfortable chairs and a nice little table with a plant.

'Come in,' said the psychologist, with a smile, gesturing for me to sit down. She seemed earthy and kind, legs folded, with her notebook at the ready. 'So, Benjamin, this was your first mission?' she said, checking the form I had completed. 'Tell me a bit about your job profile.'

I did as she asked, and she soon eased the conversation towards the epidemic. I began to recount the story of GRC and the closure of maternity, the words falling from my mouth as if I were explaining the plot of a somewhat uninteresting film. I felt nothing. I was just describing something that happened somewhere, emotionless and blunt, like a history class.

When I looked up, I saw the psychologist had stopped writing notes. She stared at me with red eyes and a wet face. It felt the wrong way around. I tried to squeeze a tear out; I needed her to know I wasn't frozen inside. As I continued to talk about the treatment centres, the dying children and how I'd felt like I was lost in a concentration camp, she began openly crying. I kept talking, distracting myself from her sniffling, but it was too much for her. She asked me to stop and return the following day. I left knowing two things: I had upset the psychologist, and I was out of touch with myself.

Eventually, I made my way with the other evacuees to the accommodation in town. I was beyond the point of tired. Once I was alone, I lay down on the cool fresh sheets of the bed and let my mind wander. There was no chance of sleep. I was still in West Africa, running along a cliff edge. After speaking to a couple of friends back home, I got up and went to meet the others for dinner.

I sat with Geraldine and MJ in a burger bar. As we chatted it became clear that everyone had come to their own realization that they would return to the epidemic response, after a break. As the meal ended a tall slim woman came into the bar. She had long straight hair trailing to her mid-back and her presence was both subtle and radiant, like moonlight reflecting off a still lake. MJ knew her, and she got up to introduce us.

Ruth was an American nurse and midwife, and she was heading out the following day to work in GRC. I pitied her immediately. 'You know there's not much happening in maternity now,' I said, trying to break the news gently that her mission was to a closed programme.

'That's fine,' she said, unfazed and smiling.

'I mean, you might have nothing to do,' I pushed, concerned she didn't grasp what I was saying.

'I've spent years in Sierra Leone,' Ruth said. 'I know I need to be there. I'll have plenty to do'. Her gaze shifted, as if she was looking past me, towards the path she would soon be taking. She had no doubt that she had to be there.

We chatted a little more about the Ebola outbreak, the impact it was having on maternity care and the urgent need for guidance in the ETCs. The conversation was brief and, just as she had drifted in, Ruth soon floated back out. I turned towards the others and thought nothing more of our meeting.

In the days following our arrival in Brussels, I would go to the MSF office to discuss what had happened and the decisions made. I joined Severine, the obstetrics and gynaecology adviser, and her colleagues to write guidance for the future management of Ebola-infected pregnant women. People often stopped me in the corridor, recognizing me from the articles I had written – a voice reporting directly from the outbreak. The organization remained at constant full speed. As a new face among a sea of aid workers, I was aware I might also be viewed as a trouble-maker. To have the audacity to suspend a longstanding project, without the backing of head office and on the first mission, I was half expecting to be called into a room and reprimanded.

Two days after my arrival, Michel stopped me as we passed in a corridor. 'Have you seen the news today?' he asked.

Actually, I was news obsessed, checking into apps and websites repeatedly for updates. I looked blankly at him. 'Which bit?'

'Another American got infected, in Monrovia.' Michel paused, as if looking at me for the first time. 'He wasn't working in the ETC. He was in obstetrics – normal pregnant women.'

Every hair follicle on my skin contracted, and a chill moved up my neck.

'You did the right thing to stop when you did,' Michel said. 'That could have been all of you.'

Perhaps I should have felt relief, but anger burnt inside me. There was never a right or wrong. What we had lacked was direct, open and honest dialogue. Our first conversation with MTV replayed in my mind, especially her words, *If you close, you send the women of Sierra Leone to hell.*

'Is it true, all the ZMapp is gone?' I asked. I had heard there was only enough of the experimental drug for a handful of patients. After treating several,* the world's supply was exhausted and it would take months to manufacture more.

Michel shrugged his shoulders, smiled and moved on to his mountainous list of tasks and responsibilities. I imagined the American obstetric doctor being told there was no more ZMapp and pondering how it would all end. I wondered what his misfortune meant for the women of Liberia, for the women of all affected countries.

It was a convenient story for the media's real-life thriller, the next instalment to heighten global paranoia, headlines screaming, *Doctor didn't treat Ebola patients yet still caught the virus*. He, like all health workers outside the ETC, would have had no idea what his level of contact with the disease was.

Lying on the crisp, white sheets of the hotel bed, I allowed myself to drift back to the last months – the people who died, the people who survived, and mostly to the teams I had left behind in GRC and Kailahun. The day we left, the ten-year-old 'President' had been due to be retested. He was, for many of us, a favourite relief on the ward round, and I'd recently heard that he was now 'cured' of Ebola and had been discharged. His departure, I'm sure, gave the team an immense boost to keep going at a time when nearly all else felt it was falling apart.

My emotions from Kailahun resurfaced. I was angry and frustrated that international powers continued to remain limp in their response. Big statements, big ideas, but very few feet on the ground. The epidemic should never have exploded – the fuse had been in clear site. It had all happened in slow motion and was totally predictable. It still was. It felt like we were screaming into a vacuum. Visualizing the beautiful hills of north-east Sierra Leone, mist rolling over the treetops, I asked out loud to the empty universe, 'Where is everyone?'.

---

* Six courses of ZMapp were shared between seven people, two died and five survived.

I had been ignorant of the global mechanisms needed to deliver a response. Now, with the comfort of distance and time, I could read about the recent financial cuts made to the WHO and the reduction in staff with technical expertise. The system prevented the orgnization from speaking out at risk of compromising their neutral status or receipt of much-needed donations. The WHO had never been intended for the operations being demanded of it. It seemed they too were victims of global unpreparedness and short-sighted decision-making.

The epidemic rampaged through communities, and with normal health services severely affected, including GRC, it was likely even more people would die indirectly than all those who had died from the disease so far. I had heard the predictions: sooner or later, the mines would be infected, then more cities, then, then, then . . . It was not rocket science, but it was complex. To save lives, we had to stop the disease. Experimental drugs and vaccines were promising, but they were inaccessible to the people needing them most, nor could they replace basic hygiene, health promotion and community engagement.

Images flowed through my mind: women with newborn babies, and the women without; the operating theatre, blood on the floor and sweat dribbling down my face; the dying children and jubilant survivors. I remembered the tense concentration and the impossible decisions. At some point, sleep found me.

*

LONDON

SEPTEMBER 2014

I arrived back in London on a beautiful autumn day; the leaves were still green and the sun shone strong through the afternoon. The world around me was comfortably familiar. I sat on the underground train from Heathrow Airport, wondering how the other passengers would react if they knew my journey, and slightly paranoid someone would somehow know and make a scene. But I was as much of a stranger in London's bustling transport system as everyone else.

I met my sister, Julia, in a café on Hampstead High Street. Her daughter, Maya, was climbing over the back of her chair and flicking orange juice with her straw. As I sat down, she looked quizzically at me. 'Uncle Benji, did you bring me a present?' With complete innocence and blissfully unaware of the world's problems, Maya's little smile and sparkling eyes searched mine for the important things in life.

'Something for show and tell,' I told her, as I passed her a bag of brightly coloured bangles.

Julia watched as Maya began inspecting the jewellery, then she glanced up at me with a look of concern in her eyes.

'Don't worry – they're OK,' I said, under my breath.

I reconnected with friends and family, going to restaurants and parties, just as I had before I left. But something was missing. I was detached. I continued to swing between talking bluntly and without emotion about my experiences, and bursting into tears without reason.

I went to visit Tara, my friend from medical school, who told me all about her wedding. 'We should get the video soon,' she said, closing the photo album spread over our laps. We were drinking red wine together, as we had done since the days of our shared student house, over a decade earlier.

Putting the photo album away, Tara pulled out a cardboard folder. 'I kept all the newspaper cuttings for you,' she said, as she opened the folder and showed me the loose papers and pictures inside. 'I couldn't believe it when I saw you on the front page of the *Metro*. I wanted to tell the whole Tube carriage, "I know him!".'

I put the folder on the coffee table in front of me. 'I needed to leave,' I said, picking at the corner of the couch. 'But now, I feel like there's so much I have to do. I feel like every moment I'm not doing *something* about Ebola is a moment I'm wasting.'

'I want to come too. When you messaged me about palliative care for the children, I felt like I had to be there. This is what we all trained for, but my work won't agree to release me.' Tara sipped her wine, looking at me over the glass.

As I walked home from Tara's place, I could feel the wine had loosened some of the knots of frustration inside me. I felt as if I were perpetually crouching at the start line for a sprint. Waiting for the gun to shoot in the air. I couldn't handle being stagnant.

My mobile phone buzzed: a queue of messages had collected while I'd been with Tara. I scrolled down through the notifications. *Any chance you want to go on a date?* one of them asked, breaking my Ebola-obsessed stream of consciousness. Maybe. Life goes on.

I had been asked to come for a chat at MSF's UK office in Farringdon, to debrief my mission and discuss what might be next for me. I always felt like a bit of a stranger there, intimidated by the constant buzz of the busy open-plan office. I thought I would be able to sneak in, like I had before, for my meeting with Brigitte, the medical human-resources officer, but as I walked through the office, a member of the communications team stopped me.

'Benjamin Black?' She ran around the desk and whispered to another member of the team, who, in turn, stood and told colleagues, 'Benjamin Black is here'.

She turned back to me, 'The MSF response has generated a lot of media interest,' she said gesturing to a wall with newspaper cuttings stuck to it. 'As one of the first UK returnees you're in a position to speak out, if you want.' I nodded, wondering what speaking out might mean. 'Would you mind telling us about your time in the field?' she asked.

I was led to a small room, where three of her colleagues huddled together. There was a window looking out to a wall and a green-leaved houseplant on a low table. A woman had come prepared to take notes, with a pen and paper in her lap. I wasn't sure what they wanted to hear, so I began to tell my story from the beginning. I felt the anger bubbling away inside me as I remembered all the details and as the images moved across my mind's eye. The clinical disconnection also returned. I stared at the brick wall as I continued speaking, and when I paused, I realized that the woman with the pad had stopped making notes. It was just like my experience with the psychologist in Brussels. The woman was dabbing her eyes with a soggy tissue and apologizing, though I felt it was me who should be saying sorry.

One of the others asked if there was anything I would consider saying to people who had donated money in response to the Ebola coverage. I sat silent for a moment, recalling the two young brothers, and the feelings of heat, humidity and desperation inside the ETC tents. I wanted to say something profound. I managed to squeeze out, 'Thank you.' The words sparked a connection between the memory and the emotion.

Finally, I felt meaningful pools begin to form in my own eyes. 'Thank you for not leaving us alone.'

Brigitte took me out of the office for lunch. We sat outside a small Italian café as men and women in business suits went rushing up and down the street. The sun shone down on us as we spoke about the mission and what might be next for me. Though I had been home for a fortnight, I asked Brigitte to put me forward for another Ebola mission in the affected region. I was uneasy with the way I had left, and hearing from friends still out there only strengthened my resolve to go back. Within a week of our meeting, an email arrived confirming my return to Sierra Leone in October.

In the weeks before I was due to return, I was invited to give lectures and interviews to a hungry public. The MSF press office would call me with lists of requests from journalists wanting to speak with returnee aid workers. I wanted to share the view from the field, but I also needed a break. I agreed to a few interviews where we thought the impact would be of highest value.

Walking down Great Portland Street to the BBC, my mind overflowed. The anger inside me had had time to collect and form a coherent voice. The images of GRC and Kailahun continually played in my mind, the faces of the two brothers staring back at me. I paused outside the BBC's New Broadcasting House, allowing a burst of rage to pass, then took a deep breath and composed myself again. The responsibility to get the words right felt immense.

In the make-up room a woman with a pouch of foundation in her hand and bright red lipstick asked, 'And what are you talking about?'

'The Ebola epidemic,' I replied, as she put a gown over my shirt.

She looked at me in the mirror, tilting her head and pouting. 'Oh, you won't need much,' she said, stepping back and sending me through to the green room.

The anchorman read the headlines to a beating rhythm for the live news broadcast. I was ushered to the seat opposite him during the segment on the Ebola epidemic. After introducing me, he turned and said, 'And you will return soon to the region. Do you feel the response has improved?'.

Adrenaline surged through my body, mixing with the rage and igniting a fire inside me. I held no bars. 'No. They have not got a handle on this.' I explained the need for a comprehensive coordinated response and global attention towards West Africa.

When I told friends and family of my plans, some could not understand why I would want to go back to the horrific scenes appearing on the news. The explanation I gave was simple: I could not *not* be there.

Friends from my first mission had already begun returning to the region: Geraldine had gone to Monrovia and Stefan was back in Kailahun. I would hear about the unfolding situation, in real time, directly from the field, while simultaneously watching the TV, seeing the terrible images streaming out. Ebola cases in Monrovia had exploded and the ETCs were full to capacity. The more I saw, heard and read, the greater my desire and impatience to return became.

The weekend before I was due to fly out, I went over to Araba's place for Sunday dinner. Araba, another of my former student housemates, was working as a GP in east London. She was also an excellent cook, and our small group sat around the table, enjoying the meal and each other's company, like a family.

'How was the date?' asked Araba, turning all the table's attention to me.

'It started well,' I said, taking a sip of my gin and tonic, 'till we spoke about what I'm doing now'.

'Not even a kiss?' Araba probed, smiling hopefully.

'Not even a handshake. But thanks for trying.'

As we were preparing coffee, I received a call from Sierra Leone on my mobile. Stepping out on to the balcony, I heard Jenny's voice. It was strange to imagine they were still there, still trying to cope, taking each day as it came.

Jenny's tone was tired and weary. 'I wanted to tell you, before you heard it from anyone else,' she said. 'Silje's sick. She got a fever yesterday and self-isolated. We took a test. It's Ebola.' She paused, and I heard her breathing over the line.

I sat on the balcony, taking in the cool autumn air, staring out over the rows of red-tiled rooftops. Behind me, I could hear Araba and the others laughing, unaware.

'We are trying to arrange an evacuation,' Jenny said.

We spoke briefly about the rest of the team, how they were managing and the general mood.

'And, Jenny, how are you?' I asked, unnecessarily, knowing there was no answer she could give. 'Look after yourself, Jenny,' I said. 'Send my love to all the team. It feels like I'm still with you.'

After she had rung off, I stayed out on the balcony for a while, meditating on the events, imagining and processing, and considering my own imminent return to Sierra Leone.

Sitting on the train back to north-west London I began getting messages from Alessandro, Juli and other previous GRC colleagues. Invisible threads pulled us together from all around the world. We were connected by our short, shared history. Someone had begun a group chat, and a flurry of messages went back and forth as we chatted and offered support to each other. From her isolation in Sierra Leone, Silje also joined us. Unified, our stamina and strength intensified.

I had spent many nights imagining how I would react if I were the one infected. I assumed the terror would consume me. Silje's response was a lesson of composure and pragmatism. When she issued a press release upon her discharge from hospital, she spoke with not only the credibility of a survivor, but also the conviction and heart of a genuine humanitarian.

17: SAME, BUT DIFFERENT

LONDON/CAPE TOWN

MARCH 2020

'I wouldn't ask a gynaecologist to fix a broken leg, so why is an orthopod telling me about infection control?' said Juli, from her balcony in Cape Town. She took a sip of wine and it was as if we were together, but we were speaking via our computers, over Zoom.

'You're a specialist in infectious diseases; they have to respect your opinion,' I said, adjusting the laptop screen. 'It's like every professor, doctor or person with a computer has become an expert in pandemics. Doesn't matter if you ever gave a toss about epidemics before this all started. Now, everyone is shouting and scrambling to plant their little flags in the terrain. I've lost track of all the guidelines being published. And they contradict one another. It's like being loud has replaced knowledge or understanding.'

'Look –' Juli put her glass down – 'there's a golden rule in epidemic response. Be consistent. Adaptations will need to be made as the situation and knowledge evolves, but these should be as infrequent as possible.'

'Yes, *we* know that. But I'm getting different guidelines posted every day, fighting to have procedures done the way *they've* decided is best. Not based on evidence, but general impressions, anecdotes and hunches. I had a colleague scream in my face because she wants everything done the way she heard it presented on a webinar last night, but the webinar was by urogynaecologists. No obvious experience in any of this stuff. Their "international experts" were colleagues who had seen anything from a handful to zero patients. It's as if there's an open platform for any self-identified expert.' I laughed, though nothing about this was funny. Amid the confusion and heightened anguish, the uninitiated clamouring voices were counterproductive. Their public profiles and expertise could be valuable, but not as back-seat drivers in a vehicle they had never driven. I poured myself a little more wine.

'Sorry,' said Juli. 'That sounds horrible. Did you manage to reason with her?'

I shrugged. 'Look, I get it. People are scared. They've never had to face anything like this before. It's not what they signed up for. But here we are, all on this learning curve together. Problem is, the extra noise undermines the efforts for a united approach. It's not that we can't disagree, but there are ways to do it without making colleagues lose their shit on the shop floor. It's as if the pandemic has become an opportunity for show time – a battle for centre stage.'

Juli gave a wry laugh.

'It's like you said,' I continued. 'They broke the rule, changed the message too many times. They changed the protective equipment, so everyone assumed it was being downgraded; they changed the case definition and testing protocols so often no one could keep up. They've dug a ditch for us all to fall into.'

'OK, go easy,' said Juli, her serious tone making an unexpected entrance. 'They're going with the evidence they have at the time. You know as well as I do, these situations can evolve quickly. Plus, we don't know what is happening behind the scenes – what politics are at play. For sure, we have done it differently in South Africa. They were quick here. Firm and decisive in lockdown. But the wider impacts are going to be massive. I'm worried about our HIV and TB patients. The kids not getting here in time, or missing their meds.'

I looked at Juli through my computer screen; I missed our evening chats. 'I feel, in the UK, the leadership have failed to engage with the wider health community. They haven't explained the challenges and rationale behind their decisions. So colleagues seek out and listen to the other voices, and, you know, too many cooks and a little bit of knowledge can be a dangerous thing.'

Juli nodded, then drained the last of her wine. 'Right, buddy,' she said. 'Time I got some sleep. Got another day of discussing PPE with the bone surgeons ahead of me. Let's do this again.'

'Sure, and let's not talk about COVID next time,' I said, waving goodbye and closing the laptop.

I took another sip of wine and thought about what tomorrow would hold for me – the feeling of déjà vu, the huge canyon of unknowns and the sad predictability of it all. I put my glass down, avoiding the urge to open my emails.

You can't control it, I told myself.

*

LONDON–BRUSSELS–FREETOWN

MID-OCTOBER 2014

St Pancras station was an ants' nest of purposeful activity. As I waited to pass through security at the Eurostar terminal, Mum and Dad stood with me, maintaining a solid composure. Only we knew where my journey was going to end: the train would take me to Brussels, but then I would continue onwards to Freetown. I was ready. Every part of me knew returning was right. As I reached the barrier, Mum let a glimmer of uncertainty show: 'Just be careful, hey?' she said, squeezing my arm.

Neither of my parents are strangers to difficult journeys. My father was a child during the Second World War, sent on a boat through rough waters to Canada as the bombs fell. My mother left Iran when she was twelve years old; her mother brought her to a boarding school in the English countryside and returned to Iran without her. It was a prophetic decision, for, some twenty years later, an Islamic revolution swept through Iran. Perhaps because of their own frightening and traumatic histories, they are brave enough to let me write mine.

In the MSF headquarters I crossed paths with Ruth, the American midwife I'd met in September. She had returned from Sierra Leone the same day, and arrived at the office shortly after me. She looked tired and wired. We sat together under a staircase and got coffee from a machine.

'We restarted maternity services in Gondama, but without the surgery,' she said, looking into her plastic cup.

I was surprised they had reversed on the decision. I felt guilt ripple through me for assuming it couldn't be done, for underestimating colleagues and reducing life-saving care: for failing.

'But we encountered the same challenges as before: difficulty know-ing who did and who did not have Ebola.' Ruth looked right into me. 'We had terrifying near misses, and deaths we'll never know the answers to.' Her coffee trembled in her hand. I could imagine those hands deliv-ering babies. I could visualize her in her element.

'There was this woman having seizures,' she continued. 'We had pre-sumed it was eclampsia. You know how it is in Sierra Leone – so much eclampsia. We admitted her inside, had her round the other patients, the staff all treating her like normal. But when she got worse, we tested her. She had Ebola. Everyone was freaking out.' She looked upwards, her face etched with disappointment. 'And still – despite everything, after all the training – still, infection control was sketchy. I was just like, "What can we do? We have to protect the healthcare workers".'

History had repeated itself: Ruth's team had endured the same ago-nizing decisions on continuing or stopping, deciding staff safety must prevail. Maternity was suspended a second time, paediatrics stopped soon after, and the entire 200-bed facility had closed down by early October.

Ruth had been yo-yoing up to the Kailahun ETC, supporting the team with their infected pregnant women. Guided by her experiences, she developed the clinical management further. Alongside the logisti-cians, she had designed a special area for labour and birth inside the ETC. It was smart, with beds on high stilts so healthcare workers didn't need to bend over the patient, reducing the risk of body fluid exposures. She had also continued collecting samples from births and miscarriages, which were giving us more information about how high the Ebola viral load was for the fetus, placenta and amniotic fluid.

Ruth's shrewd observations provided me with my the next steps. She noted how pregnant women in convalescence continued to have low-level positive Ebola tests, even if they appeared asymptomatic and recovered. She wondered if this was because they were still carrying the virulent contents of their womb. She proposed, rather than waiting for the negative test, that induction and delivery of these well women could reduce the amount of circulating virus, hastening their discharge. After delivery their viral load would drop, usually to negative.

I felt foolish for having brushed Ruth aside when I first met her, assuming she would have little to do in Sierra Leone. Evidently, we were kindred spirits, each feeling a deep responsibility to pursue the safest ways to help women living in the affected areas, both those without access to health services, and pregnant women in the ETCs. It was clear to us there needed to be a dedicated service for this latter group, and, even with our limited experience, we should be advocating to provide it.

I had been in continual dialogue with friends who had returned to the outbreak in Sierra Leone, Liberia and Guinea. We all knew pregnant women were not being looked after as well as they could be – not through any fault of the team, but because of a lack of knowledge and confidence. The feedback was for clear instructions and training on how to manage complications. If health workers, particularly the local staff, could be trained, the mortality rate in pregnant women could be reduced. Stopping an obstetric haemorrhage was my bread and butter, but, for most of those going out to the response, it was far from their comfort zone.

Ruth was exhausted. We finished our conversation and promised to keep in close contact. Without saying it, we had made a pact: together, we would see this through.

In the Operational Centre of Brussels, I began discussing the prospect of advising on pregnant cases across the region – supporting the ETCs, demonstrating how infected pregnant women need not be feared, and that their deaths need not be inevitable. The proposition received a mixed response. On the one hand, the principle was agreed; on the other, the commitment to seeing it through was not there.

Hilde had returned from Kailahun and was also in the office, so I spoke with her about it. I trusted her instincts and experience. Her advice was clear: 'Push, push, push'. In her opinion, if we didn't fight for it, it would not happen.

Working my way round the office, I talked with anyone willing to listen about appropriate training and support for the different ETCs on managing pregnant women and dealing with complications, such as haemorrhage. The lead of the Ebola task force listened between a flurry of meetings and activities, verbally giving the green light, 'as long as it is OK for the field'. I took this as a yes and began sending emails to the field hierarchy.

Flying back to Sierra Leone I mulled over the ongoing needs of pregnant women, the general health crisis and what might be different, this

time. The major change in response now, was the size of the effort. MSF
was still one of the only organizations providing direct patient care, but
our manpower was much larger. When I left West Africa in September,
the Operational Centre of Brussels (OCB) had been the only MSF section responding to the epidemic. Now, the Dutch section (OCA) was
due to take over operations in Sierra Leone, and there were rumours of
two other sections entering the response to help share the workload. The
numbers of aid workers and officials travelling to the area for Ebola had
increased massively. I got the impression Ebola had gone from being the
response nobody wanted to be a part of, to being the 'must do' of the aid
worker agenda.

Joanne Liu, the MSF International President, told the United Nations
on 2 September that member states should immediately 'deploy civilian
and military assets with expertise in biohazard containment . . . dispatch
your disaster response teams, backed by the full weight of your logistical capabilities'. This was followed by a public and heart-rending plea
on 9 September from Liberian President Ellen Johnson Sirleaf to US
President Barack Obama: 'without more direct help from your government, we will lose this battle against Ebola'. Within weeks, the UK, US
and France had announced ambitious responses to the outbreaks in Sierra
Leone, Liberia and Guinea, respectively. Despite the grand and trium-
phant claims of the UK entering as heroes into Sierra Leone, it would
take time before their presence was seen on the ground. China and Cuba
also committed significant assets to the Sierra Leone response.

The United Nations was also ramping up its intervention. On 18
September, a Security Council debate was held – only the second time
in its history a debate had been devoted to a health concern, the other
being for HIV/AIDS. An MSF team leader, Jackson Naimah, addressed
the Security Council from Liberia. Describing the overfilled ETCs, he
said, 'We have to turn people away . . . Right now, as I speak, people are
sitting at the gates of our centres, literally begging for their lives . . . left to
die a horrible, undignified death'. A unanimous decision, reportedly the
first ever, was taken to adopt a resolution to deploy an emergency health
mission, as the outbreak constituted 'a threat to international peace and
security'.

The United Nations Mission for Ebola Emergency Response
(UNMEER) was established the following day, an unprecedented UN

response for an unprecedented and complex crisis. UNMEER headquarters were outside the affected countries, in Accra, Ghana. It was
tasked with leading and coordinating the multitude of UN agencies in
order to end the epidemic, though there were concerns the mission could
suffer from the bureaucratic and clunky systems for which the UN was
notorious. On the same day, Sierra Leone began a three-day lockdown,
a heavily militarized house-to-house effort of health promotion and to
identify the infected. Over the border in Guinea, a team of health workers and journalists raising awareness of Ebola were found murdered:
eight bodies, three with their throats slit. Hostility, confusion and disease
denial continued to surge alongside the response.

The attitude towards aid workers heading to the Ebola-affected
countries was changing too. Negative media stories and paranoia had
reinforced misplaced beliefs in isolationism for protection. There were
people who believed my returning to be selfish, putting them person-
ally at risk. My brother-in-law told me his work colleague had said, if
I returned, she wouldn't share office space with him. This was totally
illogical.

In Brussels, I had met one friend who, on returning from an Ebola-
affected country, had been thrown out of his apartment by his landlord;
another's family had refused to see her. As responders we were being
viewed as potential vectors of disease, and stigmatized.

The unfortunate infection of a returning New York doctor from an
MSF project in Guinea heightened the public hysteria, despite reassurances that risk of further transmission was virtually nil (there was none).
Unbeknown to me, as I flew into Sierra Leone, an MSF nurse from the
project I was joining was flying back home to Maine, US. Kaci Hickox
was detained in a tent and quarantined against her will on arrival back in
the US. The New Jersey Governor responsible, however, found himself
publicly humiliated by Hickox, who went viral (only in terms of media
response), flouting his conditions and threatening to sue him.

My flight landed in Freetown at night. As we descended the steps
on to the tarmac, I saw the iconic MSF symbol on some of the other
travellers' bags. A small group stood together. I went over and introduced
myself. They were all heading to the same project as me, in Bo – the
same ETC I would have gone to if I had not left previously, and where
Silje had been working when infected.

The following morning we travelled from Freetown directly to the ETC by helicopter. Flying over the patchwork of green fields and small villages, the land below looked serene, and puddles from the daily rains sparkled with reflected sunlight. The disease was spreading through these lands. In Sierra Leone, roughly five new infections were occurring each hour. Freetown was seeing increasing case numbers too, sparking concerns of an explosive surge, as had happened in Liberia's capital city, Monrovia, in September.

As we disembarked the helicopter, I caught a glimpse of Kathleen, the Ebola focal person at GRC, as she ran to get on board for the return to Freetown. She had remained behind to support Kailahun when the rest of us had left. Even after her long months in the field, she still maintained her statuesque composure and look of total conviction.

The new arrivals and I sat with Marc, a smart Canadian doctor and the new project coordinator, for a briefing and to discuss our experiences. I was the only one who had previous experience in this outbreak, though Marcio, a Brazilian infectious diseases doctor with wild curly hair, had worked years ago in a smaller outbreak in Uganda. Marc had been copied into the emails I had sent requesting that I be given the role of training and supporting maternity care in the ETCs. He was enthusiastic, and felt we had enough doctors in the project that I should be able to help the other regional teams. We sat together and discussed the logistics of the role, creating a draft schedule.

The ETC was outside Bo city, in the small agricultural town of Bandajuma. The design was markedly different from Kailahun. The High Risk area was surrounded by a tall chain-link fence, and inside were five long Rubb Hall tents, lined up next to one another in military style. The Low Risk area was a solid concrete structure. To get to the treatment area, you had to walk along a curved slope, round the helicopter pad. There was no shade, which in the West African midday sun was punishing.

As I made my way in I was warmly greeted by local colleagues who recognized me from GRC. Since its closure, many had been re-employed into the ETC. There was an immediate bond between us because of our shared experiences, and they seemed pleased to see a familiar returnee among the many new internationals. The distance between national and expat that I had felt during my first mission evaporated. We were all in this together. Although, the stakes of the outbreak were immeasurably higher for my local colleagues than they could ever be for me. It was three months since the state of emergency had been declared; markets were empty, fields were not being ploughed, the economy and social cohesion were faltering and schools remained closed.

I changed into the familiar green scrubs and big damp wellington boots then entered the Low Risk area, where patient names were listed on a whiteboard. Standing in front of the board, hands on hips and looking sharply at the situation, was the South African paediatrician Juli – my first friend from GRC. Juli had arrived in Bo two days before me, she turned around meeting my eyes, her jaw unclenched allowing a smile to spread across her face. Seeing her here, it felt like we had never been apart.

On that first evening, I joined Juli on the veranda outside her bed-room, we lit candles and put Juli's eclectic music on in the background. This became a recurring event, our evening debrief. Juli told me about all that had happened in GRC after I had left, and the eventual closure of the hospital. Since returning, she had been finding the influx of new expats for the response a challenge, referring to the EOAs ('experts on arrival') – medics who had completed a two-day course on Ebola, who would stride into the mission believing they knew it all, ready to make immediate changes. Juli was no one's fool. She would return the EOAs to ground level, reminding them how local colleagues had been working with Ebola for months already.

The most pressing concern for Juli was patient numbers. Part of the fallout from Silje's infection had been a decision to gradually build up the numbers inside the ETC. The centre had a capacity for over a hun-dred patients, but at that moment there were around thirty, with two of the tents not open at all. Juli's position was clear: we needed to upscale quickly to relieve the pressures on the community and offer comfort to those infected. Leaving infected people outside was exacerbating the epidemic, and having unfilled beds was unacceptable. I agreed. Once patients were in the centre, the strict infection control practices were already there, whether we had one or a hundred Ebola patients. When it came to combating the epidemic, breaking the chains of transmission was a cornerstone.

Juli, in all her feisty glory, was instrumental in the quick expansion and opening of the rest of the centre. Soon, rather than one whiteboard of patient names, there were three, then five. We in the ETC didn't get to see most of the lives saved. Juli's determination to get the disease out of the community will have saved many from the direct and indirect damage the outbreak was unleashing beyond the isolation centre's fences.

Soon after my arrival in Bo, Stefan called from Kailahun requesting my assistance with two pregnant women who had tested positive. The team was nervous about their management. It was agreed I should travel back to Kailahun to train the team, and support them in managing the births.

This was exactly the situation Ruth and I had planned for, and we were in constant contact now, sharing thoughts on ways to simplify the protocols. There were key problems faced in the treatment of pregnant women, and the complexity of working in PPE meant stark choices had to be made. No one could claim to *know* what the correct management was, as it was all unchartered territory, but Ruth and I relied on our clinical judgement and small, but not insignificant, experience.

Ruth had focused attention on the most hazardous time for the pregnant woman: the moments immediately following birth, when the risk of bleeding is greatest. We had agreed, as no baby had survived, that we need not concentrate on fetal wellbeing, but should focus our full attention on maternal survival. We were mindful of our time limits – it took at least fifteen minutes to put on the PPE, with a maximum of one hour that could be spent in the suit while under the African sun. However, this time limit was often shorter in the maternity setting, due to the large amounts of body fluid and stressful circumstances. The combination of these factors encouraged us to focus our time not on the birth, but on post-delivery. This meant reluctantly accepting that women could end up delivering their baby, usually stillborn, alone. Not a palatable decision. It felt immoral. However, this was where we were, and we had to make hard choices to utilize our time for maximizing life-saving activities.

Efficiency, forward thinking and reducing the time needed to perform tasks were central to our plans. In a strange way, the women inside the ETC were delivering in a remote setting. While they were surrounded by medical teams twenty-four hours a day, they were isolated, untouchable, and no intervention could be performed rapidly. We therefore extrapolated from other remote settings where innovations had been used to save mothers' lives. For instance, we left medications to prevent haemorrhage with the patient to self-administer, as is done with Himalayan communities.

There were also concerns with the ongoing risk of transmission from breast milk, which we knew from performing virological tests remained Ebola positive even after the woman herself had survived. What we didn't know was whether it was live contagious virus, as no cultures had been grown. Relying on our experiences of inhibiting lactation in women with HIV or following stillbirth, we established protocols. Part of the management required finding a way to either suppress or safely dispose of the breast milk, and we also had to ensure good breast care to reduce the chance of painful engorgement and infection.

I was thinking over all of these things as I travelled to Kailahun. The journey was much easier than before, since the rainy season was almost over and the roads were no longer pools of mud. The morning sun hovered low in the pale blue-grey sky, a perfect yellow circle. Banana and palm leaves hung over the mud tracks on both sides, coated in the thick orange dust thrown up by the passing vehicles. This was my third time making the journey, and the landmarks were becoming familiar, triggering memories. I wondered how it would be to see the staff in Kailahun. I hadn't been in contact with them since the evacuation. Since Morris died.

Arriving back at the Kailahun resort, now an MSF-only compound, was surreal. Flashbacks to the fateful morning of evacuation and those long tense evenings leading up to it hovered in front of me. The new medical team leader and I sat in the courtyard to discuss the objectives for the time I was going to spend in Kailahun. I wanted to ensure a safe birth for the pregnant women, and to train the ETC workers on how to care for them and manage complications. We also began discussing the need for contraceptive options to be made available to all women leaving the ETC.

The Dutch section of MSF, OCA, had taken over the running of the ETC. It had undergone renovations since I was last there. Even though it had only been weeks, it was as if returning to a childhood home as an adult – all familiar, but disorientatingly different. The flow of staff movement into the ETC had changed, and an extension had been built in the High Risk area for convalescing patients. These patients were generally well, waiting until they were negative on blood test so they could be discharged. They knew they would become survivors. Together, they lay out in the sun, braiding hair, chatting or listening to the radio. The area was fondly referred to as the 'beach'. The atmosphere was one of chilled-out recuperation.

I wandered through the Low Risk area of the ETC. It was a strange feeling. Besides Stefan and Grazia, the Italian epidemiologist, I did not know the international team members. The national staff, though, whispered indiscreetly to one another.

'Dr Benjamin?'

Beaming faces soon surrounded me.

'Why did you never say goodbye?' they asked.

It was a difficult thing to explain. Why hadn't we gone and said goodbye before leaving?

I sat together with the national staff and we spoke about what had happened, about Morris and others who had perished since that time. It was humbling to be back, and to be welcomed by those who had remained throughout. I explained why I was there and that I had been discussing with Ruth, and MSF, safer ways to care for pregnant women. Ruth's name was met with delight – they recalled her with affection and were excited to discover we were a joint force.

18: BELLY WOMAN

KAILAHUN, SIERRA LEONE

OCTOBER 2014

The ETC team had a range of skills, from community health officer to nursing assistants. At my first training session, I asked around the group how many had trained in maternity; a few cautious hands went up. But when I asked who had delivered a baby, every member of the group nodded. Grace, a local nurse who had been working in Kailahun ETC for months, told me she had delivered a baby with Ruth in the previous week and wanted to get more experience. Her enthusiasm was underpinned with strong confidence.

One of the patients was already in her third trimester and recovering from Ebola, the other was thought to be in the early second trimester and quite unwell. I asked Grace if she knew which patient the recovering pregnant woman was. There were about eighty patients in the ETC. She looked at me disapprovingly, tutted her tongue and led me along the orange plastic fence towards the far end of the High Risk area. I took that as affirmative.

When we got to the 'beach', Grace put her hands on her hips and shouted out to the twenty or so convalescing patients resting to music and braiding hair.

'*Yeah!*'

Nobody responded.

She took a deeper breath, puffed her chest out and shouted again, in a voice meaning business.

'*Ye-ah!*'

A few heads propped up in recognition.

'*Yeah. Where di be'leh 'uman?*'

A couple of women turned and pointed towards a corner of the 'beach'.

'*Eh, be'leh 'uman – dis na di be'leh 'uman docto.*'

A skinny woman with long legs and arms sauntered over. She was wrapped in a colourful lappa sarong. Her eyes looked to the ground, every now and then flickering upwards to reveal a dazzling smile trembling with shyness.

Hawa was in her early twenties. Like many women in Sierra Leone, she had a sad childbirth history. This was her sixth pregnancy, but she had only one child. Her husband had been a community health worker, helping to treat sick people in their village. When he became sick himself, he brought the disease into their home. Hawa was still counting the days since he died; this was day twenty, and the mention of him filled her large brown eyes with heavy pools, a reservoir of emotion being held back.

'*Aw di bodi?*' I asked in my broken Krio, raising my voice so she could hear from me across the fence.

'*Di bodi fayn,*' she said, as another member of the 'beach' brought a white plastic chair for her to sit on.

Calculating the gestation of the pregnancy was typically challenging and way beyond my Krio abilities. Grace translated Hawa's answers to my questions with a mischievous glint. 'If he's a boy, eleven months; if a girl, ten months.'

This made no sense to me; looking at the size of her bump, I estimated she was around thirty-four weeks pregnant. When Hawa had first been admitted to the treatment centre, the fetus was moving, but she hadn't felt anything for a few days now. There had been no recorded case of a baby surviving when born to an infected mother, in this or any previous epidemic. The vast majority were stillborn, and the few liveborn had all died within their first month.

We discussed what had happened to her over the past few weeks – getting sick, being admitted to the treatment centre and now getting better.

'Tomorrow we'll take the blood test to see if you still have Ebola,' I said to her and Grace.

Hawa smiled and looked to the floor.

'Grace, let's explain why I've come to see her,' I said, in the most delicate tone I could muster. 'Even if Hawa is free of Ebola, the pregnancy remains infected. The placenta, amniotic fluid and fetus have all accumulated the virus. Hawa might be negative, but the pregnancy is still potentially contagious.'

Grace nodded, indicating for me to continue.

'The options are to induce the labour, delivering the baby and placenta, once we have the blood test result. Or wait till labour begins naturally, but still give birth inside the ETC.'

Grace translated the predicament across the plastic fencing to Hawa, who sat upright, carefully listening, as if a student attending class.

The stillness of the baby within her somewhat simplified Hawa's decision.

The following day, I had the pleasure of telling Hawa she was Ebola negative. She grinned with relief. Behind the smile, though, remained the fear of ending the pregnancy. I showed Hawa around the delivery area Ruth had designed, explaining how the induction of labour would work. I wanted her to understand precisely what would happen.

Knowing the work environment we faced, and its unique challenges, we created non-standard plans to mitigate the risks. When I gave Hawa the first tablet to begin preparing her body for labour, I also gave her a small packet with one of the medicines for controlling a haemorrhage. 'You take this as soon as the baby comes out,' I told her. Knowing she could deliver at any time, and the high risk of bleeding, I would rather trust her to take the medication immediately after birth than wait for us to be present.

While awaiting her contractions, I prepared the 'maternity box'. This was a cardboard box, which, like every other object, would not return from High Risk once taken inside. Creating the box was a training opportunity for the staff on what to use and do if faced with complications. It contained all the emergency drugs already drawn up, intravenous fluids and infusions ready prepared, apparatus for inserting lines, urinary catheter and items for sanitation and hygiene. If you had a problem, this box would mean you had everything you needed at your immediate disposal. Once in PPE, time is everything; looking around for equipment in an emergency, or running out to call over colleagues to fetch things is energy wasted and precious moments lost.

Early the next morning, my mobile phone rang. 'Hawa says the contractions have become strong,' said a nurse from the night shift. 'She feels the baby will come soon.'

I quickly dressed and headed for the ETC, where the nurse was wait-ing for me. Together with another Sierra Leonean colleague we entered High Risk with the ready-packed maternity box. Hawa was silent in the maternity room, but her facial expression gave away that she was close to giving birth. As an obstetrician, there is the temptation to internally examine a patient to assess how the labour is progressing, but, as I told the others, 'Inside Ebola High Risk, you keep your fingers where you can see them'.

I ensured the two intravenous lines I had inserted yesterday were patent, and lay out all the emergency drugs and infusions in anticipation of a haemorrhage. Outside the sun was rising and the day was heating up; after almost an hour inside the High Risk area we were becom-ing dehydrated in the heat of our PPE. It was time for us to get out. I repeated to Hawa exactly what to do and put the drugs in her hand.

There was a small queue to get through decontamination, so we had to wait, our scrubs sodden with sweat. I had grown to enjoy the relief of the chlorine spray as it descended down on to me. It reminded me of the posh women in north London, who would have their partners spray their brow with cooling cucumber mist while in labour.

As I sat down to drink water with rehydration salts, my scrubs not yet dry, a female patient from the 'beach' shouted across the fence: the baby was delivering.

The evening shift and morning shift had changed over and I called to Grace, who had just arrived, to see if she would join me, together with a fresh hygienist. It was vital to have a group of us, watching over one another for safety. We donned the PPE, and I stared into my own eyes in the dressing area's mirror, correcting my facial hood and masks to ensure no skin was showing. I looped the straps round the back of my head and pulled them tight, but not too tight. The adrenaline was flowing freely through me. I was excited to be in this position, to have the privilege of offering obstetric care and training at this time. Equally, I was nerv-ous. The situation was thwart with hazard and I was aware things could quickly deteriorate.

Grace and I were soon ready, but the hygienist took her time. It's not appropriate to rush someone getting ready to go into the High Risk area, but, conversely, every second in PPE counts and sweat was already drib-bling down my back and arms. Furthermore, Hawa was delivering alone inside the wooden shack and I was concerned about haemorrhage. I was keen that we lost as little time as possible in case she was bleeding out.

The PPE immediately slipped me into an alternate reality, all senses muffled, but my mind remained focused. We left the dressing area and began the dance of entering High Risk, our movements like a waltz. I lifted the rope off the metal pole, let the others pass me into the no-man's-land between Low and High Risk, and then put the rope back over the pole, sealing the border. After a few metres, we did the same again to make our way through the 'suspect' and the 'probable' zones. Normally, we would stop along the way to check in on patients, but this time all three of us glided through the one-way system on autopilot, opening and closing gates, to get to Hawa.

The sun shone down on us as we moved across the ETC; with little shade, I could feel the heat burning through the layers of rubber and plastic covering me. When we got to the entrance of the delivery room there was no sound coming from within. Without a word, all three of us paused for just a moment, sucked in a breath, and went to do our job.

Inside, we found Hawa crouching on the floor below the stilted delivery bed. She must have collapsed, I thought. As I shuffled over to help her up, I began absorbing the rest of the scene around us. In the training and advice I gave to ETC teams, I had certain rules, one of which was 'never hurry'. Never rush. And, when you think you need to move quickly, when the adrenaline is pumping hard, that is the cue to slow down. I lived by my own words; without them I could have missed the stillborn baby and placenta lying on the bed above her.

Hawa looked like a small child, cowering in fear. Her eyes were wide open, she was shaking and tears were running down her cheeks. There was a small trickle of blood coming from under her. In her hand was the empty pill packet.

We moved like clockwork. Grace spoke to her with reassurance as I got the other drugs. I gave her the prepared injection to prevent haemorrhage, and connected the IV infusion, already hanging and primed. We cleaned her and gave her fresh pads, while the hygienist dutifully watched over us to make sure we were not exposing ourselves to risks. The hygienist had brought the chlorine pump and began to clean around us, intermittently washing our gloves of the blood and fluid.

On the delivery bed was the infant, cord and placenta, all attached together as one. My first reaction was to be sure there was no sign of life. I rested my fingertips on the baby's chest: nothing. I scooped it all together inside an absorbent sheet and moved away to the other side of the room, behind a partition. The baby was pale and, from the appearance of the skin, had died a few days earlier. I took samples for calculation of Ebola virus, from inside the mouth and from the amniotic fluid, and placed a small piece of placenta into a specimen pot. Grace asked Hawa if she wanted to see or hold the baby; she did not. With the hygienist, we sprayed the body, cord and placenta in chlorine and placed it into a child-size body bag. I carried him to the morgue.

Together, the three of us meticulously went about disposing of all the medical equipment. We cleaned and decontaminated every place and object we had touched. Once wiped clean, Hawa returned to the bed she had earlier fled from. We gave her food and something to drink, telling her how well she had done. We checked she wasn't bleeding and explained to her what to do if there were any concerns. We would return to her in about four hours to remove the infusion of oxytocin. We made one last survey to check we weren't missing anything, and then we left. Hawa was already looking like a different person, smiling with pride, knowing she had survived.

Outside, we observed each other to check there were no breaks in our PPE, then sprayed one another's gloved hands with the high concentration chlorine and asked if we were each OK. Together, like a group of victorious soldiers returning from the trenches, we made our way out.

While waiting to return to Hawa, I held a training session for the morning team. Their enthusiasm went far beyond the delivery and care of infected women. They wanted to understand how to look after any pregnant woman and manage the complications that were all too common as a cause of death in their country. It was evident that the training had the power to extend beyond the outbreak. It was an opportunity to invite all cadres of healthcare worker present to understand the basic principles of emergency maternity care. Their motivation was without question; whether they would have future access to the resources required, though, was much less certain.

Each team entering the High Risk area was asked to check in on Hawa. When I returned to her, I found the bleeding had been minimal;

the drugs had worked. After unplugging the infusion, and again telling her how impressed we all were with her, we asked if she had any questions. She wanted to know if she could return to the 'beach'. Absolutely.

The following day, Grace and I repeated Hawa's Ebola test. It remained negative. She could go home. The news was met with both relief and sadness. Hawa knew her husband and child had not survived, and now she had birthed a stillborn baby. The trauma did not stop with survival. She would be returning to an uncertain future. There was no guarantee she would still have a home or any belongings, which may have been either destroyed or stolen, and she no longer had her husband or his income to rely on. She might not even be welcome back in her village; fear and suspicion of survivors was an ongoing problem.

Hawa went through the routine discharge process. Led to a shower inside the High Risk area by two colleagues dressed in full PPE, she removed all her clothes and was encouraged to wash thoroughly with chlorinated water – particularly to make sure she washed her hair, where infected matter could get stuck. Following the first shower, she was passed a bucket of water to wash again. A 'clean' assistant, who had touched nothing inside the High Risk area, would then pass Hawa her new clothes and flip-flops. On instruction, she walked with arms crossed over her chest, touching nothing, and was led to the exit of the High Risk area. No further decontamination needed, she was reborn back into outside life.

Across from the ETC was a psychosocial area, where counsellors and health promotors gathered. I had built a good relationship with these teams from my previous times in Kailahun, and had been in discussions with them about the practicality of introducing more comprehensive contraceptive services for survivors at discharge. This was a subject they were keen to move forward and implement. The men and women working in psychosocial care led the survivors through the process of discharge and reintegration, often accompanying them back to their villages to help with the transition.

Hawa looked fragile in her chair in the psychosocial area. I told her again how well she had done, how proud she should be of herself. Though we had been ordering the drug used to suppress breast milk, it had not arrived yet; instead, I had a breast pump for her. Together with Aminata, the counsellor, I explained how to use the pump and dispose of the milk. These are difficult conversations with any mother who has suffered a stillbirth. But, although Hawa had lost immeasurably, there was also celebration in her survival and return to the living world. The conflicting emotions twisted within us all. As I said goodbye to Hawa, I took pleasure in shaking her hand, skin to skin.

The samples I had taken from the fetus and placenta all returned highly positive results for Ebola, despite Hawa's blood test being negative. The significance of these results, though, was murky. The standard test being used in the outbreak was a form of polymerase chain reaction (PCR), where a portion of the virus's genetic sequence is amplified and detected. The virus need not be alive nor intact for the test to confirm its presence, as long as those few chinks of the genomic chain are present. There are advantages for using the test: it can be run over a few hours and it is safer for laboratory workers, as the sample can be deactivated before testing. *But* the interpretation of the result is that the Ebola code is present regardless of whether that code is on dead virus, a fragmented strand, or actively contagious disease. To know if the detected virus was active, a culture would be required – a riskier procedure and unavailable in the field. Naturally, we were not taking any chances, but the fact remained that we were making a calculated assumption on infectivity.

While in Kailahun, I continued to hear about pregnant patients inside the other ETCs in Liberia and Sierra Leone. They worried the teams, regardless of gestation; in some cases, it wasn't even known if a woman was pregnant, miscarrying or menstruating. I would support them by phone or offer to travel to provide training and oversee the delivery.

Monrovia was problematic. Sometimes I was called to give advice late into a developing case, and I always returned to the same issue: train the national staff to manage these cases with confidence. It was our experience that pre-emptive treatment saved lives. Once a pregnant woman began bleeding, and the floodgates opened, it was much more difficult to stop it. It felt unacceptable to either do nothing and hope for a swift resolution, or decide to act only once complications had arisen. The international staff who called agreed on the need for training and support, requesting that I attend to deliver the training. However, the higher management levels, for reasons I never understood, blocked any visit. There seemed to be an attitude of *We can handle it*.

On one occasion, in November, I received a call from a German doctor in Monrovia, asking for advice on a woman bleeding. The woman was a probable case of Ebola, but they were still waiting test results to confirm this. She had entered the ETC the previous day and was known to be twenty-four weeks pregnant. No specific preparations had been made for her and she had gone into spontaneous labour overnight. Following a stillbirth, she had passed the placenta and had been bleeding ever since. She was still conscious. I asked what had been done to try to stop the bleeding. The doctor told me they had given a small amount of misoprostol, to contract the uterus, and a bag of IV fluid. I explained it was paramount to take fast action, stopping the bleeding before she entered a state where the body becomes unable to clot blood.

A couple of hours later I got another call for further advice. The woman was still bleeding and was now unconscious. I went over with the doctor what had been done since I last spoke to him. The medical team leader had not permitted the team to follow the instructions I had given. He had not allowed them to pass a catheter to empty her bladder, helping the uterus to contract, stopping bleeding. His safety concerns were unfounded; a catheter is a soft rubber tube, which could not breach PPE. I felt a rage burn inside me. Ebola might have sealed her fate, but she had been denied the chance to prevent haemorrhage, and now death was inevitable. I reassured the doctor and advised him to continue with the other measures. I would contact the team leader myself. The woman died shortly after our phone call.

The following day I received a reply from the medical team leader (MTL). It was a kind and thoughtful email, thanking me for the advice. I have no doubt each person was there to do their best, but the final line was telling of something else: *Not surprisingly the poor girl died . . . that's Ebola.* His blind, exhausted acceptance held a mirror to my own assumptions; that colleagues would also view maternity care as critical within the emergency. The frustrations churning inside me from her case clarified my own stance. This was not *just* Ebola; it was a maternal death from a preventable cause. She may have died from Ebola, but she need not have bled to death from childbirth.

19: BANDAJUMA

BANDAJUMA, SIERRA LEONE

NOVEMBER 2014

Returning to Bo, I reunited with Juli and the rest of the team working in the large Bandajuma ETC. Each day I would first take a long look over the increasing number of whiteboards with the lists of patients' names. We were climbing to the peak of the epidemic and, with such a high turnaround of admissions, discharges and deaths, it could be difficult to keep track of all the patients. Suma, the manager who had commanded respect among the team in GRC, became one of the coordinators managing the allocation of tasks and the arrangement of patients, leading the clinical team. His soft voice hid the directness of his commands. Among all bustle of the ETC, Suma was still able to run a tight ship.

With Juli and Suma taking the lead, a code was devised to rank the patients according to severity of illness. During November, the red marker pen, for severe, had been getting a lot of usage.

If I was covering the morning shift, I tried to organize the medical team as early as possible, so we could maximize what we got done before the sun rose high. I generally aimed to have the ward round completed by 10 a.m. First thing, we would gather together and look over the whiteboards and individual patient charts, making a rapid assessment of who our sickest patients were. As far as possible, we tried to keep the most critical together, to make nursing them easier, as these were the patients most likely to require intravenous access and more intense nursing duties. Their bay became a mini ETC-ICU.

Broadly speaking, the patients were either self-caring, requiring assistance or end of life. I was keen for local colleagues to lead as much as possible. They needed to be the decision makers and understand the principles of care. Expats would continue to come and go, but the national medics would be the experts with the hands-on experience.

One of the key functions of the ward round was to determine if a patient was ready for a blood test to check if they were still Ebola positive. Timing was everything. It was important to minimize unnecessary blood tests, as we did not have the capacity to perform more than about ten per day. Testing a patient too early wasted the opportunity to test someone else, but leaving it too late kept a bed filled with a patient who no longer needed to be inside the ETC. Together, we would discuss who should be tested the next morning. Increasingly the Sierra Leonean community health officers were encouraged to take the decision.

I tried to balance conducting the daily ward round according to patient need. The majority of patients could be reviewed without PPE. Taking the boxes of patient notes, we sat at the fence, calling over those who could walk. This was preferable. The patients could see our faces and we could talk without the time and heat pressures of PPE. It also allowed us to focus our time inside the High Risk area on the sickest patients, performing procedures and tending to the young and elderly. Our PPE stocks were precious too. We needed to make the most practical use of what we had.

I enjoyed these outdoor rounds, and the opportunity to observe my colleagues as they grew in knowledge and confidence, prescribing medications to help manage symptoms, giving advice on hygiene and deciding who to test. It was from this area that I counselled any pregnant or breastfeeding women when longer discussions around difficult subjects were needed. On our patient list, we would note which patients had improved and were able to come to the fence, and which ones had not managed to find their way out of bed.

Inside the High Risk area, as in all the ETCs, we worked our way round the one-way system. I entered the 'suspect' area with Sulaiman, a young CHO I had been working with at the fence. Our first patient here was an ETC nurse's daughter. Ebola was not affecting strangers here; it happened to colleagues, family and friends too.

We continued into the area for 'probable' patients; their Ebola test results were still awaited, but their symptoms and contact with the disease were sufficient for us to make a calculated judgement. Among them was a two-year-old girl, who was lying on a bed, working hard to breathe.

I gently woke her, sat her up and, with the help of one of the nurses, assisted her to take a few sips of water. With so many patients to see, we could not spend too long with her. I made a note to insert an intravenous line with fluids, and moved on.

The final area was designated for patients confirmed to have Ebola. It was a series of long white tents, like an army barracks of contagion. While working our way through the patients, we were alerted to a commotion outside.

'Hey, hey, hey!' the staff from Low Risk called, waving and pointing for us to investigate what was going on.

Sulaiman and I plodded over in our heavy wellington boots. A woman was wandering around naked and screaming. She knelt down in the area between High and Low risk, then lay on the concrete in the glare of the sun, rolling around and moaning. It was times like this I feared the most: the unpredictability of a confused patient with a lethal disease. But the woman was not aggressive; she was distressed.

Together, Sulaiman and I protected her head from the hard ground, then we carried her to bed – hot work in the sweat-proof suits. We observed each other as we moved her, watching for any hazards, every step coordinated by our eyes.

'Are you in pain? Does your body hurt?' I asked, when we finally had her in a bed.

She pointed with her fist to her chest. 'Father dead. My mother dead. Sister dead. Children dead . . .'

I had nothing to give for a broken heart, just a gentle hand on the arm, a blanket and a sedative.

With so many sick patients, it was easy to lose track of time. The work was endless: help drinking for one, intravenous line and fluid for another, cleaning away vomit and diarrhoea, offering comforting words and pain relief, diagnosing and treating other illnesses, straightening out the bodies of the dead that we discovered on our way. We had become masters of task shifting and job sharing.

It was vital to take note of who had died and where they were, so their body could be removed by the hygiene team. Patients often became confused prior to death and it was not uncommon to find them lying on the floor or in a different patient's bed. Patients sometimes had identical names, so all patients also wore wristbands carrying their unique identification number. Recording an incorrect death and informing the wrong family was a very real risk, which would do nothing to build trust in the community.

At one time, we had five women named Kadiatu Koroma. One Kadiatu died in another Kadiatu's bed. In feverish sweat and delirium, her wristband had slipped off. There was much cross-checking and confusion before we all agreed we knew who had died and who was alive.

Once Sulaiman and I had been decontaminated and had exited High Risk, we heard that three more patients had died since we began the round, including the two-year-old girl. Death was a daily occurrence in the ETC, but so was survival, and every day a group of survivors would be discharged to the banging of drums, the blowing of horns and much dancing, reminding us that we were also in a place of life and resilience.

Filling the beds emptied by death or discharge were patients arriving in ambulances from all over the country, the origins of their journey informing us of the epidemic's spread. Increasingly, we were receiving patients from Freetown. Other organizations were now setting up alongside MSF, but it would take weeks for them to become operational. In the meantime, the continued arrival of the ambulances and what their shipment represented was most disturbing.

Those weeks between October and December blurred together; each day was another catalogue of difficult choices, ethical conundrums and frustration at global hesitance. Reading the daily news, I searched for stories exploring the true face of the outbreak, the experience of the villagers crammed inside the ambulances, rather than the paranoid ramblings of a Western politician.

Receiving the ambulances was often stressful. Those who were lucky enough to make it to the ETC emerged bleary eyed after the long, hot journey down bumpy roads. Their stoic expressions said nothing about what they had seen. Families and communities were crumbling. Women watched as their husbands died, then, because they had been unprotected, they succumbed to the same illness, knowing, if their children tried to help them, they would become the next link in the chain. Every admission was a tragedy not being told.

The new patients would be met by strangers dressed in yellow suits, and led to a bed, where they were given a blanket, toothbrush and some food. There was an unwritten observation among those of us who had been around a while: the patients who arrived and immediately lay down were usually the ones who didn't get back up.

Drivers, dripping in sweat, were keen to unburden themselves of their human cargo. They often had long return journeys home, or needed to find a place to sleep for the night. We would know in advance from the central command centre how many patients to expect – this was negotiated with Marc, our project coordinator, who knew what our capacity each day would be. On one particular day, we were expecting an ambulance with four patients already confirmed to have Ebola. But when it arrived and we opened the doors we found five.

Juli had dressed in PPE and gone with the hygiene team to receive the patients. I stood on the other side of the fence, collecting patient information so it could be quickly transcribed into patient folders and wristbands. We tried to make the admission process as smooth as possible.

Juli shouted across to me, her voice distorted by the face masks covering her lips, 'There are too many patients'.

Communication in these times was always fraught. The driver wanted to leave, but we couldn't move the patients without knowing who they were, if they had Ebola or were suspected of Ebola. The nurse escort had the details of four patients. She held up the papers for me to read through the fence.

Juli peered into the ambulance. 'Ah, God!' she shouted. One man was lying along the bench, bleeding from his mouth and nose. The blood had smeared across his face, hands and on to parts of the ambulance interior. There was an elderly woman, two young children and another woman in her late twenties. After frantic document checking, shouting and sweating, we understood who each of the passengers was.

The woman in her twenties was the mother of the young children – an eight-year-old boy and his six-year-old sister. The children had already been sick for a week, but their mother was in good health. They were from Freetown and she had been told she could stay and care for her children inside the ETC. Juli and I knew this wasn't a possibility. The children both had blood tests confirming they had Ebola, but the mother didn't.

'What should we do?' shouted Juli from behind the chain-link fence.

'She's not been tested,' I shouted back, looking at them all. 'We can't send her with the kids to "confirmed".'

The woman stood by the ambulance doors, wearing a pair of latex gloves and her house clothes.

'She probably needs admitting too; she's been exposed,' I added. 'You take the others and I'll triage her for symptoms.'

We all thought she understood, but as Juli took the children through the mother began following.

With a coldness I did not know lived inside me, I shouted over the fence, 'Madam, no! Madam, you cannot go with them.' The concentration camp notion haunted me again – the guard separating a mother from her children. No emotions, just following protocol.

Juli took the others into the High Risk area, and I sat two metres from the mother, on the opposite side of the orange fence in the triage area, to discuss what had happened and to identify signs of infection. She told a sombre story. Her children had become ill in Freetown. She had taken them from clinic to clinic, and was often turned away. She had the foresight to wear a pair of gloves while looking for help. Finally, she was isolated with the children, deprived of food and water, and left alone. Once her children's blood tests had confirmed they had Ebola, she continued to look after them, as no one else would come into the holding room.

'How do you think your children got infected? Was someone else in the home sick?' I asked, as I made notes.

'No, no one at home has been ill,' she said. 'They play outside, behind the houses; some dead body was there.'

Her risk of exposure to the virus was huge. I was certain she would have symptoms suggestive enough to admit and test her inside the ETC, but she denied feeling ill at all. Her only symptoms were those of a concerned mother.

After giving her something to eat and drink, I explained what MSF would provide for her children.

'I know who you are,' she interrupted. 'I wanted my children here. I know you will care for them.'

I knew that when I had shouted, *No, Madam, you cannot go with them!* it may have been the last time she would see her children alive. I carried her trust on my shoulders.

We couldn't admit her, but given her history of exposure, we decontaminated her like a survivor, through the discharge shower, and gave her fresh clothes. Before she left we made sure she knew how to call us for updates, what to do if she became unwell and how to visit her children. She returned daily and never developed any symptoms of Ebola.

Within forty-eight hours of entering the treatment centre her daughter died, but her son recovered. As with most of the children, he was cared for by other convalescing patients. He was discharged two weeks later, accompanied by all the drums, songs and mixed emotions of a survivor, as he reunited with his mother.

Over those months, there was a continual expectation for the international response to take lift-off; mostly, though, there was only the sound of engines blasting. The British news had written triumphantly in September that £225 million would be spent on curbing the epidemic, including six new ETCs, providing 700 Ebola treatment beds and the potential to treat up to 8,800 patients over six months. By late November, the UK response had only one ETC partially open, being managed by Save The Children, eleven treatment beds were available, and a total of twenty-eight patients had been treated.

While the UK ETCs were being built, we continued case management. Outpaced and chasing the tail of transmission, all the available ETCs were providing only 60 per cent of the beds needed. MSF had agreed to mentor other NGOs entering the response, including International Medical Corps and the Irish charity, Goal. Four of Goal's senior team were integrated into Bandajuma ETC, where they learnt our daily routine. Among them were two nurses: Rachel, Irish and bold, and Gillian, Canadian and quirky. They both radiated dynamic energy, were eager to absorb everything happening in the ETC and were open to troubleshooting for a way forward. Over the course of their time with us, we all became close friends.

The Sierra Leone government had agreed to reward those employed in the Ebola response with a financial incentive; it served as recognition and encouragement to keep working. The so-called 'hazard pay' was worth £63 a week. It often did not reach the frontline workers, however, and, as frustration at the disappearing funds grew over time, hostilities increased. By mid-November, no hazard payments had been received by the staff of Bandajuma ETC, though their MSF salary was paid. A decision was taken without warning for an immediate strike of over four hundred staff. Gang mentality rapidly swept through the ETC. Colleagues told me in confidence they wanted to work and look after the patients, but had been threatened with violent consequences if they did. This left us incredibly short-staffed, with over sixty patients and only a handful of international medical and hygiene staff. The Goal team demonstrated their competence, stepping up and sticking out the wildcat strike to help us continue providing care while the national staff negotiated a settlement. The strike also exposed how vulnerable we were without the massive machine of local workers supporting the organization.

20: PREGNANCY PREVENTION

'It's a quick procedure,' I said, crouching on the floor in one of the small cubicles in the pre-operative waiting area. Katie was already in the hospital gown. 'I read over your notes; this is your third pregnancy, right? And the abnormality was detected when you had the scan?'

Katie nodded in acknowledgement.

'I'm really sorry.' I looked up at Katie, who appeared to be about to say something.

'I'm going to be sick.'

I darted out of the way and grabbed a grey cardboard vomit bowl for her.

'Ugh,' she groaned. 'Will this go away after you've done . . . the thing?'

I went from cubicle to cubicle, meeting the twelve waiting patients. Each had her own story, her own reasons for being here. There was a skinny student sitting school exams and a Romanian woman who spoke no English; a morbidly obese girl who'd thought she had a working contraceptive; and a mother of five who was living in a women's refuge, fleeing her abusive partner. Each meeting was conducted with sensitivity. There was nothing to be taken for granted here. We discussed the procedure, and I offered the different contraceptive options available.

As I worked my way through the cases, stopping the progress of pregnancies, I considered Sierra Leone, Central African Republic and all the other places I had worked where choice was restricted, and I remembered the girls and women who had died in their desperate search for control. These surgical lists bring me a mix of feelings. I had always been pro-choice for every pregnant woman, but it was not till after working overseas that I felt the calling to participate.

I walked with a feeling of lightness in my step after the surgeries were completed, and I popped into each cubicle to check on the women, answer their questions and consider their futures.

Katie had her husband with her, and they held hands, both with tears in their eyes. I was acutely aware that I was the one who took the pregnancy out; I wondered if they hated me.

Katie leaned towards me. 'Can I hug you?' she asked.

I was startled. No patient had ever asked to hug me before. It was an uncomfortable request. I wondered whether it was even allowed. She clutched me tightly and I felt her body shudder with emotion. Any doubt drifted out of me.

*

BANDAJUMA, SIERRA LEONE

NOVEMBER 2014

It had been over three months since the suspension of obstetrics at GRC. I relived those decisions constantly, replaying them in my mind, knowing I had participated in reducing healthcare access in a country, and at a time, demanding the opposite. Now, I searched for solutions.

Formulating guidelines for treating pregnant women infected with Ebola was not difficult, once we had figured out a standard package. The greatest challenge was finding willing partners to give these women the chance of survival. Meeting the needs of women in the general population with obstetric complications remained much more challenging.

The fundamental barriers had not changed since June. Although receiving Ebola test results was quicker than before, they were still not rapid – a turnaround of at least a few hours. Furthermore, we now knew that, even if we tested a pregnant woman's blood and she was negative, she could continue to carry high levels of viral particles in her amniotic fluid, placenta and fetus, despite having recovered from Ebola herself. I spent many days pondering a way around these dilemmas and discussing the problems with Sierra Leonean colleagues and international staff. The outbreak remained uncontrolled and widespread, and we struggled to come up with a solution that would be palatable to the higher powers of our overstretched organization. When GRC closed it had been explicitly advertised as a temporary measure, yet the gates showed zero sign of reopening.

In October, the United Nations Population Fund (UNFPA) published a call for action, declaring that without access to emergency obstetric care a potential 120,000 pregnant women could die across the three most affected countries. In November, the call was widely reported in the media after ActionAid claimed one in seven pregnant women could die in childbirth, a twenty-fold increase from pre-Ebola levels. The predictions were based on the closure or abandonment of facilities, and the joint fear of women attending a facility potentially riddled with Ebola or of healthcare workers fearing the pregnant woman with her Ebola-like symptoms and soup of bodily fluids. These shocking statistics made headlines, but were no different from the risks in other humanitarian emergencies if no assistance arrives.

Colleagues who were pregnant, or those who had relatives who were, asked what could be done to ensure their safety. During antenatal consultations we identified women for whom delivery near a functioning obstetric operating theatre was going to be vital. There were still some parts of the country the outbreak had not yet reached and we began transferring women in the latter part of pregnancy. It was not a popular intervention and some chose to stay in Bo and take their chances with local facilities. A nurse I had worked closely with at GRC was in her third trimester; she had diabetes and a previous caesarean section. Another nurse was pregnant with twins, the first presenting by its feet. We sent both of these women away to deliver in a hospital outside the epidemic area. Our colleagues were, in many ways, the lucky ones. Childbirth, though, is unpredictable, and even the most uncomplicated of pregnancies left me anxious.

As we had begun developing guidelines for the provision of different contraceptive options for Ebola survivors, I had questioned why we weren't offering these to all women. If we couldn't offer obstetric services, we could at least reduce the requirement for them.

I put together a proposal and spoke to the head of the emergency response. My enthusiasm was not reciprocated. He was a wise and experienced aid worker, with many years working in humanitarian response; I was a novice in comparison. While we were able to have a frank conversation on the current reproductive health issues, when I suggested that we begin a family planning project the tone of the conversation diverged.

'This is an *emergency*, Benjamin. Family planning is *not* an *emergency*,' he stated.

I disagreed.

Pregnancy, at that time, could be viewed as a life-threatening condition. Contraceptive access therefore had the power to be a life-saving intervention. In my eyes, its provision *was* an emergency.

Meanwhile, support for female Ebola survivors having a broad range of contraceptive options at discharge remained strong. The initial suggestion to simply offer condoms (as we did for male survivors) was rejected, as it had connotations of prostitution if the woman was unaccompanied. I created a short training package and protocol for contraceptive choices, with infection control measures specific to the ETC. Ruth, Severine and her team all added their own touches and agreed that scaling up would be ideal. Many of the former GRC staff were experienced in providing contraception, including implants and injectables. As implementing partners, they brimmed with enthusiasm to put their skills back into use.

The conversation, though, always circled back to one thing: 'What about us? What about our children?'.

It was a valid point.

The closure of schools heightened concerns that teenage pregnancy rates would increase.* This was further fuelled by the economic downturns of the epidemic, with sex being exchanged as a commodity. Marie Stopes, a major provider of contraception in Sierra Leone, had data showing an over 90 per cent drop in women accessing their services between May and August. It was later estimated that there was a 44 per cent to 172 per cent increase in unplanned pregnancies during the epidemic. The country's restrictive abortion laws compounded the risk that this would lead to an increase in unsafe pregnancy terminations.

In trying to push the women's health agenda, I was discovering the power dynamics within MSF, frictions between the field staff and head-

---

* UN Development Programme (UNDP) reported a 65 per cent increase in teenage pregnancies in Sierra Leone during the Ebola epidemic.

quarters, and between the different OCs. Needless to say, I, like many before and after me, did not often get it right. But, in upsetting the chain of communication, I was also uncovering the alternate routes within it.

The turnover of international staff is often rapid, particularly in a response as large and intense as the Ebola outbreak. I took the family planning discussion to the MTL and PC. For them, there was no concern. If I was willing to sort it out, they were behind it. The learning curve was knowing what to say to whom. Communication was not only a delicate balance, but also a very sensitive matter, where individuals became annoyed if they felt under- or over-included. Frankly, it was a huge challenge and a life lesson in the art of covert negotiations.

With the other four OCs becoming increasingly involved in the response, and the handing over of ETCs in Sierra Leone to OCA, a whole new hierarchy entered the field, presenting another opportunity to open the door to wider and more formalized contraceptive access.

I approached the incoming head of mission and the headquarters team, explaining I already had clearance to provide contraception in the ETC. They were very supportive, and nobody asked if it extended to general healthcare. I saw no reason to volunteer that it didn't.

Hurriedly, I put together a standard operating procedure that incorporated both ETC and non-ETC contraceptive procedures, and got the greenlight. In keeping the move towards non-ETC healthcare at a low profile, it seamlessly slipped through the net.

A 'no-touch' policy had remained effective for all international staff entering the response. Occasionally, the rule was broken – generally late at night, after too many beers. However, for Sierra Leonean colleagues at home and present for the long run, it was not realistic. Rather than keeping our heads in the sand, we had the resources to help protect each other – not specifically from Ebola, but from the risks of unprotected sex and unintended pregnancy.

Initially, male condoms were supplied in easy-to-access, yet discrete locations, such as male and female ETC changing rooms. The reaction of the ETC staff to the progressive policy was welcoming, exemplified by frequent requests for additional supplies, including demands for female condoms to be included. Regularly, a coy male or female colleague would call me aside, informing me the box was empty, or requesting a few extra.

The condom supply was accompanied by health promotion activities, particularly around the importance of maintaining a no-touch etiquette at work, and reminders that condoms would not stop Ebola transmission with an infected person. Nonetheless, it represented a positive shift in mentality and created an open space for candid dialogue.

MSF was running a staff health clinic in a repurposed house close to the ETC. The clinic provided basic-level healthcare. It also served to screen for Ebola when workers became unwell, as they were, by virtue of their jobs, a high-risk population. The clinic served a population of approximately a thousand MSF employees and their dependents. Many former GRC workers were also eligible.

In order to implement the full range of contraceptives at the staff health clinic, strict infection control procedures were necessary to counter the risk of inadvertent Ebola exposure. The system relied on 'no-touch' questioning for symptoms of Ebola, temperature checks, a one-way flow of movement through the clinic and a strategy for transfer into the ETC, if deemed necessary. We kept a register of all contraceptives supplied, and to whom, our main worry being, if a client later became infected with Ebola we should be able to trace if we had had contact.

Everyone working in the staff health clinic was ex-GRC, giving a sense of familiarity, but also leaving me wondering how they viewed me – the guy who ended GRC obstetrics and began the cascade towards its eventual total closure.

We would gather around a large wooden table and begin each day with a communal prayer – Muslim and Christian together: 'Dear Father, we love you, we need you. Help us in this time. Father, we beg you to not forget us as those around us perish. Father, protect us from the disease moving around us . . .' The words were spoken in earnest, like a child talking to their father in a time of despair. We all knew of friends and colleagues who had died; coming to work each day was a reminder of our vulnerability. We always ended in quiet meditation, palms up to the sky as *Al-Fatiha* was recited. No touching, but we were bonding nonetheless.

Fatmata, the head midwife from GRC, was now working as the staff health midwife. We would often discuss the management of our pregnant colleagues, and reminisce about the GRC days. It was only after I had been in the clinic a few times that she brought up the facility's closure.

'Dr Benjamin,' she said, adjusting herself in the wooden chair, 'you know, when GRC stopped, we were all very angry with you. We knew it was you who had said we should not have any more patients. We spoke about it, the others and me – we were so angry. We were worried for our jobs and our families. We all blamed you'.

Sweat beads collected on my forehead. I had always assumed this was the case. Everyone else had been too polite or concerned with offending an expat to tell me bluntly. I still had not resolved within myself those decisions and their implications.

Fatmata paused to gather herself; it was an unusual show of emotion for a woman hardened through her country's tough history. She looked to the floor and lowered her voice: 'Then we started hearing more and more about the others getting infected and dying in the clinics, the infections at the maternity hospital in Freetown. We spoke about it and we knew – you saved our lives. We were angry with you, but now we are thanking you.'

I swallowed and thought how we will never know of the lives which might have been saved had we stayed open. There were no answers to the fundamental questions of what we should have done at that time. But Fatmata's frank confession gave me the conviction that, more than ever, we were together in this mess.

Fatmata and I began putting together the system for contraceptive access through the staff health clinic. We began a registry and discussed how we would work towards restarting maternity services. Without the backing and motivation of Fatmata and the rest of the staff health team, getting the initiative started would have been far more difficult. Other NGOs were also working to provide contraceptive services and to raise the public awareness of the needs of women in the region. We contacted these organizations to see if there were ways we could learn from and support each other. We were all aiming for the same goal, while working in an unfamiliar landscape.

Posters went up all around the ETC – at the entrance, in the kitchens, the hygienists' area and with the guards. We wanted to make sure everyone was aware. We held small meetings and asked colleagues to spread the word that contraception was available through the staff health services.

As the news spread, more and more colleagues began asking if they could bring their neighbours, nieces, friends. I knew the limits of the generic policy would not allow it. MSF was not psychologically in a place to move forward with a mass contraceptive campaign. I did not want to risk drawing scrutiny, which might lead to the cessation of the small effort we were making. Equally, I did not feel it was morally acceptable to deny access to contraception when we knew the risks of pregnancy were excessively high. I concluded that we could not refuse any requests. I rationalized that my time in Sierra Leone was nearing completion, anyway – I already had a departure flight booked; if I over-stepped boundaries and was expelled from the mission, it made little difference to me. It seemed a reasonable gamble.

Initially, I only told staff they could bring other women and girls if they asked me directly. As confidence and conviction grew, I boldly announced at team handovers and meetings that the contraceptives were there for anyone who needed them. At the clinic, the nurses were asked to allow any person requesting contraceptives access, assuming there were no infection concerns. There was absolute agreement. The nurses were so much in favour of promoting pregnancy avoidance that every woman of childbearing age would be asked, regardless of why they were at the clinic, what they were going to use while the outbreak was ongoing.

Our biggest regret was our inability to become a major healthcare intervention. The small-scale provision of voluntary contraceptive options at the staff health clinic could have been an early prototype for development and expansion. Door to door antimalarial campaigns to reduce the non-Ebola burden of disease and fever were successfully implemented by MSF. With anthropological and cultural guidance, we could have engaged with communities to a similar level of visibility, increasing access to contraception for the most afflicted areas.

There is much to be proud of, and much to be ashamed of, in the Ebola response. The contraceptive service was a lifeline for those within reach, and life affirming for the staff who proudly made it happen. However, efforts to reach the wider population never progressed beyond an idealistic vision.

21: THE CAVALRY ARRIVES

BANDAJUMA, SIERRA LEONE

DECEMBER 2014

As the epidemic progressed, the response also evolved – though, which led and which followed remained unclear. At team meetings we debated the double-edged sword of providing quality care with limited resources. A stark choice: focus on treating infection or stopping transmission.

Accusations of flouting medical ethics were countered with retorts of not seeing the epidemic's trajectory. The intensity of the work environment shortened our fuses. The furious passion to resolve the scenes we witnessed risked creating tribal divides among us. These internal disagreements were exposed within the academic literature and circulated in opinion pieces, later resurfacing in retrospective analyses of the response.

In truth, the epidemic morphed. When the dragon began breathing fire on villages, we chased her tail. As the flames receded, we built water cannons, ready to shoot.

The first months of high patient-to-healthcare-worker ratios forced impossible choices. Ella, the Kailahun health promotor, described it best in September: 'We know we should be doing more, but we don't have the resources, we don't have the capacity, we don't have the staff. Some days it feels like it doesn't matter how hard we work because there aren't enough of us. We're fighting a forest fire with spray bottles'.

In December, the international muscle finally flexed, in synchronicity with declining transmission. The reality for those entering the outbreak now was a far cry from the situation during the months before.

Our knowledge of the disease had grown, as had the treatment options available. Those who criticized from outside the field, or applied the rules at one point of the outbreak to a different time or place, missed the nuances of the multiple changing dimensions. Similarly, those who had witnessed one part of the epidemic needed to adapt to the shifting sands around them.

This was seen both at individual and organizational levels. As more agencies entered the field, the egos and insecurities of each player were unveiled – the more established actors fighting to hold their turf, and the novices looking to make their mark and prove they could *do* Ebola. I recalled lectures and papers on humanitarian response and the infighting of NGOs to raise their flags a little higher than their neighbours', losing their vision of what they had arrived for in the first place.

This became more common as the numbers of patients began to drop alongside the rapid expansion in the number of ETC beds available. Undoubtedly, responders came armed with good intentions. The reducing workload, though, led to boredom and frustrations for the newer arrivals. We joked about the 'Ebola tourists', who spent their time in the field, it seemed, being photographed in the distinctive yellow PPE, and uploading the pictures to their social media accounts. Others were gathering data to write papers while the world was thirsty to publish anything on the topic.

It is widely held that the eventual UK-led response had a significant and rapid impact on the Sierra Leone epidemic. Mathematical modelling predicted that the increased availability of beds potentially averted a further 57,000 infections (including 40,000 deaths). However, had those beds been present just one month earlier, the total number of cases could have been halved. The decline in cases was not a zero-sum to beds available. The natural curve of the epidemic likely moved alongside community recognition and response, acceptance and changing practices (such as safer burials), and the wider isolation capacity. Just as a perfect storm collected to create the dragon, a symbiosis of collaborative factors augmented the quenching of her flames.

Over time, the tiredness of my first mission crept into the second. As my departure date drew closer, I felt the heaviness of physical and psychological exhaustion upon me. The thought of wearing PPE increasingly repulsed me – not out of fear, but out of pure fatigue, excessive sweating and heat. Once, I exited the High Risk area after a gruelling morning, and my scrubs, sodden with sweat, fell to my ankles from the weight as I was decontaminated. Unclean, I just stood, legs wide apart, till the regimen was over and I could regain my dignity.

I returned to the old Bo Base, about a ten-minute drive up the Kenema highway from Bandajuma, to work away from the ETC. It was both comforting and eerie to be there. I loved its sense of familiarity but it also reminded me of the GRC days. Over my laptop's screen I saw the ghosts of recent missions past.

The hum and cooling breeze of a rotating electric fan blew across my neck as I sat at a desk making plans for my return home.

'Hey, you!' an American twang came from behind me.

Turning my head, I found MJ standing there, looking just as she had on my first day in Kailahun: radiant, beaming and buzzing with energy.

MJ had returned to Sierra Leone a day earlier to support a new training and support project, focused on preparing NGOs entering the field, guiding them as they opened their ETCs. In less than five minutes she was trying to sign me up. The thought of being back on mission with MJ was incredibly tempting, but I knew, too, my stamina was waning. As we chatted, Kate, an Australian nurse who had been stationed over the border in Guinea, came to join us. She too was working to set up the new programme. Before I knew it, another American and seasoned aid worker, Paul, the project coordinator, was sitting with us and I was being filled in on their plans. It was an initiation.

As we chatted I realised this training and support project could provide an opportunity to get messages about reproductive healthcare to a much broader audience. I emailed Ruth to tell her about it and she was immediately on board, and had already begun making her own plans to return to Sierra Leone.

That evening, I sat with Juli on the terrace outside her bedroom – our regular evening ritual. 'I know they say we shouldn't stay too long, and I am tired, but it's exactly the opportunity we've been looking for – sharing experience with other organizations.' I paused as I lit the candles on the table. 'What about you? What do you think you'll do after this?'

'I want to stay,' Juli said, swigging from a bottle of cider. 'Extend for a bit longer. I don't see anything to go back for right now. I already missed the start of my fellowship, I have to see this through.'

'You're a machine, Juli,' I said, in awe of her stamina. 'I don't know – I want to keep going, but need a break. It would be nice to have some *touch time* too.'

'Did you have someone in mind?' Juli asked.

'Maybe. Not sure dipping in and out of an Ebola epidemic is going to be the time I find love, though.'

'You won't know unless you try,' said Juli, taking my phone off the table. 'You got a photo?'

'What kind of stalker do you think I am?' I said, opening up Facebook.

As we continued chatting about life, love and career, we observed a couple of black mice slip into the kitchen opposite us. Dryly, we noted that despite all the Ebola hype, Lassa fever might still be our undoing.

Paul, the PC, contacted me to see what I thought about joining their team. It was an opportunity I could not refuse, but I had one condition: no more PPE. I needed a break. I needed to stop profusely sweating. If Paul could grant me that, I was in – a proud part of the Ebola training and support team. By extending my contract I could also continue supporting our fledgling family planning project and be on hand for maternity cases.

Paul, Kate, MJ and I began planning a programme for aid agency team leaders. Several of the major NGOs entering the field were to send representatives for the five-day training, following which we would get them out to MSF ETCs to gain hands-on experience. Paul and Kate allocated the schedule, agreeing to squeeze sexual and reproductive health among the sessions I was preparing.

We had planned to start the course in early December, but the team from Goal were moving forward with their own ETC in Port Loko, a province adjacent to Freetown, and they had requested MSF's support for the critical first days. Opening an ETC was a complicated operation, as Save The Children had learnt to their cost. Their intervention had already suffered a staff infection, and they'd been accused of opening when unprepared, resulting in a reduced ability to respond. What should have been a jewel in the UK response had been marred by negative press attention. Goal did not want that to happen to them.

MJ and I set out in the early morning, travelling several hours upcountry, together with Craig, a heavily tattooed Canadian logistician who I'd met in Kailahun, who had recently returned to Sierra Leone. We crossed through the numerous checkpoints, eventually pulling into a campsite off the highway in Port Loko. The tents were being shared as accommodation for different organizations, the air-conditioned units divided into individual cubicles. The beds were similar to those we used for patients inside the ETC; I recalled the many times I had peered through my mist-filled goggles at the weary confined to these beds.

The Goal office was a ten-minute walk down a mud road. There were old crumbling buildings scattered along the way, and small groups of children played while stray dogs slept in the late-afternoon heat. As usual, before entering or leaving any building, our temperatures were checked with infrared thermometers. Merely crossing the road to another building required another temperature check. Though I went through this routine about twenty times a day, every single time, panic rose inside me. The thermometers were shockingly unreliable. Held like a gun between the eyes, when the trigger was pressed it would beep and an apparently random number would appear. Walking in midday sun could push someone's temperature up. Everyone soon learnt that, if you had a high reading, you could repeat it and you'd probably get a different number. The guards would be happy they'd done their job, and you would be relieved to be past the gate. I was occasionally recorded as being burning hot, only to be rechecked and found to be death-defyingly hypothermic. Most disconcerting, *this* was supposed to be our safety measure.

The Goal set-up was impressive. Their offices and staff accommodation occupied what appeared to be an old boarding school. The first team of NHS volunteers had arrived fired up and ready to go, but the ETC was not yet completed. There were training plans, team structures and protocols to put together. It was a massive undertaking and the field coordination team was working in overdrive. Goal had stepped forward with all the courage, but not the experience, of MSF. But they were here and they were dedicated to halting the epidemic around us. Where MSF strutted with superiority, Goal moved with humility.

The NHS volunteers were used to working hard and being busy. Boredom and frustration can be dangerous for an intelligent crowd. MJ, Craig and I discussed with the coordination team ways to manage the situation, concluding that they needed to give their colleagues purpose. Even if they weren't in the depths of the High Risk area, they would be fulfilled. It was an important exercise in managing expectations, and, for some, their pride.

While there was mounting external political pressure to get ETCs up and running, the reality was that repeating the errors made by previous

NGOs could worsen the situation and hinder the response. Opening prematurely would please the bosses back in Europe, but do little to help conquer the outbreak. Like all things in Ebola, I advised the usual principles: staff safety first, don't rush, be prepared and be efficient.

The UK-built ETC was mega-sized, a complicated fortress being erected by the Royal Engineers. Unlike the simple tents of Kailahun, this took longer, and the design plans were to be followed with military precision (unsurprisingly). Though we and Goal pointed out faults and impracticalities, nothing could be changed till the Royal Engineers' orders had been followed and the keys handed over. This hot-headed rigidity and lack of pragmatism led to longer lag times in construction and the knowing unveiling of an imperfect ETC.

As afternoon turned to evening, Craig and I shared a couple of beers with the Goal team. It did not take long for us to find common friends and shared interests. The excitement and anxiety were palpable whenever conversation returned to the new ETC. When Craig and I walked back along the mud road to the campsite, a thick and heavy night blackness surrounded us. Craig was in full monologue on his thoughts and aspirations, which kept my mind off the mysterious cracking of twigs and rustle of leaves in the darkness. A sudden sound of rushing feet came right at us, and I made out three wild dogs in the gloom. Little barking noises passed from one to another. I grabbed Craig's hand and pulled his muscular arm around me so I could shelter in his solid frame. The dogs, oblivious to us, ran straight past. Letting go of his hand, I apologized, and Craig continued unperturbed with his monologue. Thankfully, the night was dark enough to hide my burning cheeks.

As I lay on my bed, Craig's shadow moved around in the cubicle next to me, and I could hear Mohamad, our driver, snoring softly. I stared up to the top of the tent as my mind went through its routine of processing images and thoughts. It was cold from the air conditioning; I curled up into a fetal position to warm myself. Closing my eyes, I saw the faces of the two young brothers, the rows of beds in Bandajuma, and debated the unresolved ethical dilemmas of GRC. I lightly touched my forehead with the back of my hand. It would be another restless night.

The early morning light shining under the canvas and the crowing of cockerels brought me to wake. MJ had already gone for her morning run; Craig and Mohamad were still sleeping. I stood in the wet air between the tents, taking a moment to stretch and breathe before heading for a shower.

The Goal team had put together an intense programme. We observed them training their newly employed staff in infection control and how to get the PPE on and off. The UK volunteers teaching the course were largely new to the field, but, if you didn't know otherwise, you'd think you were watching accomplished experts in the art of Ebola management. Between sessions they would ask us for feedback, open to suggestions and changes.

While watching one of the sessions my phone began buzzing. I stepped outside into the sunshine. It was Sarah, the sexual and repro-ductive health adviser for one of the newer NGOs. They had recently started operations and she wanted advice on a pregnant woman.

We had spoken before, having conversations around women's health, the importance of family planning and the management of pregnancy. A week earlier, we had talked through the methods for induction of labour, managing haemorrhage and the risks of continued pregnancy in survivors. Sarah was also a gynaecologist; nothing I told her would have been new, but putting it into our current context, as a colleague, was reassuring. I had sent her all our documents and made plans to try to meet in the future.

Sarah's thick French accent sounded unusually high and rushed; she seemed distressed.

'Slow down, start from the beginning,' I said, trying to hear her over the sound of cockerels, mopeds and construction.

'We have this woman – three, maybe four months pregnant. She's been with us over a week and she's now a survivor.'

'Yes, I remember we spoke about her. You thought she would be OK. Did you counsel her about the pregnancy?'

The advice in early pregnancy was to pre-empt a miscarriage, the most likely outcome; preparation should be in place for managing bleeding or retained placental tissue. If the woman survived Ebola and remained pregnant, management became more complicated. Pregnancies stayed highly positive, even if the miscarriage occurred several weeks after the mother was 'cured', and there was virtually no possibility of a healthy live birth. There were also further risks to consider: community workers being exposed if delivery took place in an uncontrolled setting, and unreliable access to healthcare if the woman were to have complications later. We advised counselling and offering all women survivors the option to interrupt the pregnancy before leaving the ETC. If she chose to continue with the pregnancy, she would need to stay in or close to the ETC so the infected body fluids could be managed in a safe area when she eventually miscarried or delivered. Sarah agreed with our stance, and had discussed the options once the woman tested negative.

'She wants to finish the pregnancy. Doesn't matter if it is a miscarriage or still going, she wants to finish and go home. She understood everything very well. She told me she has had enough and does not want to continue the pregnancy.'

'OK,' I said, picturing myself having these same difficult conversations.

'Everything was ready. I had the tablets in my hand. I was on my way to give them. The woman is waiting. She is preparing to go home after this awful time. But *they* stopped me. They stood in my way and said they are anti-abortion.' Sarah's voice was getting faster. I closed my eyes to give her words my full concentration. 'I'm the gynaecologist,' she said. 'I spoke with her, offered her everything. She told me what she wants. Now, these men are standing in my way, saying, "We won't allow it." It's not up to them! *Merde!*'

Apparently, there had been team discussions. Sarah was trapped in an ethical debate on allowing termination of pregnancy. These non-specialist, and largely non-clinical, European men were preventing Sarah, the gynaecologist, from seeing her patient. Fuming and swearing, she asked, 'Will you speak with them?'.

The situation was further complicated as there were consultants with links to the WHO involved. I worried that if this was not handled sensitively it could have wide-reaching and detrimental repercussions for many other women facing difficult and uncertain futures.

Regardless of one's stance on a woman's right to choose, the context before us needed special consideration. Infection control, chains of transmission, maternal wellbeing, fetal viability, human rights, psychological and economic trauma all collided together. And in the centre? A person, waiting.

As someone external to the confrontation, it seemed reasonable I attempt some mediation.

I spoke to the lead doctor and it turned out we knew each other. He was a distinguished medic, admired for his knowledge and generosity. I held him with fond admiration from previous meetings. We ran back over the scenario, and, while I did not share his moral concerns, I appreciated his ethical dilemma. It was a good exercise in testing the advice we were giving: was it reasonable?

We discussed taking an ultrasound scanner into the High Risk area to diagnose miscarriage. I explained this was fraught with problems. We would first need to find an ultrasound machine, which would then become Ebola contaminated, limiting its future use. The evidence to date was overwhelming in suggesting the fetus would not survive. Even if there was a fledgling heartbeat now, this did not equal a viable life existing outside the womb months down the line. Lastly, it told us nothing about infectivity. We explored performing an amniocentesis to test the fluid for Ebola. This too had problems, since it involved an invasive procedure and would not change the pregnancy evolution. Furthermore, it could be hazardous to the person performing the procedure. Our understanding remained rudimentary; we did not know if it was possible to have a negative amniotic fluid result with a positive placenta or fetal blood, nor how to interpret the results with regards to level of infectivity (through culturing the sample to see if the virus was alive or dead). Throughout the discussion, there was a shared respect of opinion. Never did it disintegrate into a debate or battle of wills. We walked through the various concerns, reasoned with and questioned one another. We started and ended on good terms. 'You'll have to decide for yourselves,' I said, 'but, for me, the choice is hers'.

I later heard from Sarah that the woman had received the medication the following day. She delivered the pregnancy soon after, without complication, going home the next day, free to step forward with her autonomy intact.

The Goal team had allocated a few hours in the afternoon for MJ, Craig and me to deliver training, which was also an opportunity for their team to ask questions. We had prepared a session on difficult situations, logistical dilemmas and clinical scenarios. I gave a specific talk covering the management of pregnant women and the importance of family planning.

The team sat mesmerized, either with total fascination or a look of terror. We discussed their many questions, and tried to give real-life examples. The doctors in the group struggled the most, since much of the medical work in Ebola was closer to traditional nursing roles. It was vital to grasp the importance of team work and maintaining fluidity in jobs and responsibilities, but there was discontent at the idea of not maintaining a 'doctor makes all decisions' environment. The trouble lay with patient ownership. The doctors needed to adapt from saying and thinking 'my patient' to 'our patient'.

In discussing the management of a woman with Ebola in labour, our standard advice was to avoid invasive procedures – for example, a caesarean section. They were unlikely to result in the woman surviving and the risk of healthcare worker infection would be unacceptably high. A couple of the doctors were unconvinced, saying such things as, 'If I want to do a caesarean on my patient, I will do it'. These were not easy conversations to have. The necessary change in mentality, for some participants, was a struggle. What had become a way of life for me was alien to Ebola-naive new arrivals. I listened, trying to imagine if I would accept such standards, were the roles reversed. I invited fresh opinions and alternative ideas for ways to provide safe care. Nobody had all the answers. For me, when in doubt, I returned to my guiding principles: staff safety first, don't rush, be prepared and be efficient.

A few days later we returned to Bo to begin the week-long training for the NGO team leaders. It was a pivotal moment for the outbreak. Rapid expansion in bed spaces turned the situation from patients outnumbering ETC bed spaces to the other way around. Kate, MJ, Craig and I delivered the majority of training to participants representing Aspen, Save the Children, WHO and Médecins du Monde. The facilitating team was small, but we were committed to its purpose: passing on and sharing the skills and knowledge we – as an organization and as individuals – had acquired. There was a sense of change. The world was present, and interest in the outbreak was high. The motivation to stop the decimation of the most affected countries seemed, at last, genuine.

I took every opportunity to push the case for sexual and reproductive health. I wanted to ensure these future team leaders were under no illusions: their projects must have plans in place for treating infected pregnant women and providing contraception for survivors and staff. The wider impact of the outbreak, outside the walls of the ETCs, was a subject demanding overt awareness. As health organizations, they needed to consider what capacity they had for reducing the worsening maternal health outcomes, rising teenage pregnancy rates and increasing sexual violence, and providing aftercare. Family planning, safe abortion care, treatment of sexually transmitted infections and HIV all needed addressing. At first glance, these appeared peripheral to their role in the Ebola response, but for the people around them, their colleagues, neighbours and patients, they were central. It was also a vision for the future.

I returned to Port Loko with Juli, just over a week later. Juli had also made a close friendship with the Goal team, and they were impressed with her directness and ability to achieve results. After months of being in the field together, Juli and I had developed an intuitive relationship. 'Where's my twin?' Juli would shout, if looking for me. We were able to bounce thoughts and ideas off each other easily, often not agreeing, but able to bluntly put our cards on the table and find a strategy for a way forward. It was a great pairing, perhaps due to our former lives as obstetrician and paediatrician; we were both constructive and critical, with a chunky dose of cynicism and gossip.

The Goal team were hoping to open imminently. While awaiting the ETC keys, they staged simulation exercises to identify problems. Juli and I observed and made notes, taking long walks around the ETC, drawing diagrams and visualizing how it would work in practice. We took it in turns to play the patient, or nurse or hygienist, troubleshooting and re-enacting scenarios we had come across. Together, we identified weaknesses and then brainstormed for solutions.

At the end of the day, we returned to the campsite with its air-conditioned tents, hotel-style canteen and hot showers. It was becoming busier with more arrivals. Groups of young Brits sat around playing cards and drinking beer. I felt odd, out of place suddenly, hearing familiar accents.

The UK response was not uniform; it was built of partnerships with several different NGOs, each with its own personality, expectations and ways of behaving. The volunteers went out to work in the NGO's ETCs or to support other activities of the response.

I sipped a hot drink in the tent canteen, the waxy smell of canvas mixing with the plastic taste of the mug, while typing up the day's notes. I was just finishing up when an email came into my inbox. It was short, instructing me to open an attachment. There was a letter written by

British medics volunteering with Emergency, an Italian NGO. They had documented a catalogue of complaints, accusing the organization of treating patients without dignity and using medications off-license as experimental treatments, without ethical approval or proper consent.

The team threatened a mass resignation on grounds of ethical outrage. They alleged being asked to perform tasks which were neither proven necessary for the patients' wellbeing, nor safe for the healthcare workers. Two non-NHS doctors had been infected. Furthermore, the medical team felt emphasis was being given to performing time-consuming and invasive procedures over meeting basic healthcare provision. They were concerned their patients were not being hydrated properly or receiving appropriate hygiene care. Despite the innovative treatments, the volunteers had calculated the mortality rate to be higher than in other ETCs.

The WHO had published a list of potential treatments eligible for 'compassionate' use, as an emergency experimental therapy. Emergency was administering amiodarone and furosemide, and neither was on the list. They both had the potential for worsening organ failure and unappealing side effects. There had been no animal or human studies supporting their use, and while amiodarone showed some anti-Ebola effect in laboratory experiments, there were over fifty other drugs reported to have stronger supporting evidence.

The UK clinical team now demanded this stopped, or they would quit. Undersigned were the names of fourteen doctors, nurses and paramedics.

I was stunned. The thirst to join the research race, to publish life-saving findings and stand out in a popular market had been irresistible, to some. If the allegations were true, they risked breaching the principle of nonmaleficence.* I imagined the scenes described: the villager infected, traumatized and in the hands of the ETC medics. The power dynamics were immense, the fear inconceivable. My thoughts moved from the individual to the collective. What would happen when the survivors returned to their communities, telling them of the procedures they had undergone? Describing the ICU-style open-plan area, where male

---

* In medical ethics, the principle of nonmaleficence means medics should 'do no harm'.

and female patients might be exposed to one another? How would this be interpreted? Would there be demonstrations? Would all NGOs be tainted by the actions of one? Would the response falter – or, worse, allow the disease to take the upper hand? My heart pounded with anxiety, anger and anticipation of how this could all play out.

'Are you OK?' asked Juli, sitting opposite me.

'Look at this,' I said, pushing the laptop around to face her.

I continued digesting the letter's contents as she read.

'What do you think they should do?' she asked.

'Get them out. The UK should stop funding the project,' I said, still considering the consequences. 'When this goes public, it will be a disaster. I think they should release a statement directly to the press, criticizing the NGO – get in there first. Nothing can make this acceptable.'

'But, if they all leave, who will care for the patients?'

'I don't know. Emergency will have to find another team. Maybe the threat will be enough to drive a change in practice.'

There were, I assumed, practical, financial and political complexities that would need negotiating. But I was not privy to the inner dealings of the UK response. I thought it was only a matter of time before the email would be forwarded to someone in the press.

'They mustn't bury this. It shouldn't be hidden,' I concluded.

About two weeks later, the news of Emergency and their experimental treatments did hit the UK press, by which time the team had left. Emergency's evidence for the drugs was described as 'speculative, at best' and the NGO's behaviour as 'reckless'.

Emergency released a vigorous denial, accusing their critics of ulterior motives and conspiracy theories and rebuking the WHO's compassionate medications list as being for profit over efficacy. They pointed out that they had acquired Italian ethical approval, and were only halting administering the drugs temporarily while awaiting Sierra Leonean permission for a clinical trial. They threatened legal action against the 'slanderous' press, though none was taken. Most striking, they postulated that their practices were levelling the field between Africa and the West, whereas the media drew upon history and compared the episode to other times when medical studies had been carried out on populations without due consent.

Condemning the volunteer medics, Emergency wrote: 'If the NHS team had spent time looking after patients in the hospital rather than staying at home to exercise criticism, they would have had a much clearer picture of our patients' management.' The NHS team had left their homes with good intentions and integrity. They were relocated to provide care with alternative NGOs.

22: TONKOLILI

MAGBURAKA, SIERRA LEONE

DECEMBER 2014

The Belgian MSF section had handed over its two large ETCs (Kailahun and Bandajuma) to the Dutch MSF section, OCA, by October 2014. These had been national referral centres. However, as time passed more NGOs opened ETCs, increasing local bed capacity and reducing the need for lengthy patient transfers. As December progressed, the number of patients in the Kailahun ETC plummeted, and Bandajuma had scores of empty beds.

Tonkolili District, in the centre of Sierra Leone, had seen a surge of Ebola cases. Other NGOs were building large ETCs relatively close to the hotspot; however, until they became operational the Tonkolili patients continued being sent across the country. OCA decided to provide care closer and build a new one-hundred bed ETC in Tonkolili, near the town of Magburaka.

MSF had finite resources, and sacrifices had to be made. The training and support project was re-diverted to the opening of the MSF ETC, rather than assisting external NGOs. As a small group, we took the decision badly. We felt we offered something important and unique, giving experience and confidence to unacquainted organizations in the field. The Ebola epidemic had been a pivotal moment for MSF to flourish at inter-agency cooperation. There had been large knowledge transfers and training provided, particularly in Europe for incoming international teams. This was a different model for MSF, where engaging with inter-agency collaboration was a well-recognized organizational weak point. I felt frustrated; an opportunity to broaden our impact had been snatched from our hands. Ruth was also returning to Sierra Leone to continue and expand the training project; instead, she too would be sent to Magburaka.

I returned from Port Loko to Bo. The following day MJ and I were relocated to Magburaka for the opening of the newest MSF ETC.

The rainy season had broken and a fresh breeze blew through the open windows as we moved upcountry from Bo to Magburaka. We travelled via Mile 91, a busy intersection town, named according to its proximity to Freetown. The town had once been known for its bustling market, spilling over with trade, bright flashes of lappa, the yelling of children and zealous hagglers, but it was boarded up. Sprawling camps of the internally displaced had filled local fields during the civil war – MJ had worked here, back then. Now they were empty, just like the market. Mile 91 had suffered a surge of Ebola cases. The town was barren.

As we drove further away from Freetown, the tarmac road changed to mud. Small villages were dotted on either side of the track, and occasionally the driver would slow down and point, saying, 'Quarantine house'. It sent shivers down my spine. What was happening in those homes? What was their understanding? How did they get food? How were the vulnerable protected? Did it help?

A large white-and-red MSF flag came into view. Outside the gates, a few stalls sold refreshments – an opportunity for business in the Ebola economy. Following the usual rituals of temperature checks and chlorine washing, we continued on foot up a hillside. Close to a hundred daily labourers had been employed to create a clearing in the woodland and erect the ETC. We saw the large white tents and tell-tale orange fencing along the upper slope. This would become MSF's tenth ETC in the region. In sheer technical ability, it was a remarkable feat. A large treatment centre, with ambulance bay, staff quarters, warehouse and administration, all built in under three weeks.

In the centre of the ETC were two nurses I had worked with in Kailahun: an energetic Italian called Massimo and a good-humoured Australian called Emily. They were huddled around a wooden table, in deep discussion with Ruth. The ETC was scheduled to receive patients in two days. Emily and Massimo had been in Magburaka for several days already, lecturing and training the new hygienist and medical recruits. Alongside them were four of our Sierra Leonean colleagues from the Kailahun ETC, who were acting as mentors to the whole team, local and international. Their months of experience were invaluable, having worked throughout the outbreak at its original epicentre. Together, we formulated a full schedule of practical training stations for the next day, preparing the future team for ETC work.

It was dark by the time we left. At the guest house, the logistical team was gathered on a veranda, drinking beers and smoking. I knew many of them from earlier projects, but mostly their missions would complete with the opening of this new ETC. The guest house had a strange atmosphere to it; the living room had a TV set with a collection of Nigerian soft-porn DVDs, and my bedroom contained a huge double bed with bright pink satin sheets and heart-shaped cushions scattered around. Perhaps, pre-MSF and pre-Ebola, more touching had happened here.

Ruth and I sat together with our beers, two flames merging. We sailed through the events of the outbreak and our concerns for the vacuum of maternal healthcare. Though this was the first time Ruth and I had been in the field together, our shared experiences over the preceding months had united us. Ruth had worked for decades in sexual and reproductive health, she had spent years in Sierra Leone, was fluent in Krio and spoke enough local dialects to make an outstanding impression. We talked till late into the night, reliving our personal fights, and the bond between us locked. We began referring to each other as 'sister' and 'brother'.

The next morning we arrived at the site as the sky lit up with wisps of silver and gold. The little market at the gate was already in full swing. The labourers were heaving and clanking, rushing to get the ETC completed. The new recruits arrived as we finalized the day's programme. Our responsibility to ensure they were ready for the tasks ahead lay heavily on us all. They were the future health workers of the country and, while their courage to fight Ebola was admirable, no martyrs could be afforded.

They were rotated through donning PPE and walking the ETC flow, experiencing the principles of Low to High risk. They needed to begin building their tolerance to the suits, and practice doffing them safely. The practical stations included caring for patients and providing hygiene to those with vomit and diarrhoea. Massimo and I took turns pretending to be infected, requiring movement from one area to another or nursing care. All the daily duties were practised, including the inevitable management of the deceased.

A British public health doctor, Rosamund, explained field epidemiology, following which we demonstrated triage scenarios and admissions in the ambulance area. Unfortunately the place was infested with toxic Nairobi flies, and as I pretended to be a patient, lying on the floor, weak and confused, I suffered chemical burns from the insects down my arms and back. Finally we all sat together, in one big circle, a moment of unity, to answer questions and reassure.

As the sun set, Ruth, MJ and I joined the logistical lead, Miguel, for a final walk round the ETC. The first patients were scheduled to arrive the next day. It had been built at breakneck speed, a demonstration of OCA's ability and a symbol of MSF's continuing dominance over other newer actors entering the theatre. What some had taken months to do, MSF had achieved in weeks. The urgency, though, was psychological and the rush unjustified. Other ETCs had finally opened and were admitting patients. As we walked around, we documented biohazards: unguarded nails able to tear through PPE and cut skin in the High Risk area and parts of the ETC still under construction. MJ, Ruth and I raised the question of whether we should be opening if the ETC was not yet complete.

'If we don't, people will die,' Miguel said.

His reply, simply, was not correct.

The WHO reported there were now 615 beds available, over twice the number required for all patients needing ETC admission. Locally, there were operational ETCs, with several more opening within the following week.

The bed crisis, at least, was over.

Staff safety was imperative. Despite the intensive training, most had not had more than one full dressing and undressing session. Their understanding of the Ebola case definition and procedure for admitting patients remained murky. But these facts fell on deaf ears. Those who'd overseen the building of the ETC were leaving the country the next day; wanted to see it open before going home.

'We open tomorrow because I've decided we do,' Miguel stated curtly in response to our concerns.

My blood ran cold as we left the ETC, the conversation replaying in my mind. There were celebration drinks to congratulate the team on completing the ETC, and as a farewell party for the logistical and construction teams leaving the following day. I was, however, not in a party mood. I grabbed a cool bottle of Star beer and sat among a small group, too lost in my own thoughts to engage in any conversation.

There were toasts to the accomplishments of the team; it *was* a technical triumph. A weathered MSF field worker, decades of missions behind him, stood to make a speech. Beer bottle in hand, he spoke with gravitas. His words transported me back to MTV's opening presentation: *We are the best.* They were both emphasizing that *we* have the muscles, the brains and the biggest dicks.

'Look at what we can achieve,' he continued, relaying a conversation he had had with another NGO. They had run into some technical trouble and requested assistance – it was something minor, perhaps to borrow some goggles. He recalled it with delight, guffawing, able to *prove again* the superiority of MSF.

I sipped on the Star beer in my hand. Best to keep the bottle in my mouth, I thought. I felt firmly committed to MSF, proud to stand with them, but, at times like this, I also felt conflicted. My body was exhausted, while my mind ran wild – questioning, among other things, my own righteousness. I snuck away; tomorrow was going to be another long day.

The white gravel reflected the bright morning light; without half-closing my eyes, the glare was blinding. Banging and sawing came from all around, a frenzy of shouting and stressed activity. Patients were expected from midday, yet the signs were still being put up, electric circuits finalized, and impaling nails bent or blunted.

The morning medical team were given tasks to get the unit in order and stocked. There was excitement to meet the challenge, getting everything sorted up till the last second. Every labourer needed to complete the work and be out of the High Risk area by midday, otherwise patients could not be admitted. I remained anxious.

The head of mission for OCA arrived to oversee the opening. With little over an hour till show time, she asked MJ, Ruth and I if we were ready; if not, she would ask for the opening to be delayed. We were stuck. Everyone and everything around us was geared to the midday opening. Despite my reservations, I kept quiet, as did the others – this was answer enough.

As the construction team prepared to leave, the first ambulance arrived. I coordinated from Low Risk, observing the patient flow and ensuring safe PPE procedures were practised. Our first five patients were admitted, two of which were in a critical condition. As the hygienist and healthcare workers entered High Risk to tend to the patients, I watched their every move. There was no room for error. The decontamination team were also new; with each person exiting High Risk, I was terrified the worker would put their finger into their eye or infect themselves in some other way. During that first afternoon I observed three near misses: the inability to get a hazmat suit off when overheated and tired; the temptation to grab at the gown with one's hand; the decontaminator getting the order of instructions confused. These were all high-stake errors.

As night descended, we sat in a large circle and debriefed as the shifts changed. Our responsibility to these, mostly young, healthcare workers was immense. I reminded them of the guiding principles and shared my phone number. MJ was staying the night at the ETC, but once the night team had completed their first High Risk entry I headed to bed.

Over the week, Massimo and Emily left and several new expats arrived. Barely any had previous Ebola experience, but all were motivated and realistic. Ruth became the project coordinator, stepping into the role with ease.

I got to know our Sierra Leonean colleagues, who were predominantly newly qualified nurses and community health officers. Antony, a sharp-minded CHO from the nearby town of Makeni, aspired to become an obstetrician, and we spoke at length about how he could achieve his wish after the epidemic. I found it incredible he had such vision for post-epidemic; I thought Ebola had consumed every ambition, every hope. Antony's determination was like a splash of cold water, snapping me out of my Ebola-infused grogginess. 'Can I take your details?' he asked, taking his phone out of his pocket. 'In case I want career advice later?' He reminded me of my own early career commitments. The excitement your future can hold, when you consider a future possible.

The ETC was never busy; however the days were long and tiring. The team grew competent at Ebola triage and management, and we all took pride in their achievements.

Rosamund, the public health doctor, attended daily meetings at the District Ebola Response Centre, and where possible I joined her. The meetings were often tense, with the WHO, UK military, Ministry of Health and various NGOs all vying for attention, announcing clashing agendas and venting frustrations.

My time in Sierra Leone drew to a close. I had extended the length of my mission twice since arriving in October, and had been living Ebola every day since my first shift, back in June.

As 2014 ended, Rosamund and I left Magburaka together. We met
Juli and a few other returning expats in Mile 91 and continued in convoy
to Freetown. The day we left, the country was on a government-issued
'total lockdown', stopping the movement of people during the Christmas
holidays. I watched the soldiers patrolling roadblocks as we passed
long traffic jams. The epidemic was a long way from over. Emotionally
immersed, I assumed my journey within it would not be over either.

Interlude

23: FULL CIRCLE

LONDON

DECEMBER 2014 – NOVEMBER 2015

Wandering through Heathrow Airport, I expected someone to stop me, check my temperature, ask condescending questions and advise me to self-quarantine. There was nothing and I did not seek it.

If you would prefer not to see me for a while, I'll understand. I had messaged my extended relatives on a family group chat before I left Sierra Leone. I posed no infection risk, but was aware of the media's impact on anxieties.

Hurry up and come home. You can't get out of seeing us that easily. Persecution, revolution and forced migration had not weakened the web holding my family together. Neither could an epidemic.

Adjustment is different for each person. In myself, it comes fast and slow together. My mind switches instantly. I'm here or there. In or out. It gives a false sense of security, as if nothing from one side leaks across to the other. My body moves at a different pace, insists on sleeping and pausing. If my mind is a sprinter in the hurdles, my body drags me back to ponder the slow-motion replay.

A few days after getting home, I was contacted by MSF with a request to return to Sierra Leone. Along with the opening of the UK-supported ETCs, two further operational sections of MSF were beginning Ebola case management. The Swiss had opened an ETC in Freetown, and the Spanish planned another in a closed-down school in Kissy, near Freetown.

The Spanish had been toying with a pregnancy-focused intervention for months. I thought they were working towards improving access for women with pregnancy complications. However, Ebola took central focus instead and they designed a pregnancy referral ETC.

The Spanish requested I join them for the training and development phase. I deliberated. I needed a break. My gut feeling was, if I returned, it would be for non-Ebola maternal healthcare – the mass of everyday complications needing access to life-saving treatment. I maintained an opinion that all ETCs should be capable of managing infected pregnant women, rather than transferring them to a specialist centre. I was convinced a mobile support team would leave a greater footprint for the response than this pregnancy referral ETC, and for the post-outbreak future too. The project, though, was set to go ahead with or without me. I concluded I would rather be a part of it and work from the inside to meet alternative objectives than heckle from the sidelines.

Ruth became my eyes on the outbreak, updating me on progress in Magburaka, difficult dilemmas and the final assessments by the support team before its disbandment. Our emails became a continuous thread on how to meet reproductive health needs. We strategized plans for maximizing our impact once reunited in Sierra Leone. Energized by this prospect, I agreed to return in mid-January.

The UK response was sending more volunteers out and had invited me to teach on their pre-departure training. I woke early on Sunday, 11 January, to take the train to the army barracks in Worcester where the training was planned. I sipped a long black coffee and called my mother, knowing she would be awake. Oddly, no one answered the house phone. I tried her mobile.

'I'm busy,' she said, hanging up.

It was out of character. I headed to Paddington Station, and, as I wandered down the platform, I tried to call again. This time, my father answered.

'It's your grandmother,' he said in a trembling voice. 'She was found unconscious at home.'

I stood still in front of the train doors.

'The ambulance crew got her back. It took them a long time. They're all rushing to the hospital now.'

Passengers pushed and shoved past me. A flicker of conflicting commitments flashed in my mind, but my feet had already turned. I descended back into the London Underground and onwards to my family in Manchester.

In the hospital, the white bedsheets were neatly arranged around her small body, and she was breathing through means not of her own. I had seen it all before, but, when it's family, it changes your perspective; this wasn't a patient, this was my blood. I knew these would be her final breaths.

Life and death are not discreet states of being; there is a twilight through which we each must travel. Her body, spirit and mind were trying to leave, but the wonders of medicine refused to open the door.

Sitting in my childhood bedroom, I stared out of the window, as I had done many times before. I was philosophizing. We were in the midst of a major humanitarian emergency, and I was expected on a flight to rejoin the response in days. Whole countries on their knees, a region in emergency mode and individuals desperate for assistance. What was the right thing to do? Where did I belong and where should I be?

Back in September, between my missions to Sierra Leone, I had returned to Manchester for Rosh Hashana, the Jewish New Year. The festival is marked through the gathering of family. It is the start of a period of religious reckoning. A conversation with God. A time to remember, reflect and begin meditative prayer to be inscribed in the Book of Life for the forthcoming year. I silently protested, and did not partake. In the synagogue, rather than reading the scriptures, I examined the hurdles I had jumped over, recalling images from the camps, the two young brothers and the loss. My orthodox upbringing had seeped out of me years earlier. Surrounded by men draped in prayer shawls, swaying with vigour and immersed in faith, I felt like a small boat floating impossibly still in the centre of a rough sea.

Once the service had concluded, my extended family had come together at my grandmother's home – a bungalow in the peaceful suburbs of south Manchester. The fragrant scent of cardamom and rose permeated the steam rising off the tea in my glass, each breath infusing me with nostalgia for family and my Iranian heritage.

'You've done your bit,' Uncle Youssef said to me, his moustache twitching as he looked over at my mother.

Almost twenty of us sat in a circle on soft couches in the lounge. A gold and glass table in the centre was decorated with ornate silver bowls filled with sultanas, almonds and sesame biscuits. A large painting of dancing Hassidic rabbis hung on the wall, radiating a joy for religion I had lost many years ago. My grandmother, Mommon Joon, added a cut-glass bowl filled with dried figs, nestling it among the other nibbles and gold-framed family photos.

'Let's wait and see,' I said, making direct eye contact. I convinced no one, though they didn't yet know I had already agreed to return to West Africa. The room was full of untold stories of sacrifice and struggles. A family of immigrants, we had seen generations of survival against humanity's disdain for the different. My life choices were rooted in the history of that room.

Mommon Joon sat in a chair below the joyous rabbis. She blew the steam off her tea as if kissing a baby's cheek. She pierced me with her look. Despite sharing blood, we came from distant cultures. Hers was a fertile world of grand bazaars, tradition and Middle Eastern flare. Mine felt bland. But there was another cord that connected us.

'You,' she said, pointing her finger at me. 'You took me out.'

I see my family's journey from Iran like an incomplete photo album, mental images drawn from the stories passed down. I hold them inside me like a mosaic with crucial tiles blank. The partial picture I see is through my relatives' eyes.

'We asked the gynaecologist, Mr Jones, to write a note to get her out,' said Mum, as she looked over to Mommon Joon. 'He wrote a letter saying I was destitute and the pregnancy was in danger. He wrote that I needed my mother or I would die.' Turning to me, she added, 'He wrote we would both die'.

'Really? You asked and he just did it?' I said, imagining myself in the gynaecologist's shoes.

'Benjamin –' she sipped her tea and lowered her tone – 'in those days, we had a private gynae. He had looked after me for all my pregnancies. I told him the situation. It was all over the news. We had to get them out. You were her ticket'.

That was in 1981, it had been almost twenty years since Mommon Joon had first sent my mother to the boarding school in England. By then she was married to my father, a descendant of Eastern European Jewish heritage. My mother conspired and combined efforts in a ploy to reunite her family. The tables turned, her home became a refuge for them all. Mommon Joon arrived first. I was born soon after. The remaining family in Iran continued to search for ways out, as fundamental Islamic revolutionary rule tightened around them. Judeo-Kashani, a dying language once used by the Iranian Jews in Mommon Joon's birth town of Kashan, became a secret code spoken across phone lines and telegrams, helping them to evade the Revolutionary Guard and paving the way to their nerve-racking escape.

Mommon Joon remained in hospital for days, which rolled into weeks of waiting. I stood by my family as they struggled to make peace with the slow departure of their beloved matriarch.

Inside the ICU, the climate was cool and dry, controlled like the patients around us. The quiet buzzing and beeping were comforting, as was the predictable automated breathing. This was the other side to my secret door. There had been infection control concerns when the staff discovered my recent employment. I stubbed those out; this was no time for misplaced stigmatization.

Cradling her cold, delicate hand, I spoke to her in my mind. I told her to be free and leave this world. Life has limits, her time had arrived. Closing my eyes, the images of the young men, women and children from the preceding months faced me. Theirs were not good deaths. Avoidable, and painful.

In the days after we stopped admissions to GRC, we had reflected on how we had got to where we were. Had we waited too long? Taken too many risks? I don't remember who said it, but the words rung true: *It takes more courage to stop something than to carry on.* Here, in a central Manchester hospital, surrounded by the best medicine a rich country can provide, the same phrase punctured my mind.

In late February, the winter sun shone a kaleidoscope through the stained-glass windows of the synagogue. I'm not religious, but Mommon Joon was. For the first time in years, I wore the traditional prayer shawl and strapped the dark leather of the tefillin my grandfather had bought me around my head and arm. Muttering the ancient morning prayers, a moment of meditation, I approached the ark and touched the holy scrolls within. A knowing look passed between the rabbi and me. It was for her.

Together, surrounded by love, warmth encompassed us as she let go. It was a gentle passing, at the end of a good life. I felt no guilt that we suffered nothing of those across the water. My absence, though, weighed heavily upon me.

My family navigated the mourning rituals, deeply sacred both as a structure for grief and as an honour to the deceased since time immemorial. I imagined being informed her body would not be washed, no prayers would be said and she would be cremated by strangers, rather than buried by her community. The thought alone exacerbated the angst of death and guilt of the living. An empathy for the anger and resistance in West Africa stirred in me. It was a cultural connection I had overlooked.

News from Sierra Leone continued to flow back to me. Ruth and MJ had provided training for the Spanish maternity ETC. Silje, now an Ebola survivor herself, had also returned to work in Sierra Leone again. Overall, though, teams were bored and there were lots of empty beds. According to the director of an NGO in Freetown, by the end of January 2015, the various ETC teams were fighting over who got to admit the remaining patients.

Ruth joined a team exploring the country, assessing what the next response steps should be. Naturally, she prioritized maternal and reproductive health. Unfortunately, her enthusiasm was not mirrored. The non-Ebola healthcare projects she envisaged were not happening, while the direct Ebola response was flooded with funding, donations and resources. Following discussions with Ruth, I concluded that, rather than return to Sierra Leone, I should go elsewhere, get a fresh perspective in a different humanitarian context.

For a while it seemed I would be joining a maternity hospital in South Sudan – till Brigitte, the MSF-UK human-resources officer, called to say the position had been taken. I returned to waiting. I began working day and night shifts back in North London. I should have felt at home; instead I was lost. My self-identity was in question. I was psychologically fully immersed in the humanitarian response – writing articles, speaking about the epidemic and urging a move forward to meet the population's needs. But I was in London, travelling on the same old red bus as before.

I worried that time was running through my fingers and opportunities passing me by. In despair, I wrote to Severine, the OCB adviser, savvy as always, and a few emails later an invitation to provide assistance in the Central African Republic appeared.

Charles de Gaulle airport's long glass corridors stretched ahead of me. As I waited to board the plane to Bangui, a flight to Freetown was announced on the tannoy. A wave of guilt washed over me. The outbreak was not over, and a decision to move forward with non-Ebola healthcare still had not been made. Ruth and I were in a state of frustrated urgency. We wanted to see maternal health restarted. Though our concerns were shared within MSF, getting feet back on the ground was not yet on the agenda.

The Central African Republic allowed me the physical and mental distance from Sierra Leone to reflect on the last year's events, the people left behind and the responsibilities we had not delivered on. Ruth had continued campaigning hard to restart maternity services. The Belgian MSF section, OCB, were dragging their feet. Though GRC was their project, and officially not closed but on pause, there was still no sign of it reopening. Ruth wrote to me in exasperation: *It is ironic that you and I, who thought we should close before we closed, are now the ones outraged we haven't reopened.*

Ruth returned in August 2015, with the Dutch section, OCA, to Magburaka, as the medical team leader overseeing Ebola survivor health. Her main motivation, though, was to form a proposal for starting a maternal and child health project. She was fuelled with a ferocious determination.

I would email Ruth about interesting cases I was seeing in the Central African Republic, and she would reply with stories of frustration at trying to get agreement for the maternal health project to go ahead. We both shared a guilt that we had not yet found a way to continue or restart obstetric services during the Ebola outbreak. Residual fears stoked at the height of the epidemic fed bureaucratic resistance to tackling the maternal health emergency.

I encouraged Ruth to keep pushing, even when she wrote of feeling burnt out, resentful and past her limit. We both wanted to find justice, and this could be the way. Ruth was glad for me, that I was satisfied in the Central African Republic. As my relationship with the team solidified, I considered asking to stay for longer. But I was being an unfaithful partner. I had promised Ruth, if MSF gave the green light to restart a maternal health programme in Sierra Leone, I would drop everything to join her. There was nothing that stung more deeply than those memories of GRC, and the desire to return.

The Ebola outbreak, though waning, was not over, and the public health emergency remained critical for swathes of the population. In the world outside, large international conferences were taking place, where there were discussions of the 'lessons learnt' and applause for the response. Sitting in my mud hut in the Central African bush, I read the excited and self-congratulatory reports. Time though, would be the best judge of which lessons had been learnt, forgotten, wilfully ignored or recycled for the next emergency.

Stationed near the border with the Democratic Republic of Congo, I worked with a small international team and the Ministry of Health. One afternoon in August we were called to gather in the compound. There was an extensive epidemic of measles which had spread from across the border. Pregnant women were often attending with high fevers, dry coughs and patchy rashes splashed across their skin. A vaccination campaign was being planned, but was proving logistically challenging due to transportation constraints and the endemic insecurity.

'We have another problem to consider,' said Jon, the medical team leader, a senior nurse from Senegal. He looked around the small team and then to his notebook. 'There have been some unusual cases over the border in Congo. There's a suspicion of Marburg disease. A team from MSF is going to investigate whether we need to prepare for an outbreak.'

Marburg disease, another viral haemorrhagic fever, is a close relative of Ebola. We sat in the centre of our compound discussing whether we should prepare for receiving cases.

'Is anyone here able to explain about managing haemorrhagic fever?' Jon asked, looking squarely in my direction.

I felt a buzz of adrenaline at the thought of being back in awful PPE and returning to the strange comfort zone of a haemorrhagic fever outbreak. It was a false alarm and came to nothing, but it flicked a switch inside me.

I left the Central African Republic before the start of September 2015. I'd learnt a huge amount from my time embedded in a country with deep divisions and political turmoil. Ruth had been right to push me to seek a different humanitarian mission.

It was not till early November that OCA gave the green light to go ahead with forming a 'post-Ebola' maternal and child health project, to be based in Magburaka, not far from (the now decommissioned) Tonkolili ETC. The inertia had been exasperating. Ruth had threatened to resign, and I had considered returning to the Central African Republic. However, once we knew MSF was with us, we knew we would have the resources to implement a project we had been discussing for months.

On 7 November 2015, Sierra Leone was declared free of Ebola by the WHO. I met Gillian, one of the Goal team nurses in Covent Garden, London. 'What should we drink to?' she asked, raising her cocktail.

'Remembering,' I said as we toasted our glasses.

In the eighteen months since that fateful miscarriage in Kenema Government Hospital, a further 8,704 cases had been confirmed, including 3,956 deaths, of which 221 were healthcare workers. The true numbers, though, were unanimously agreed to be exponentially larger.

The World Bank reported the toll from those who died in the line of duty would continue to severely impact the delivery of healthcare in all three of the most affected countries. Sierra Leone's maternal mortality was predicted to rise by a further 74 per cent from its pre-Ebola levels. An unacceptable public health crisis continued to loom, and it was not Ebola. This emergency sat in my mind as I prepared for my flight back to Freetown.

Part 3

24: A NEW BEGINNING

I ascended out of Bond Street underground station into the bustle of Oxford Street and pulled my beanie on to my head as I pushed my way through the tourists and office workers on their lunchbreaks. I was already late for the meeting. A researcher had been asking to interview me for months; if I didn't sit with her now, I never would.

I rushed into the Royal Society of Medicine, looking scruffy in my usual jeans and hoodie, stepping out of the London commotion and into the hushed, reserved world of suits and stern looks. Jill was waiting for me in the coffee lounge, a room of deep leather sofas that looked much more comfortable than I could ever be. She was tall and slim, and held the perfect posture of a professional dancer.

'Thanks for coming,' she said, positioning herself opposite me with a notebook and pen in hand. 'I want to ask about your experience of being in the outbreak and returning home.'

Jill asked about stigmatization I had encountered on returning and the overall emotional journey. The questions were standard, nothing unexpected. Though I had spoken about it all before, knowing I was returning to Sierra Leone gave my answers an unintended rough edge. There was a bitterness haunting me – resentment at missed opportunities and indifference remained closer to the surface than I had realized.

I had not let go of the residual shame that I felt for abandoning the team at Kailahun, the mixed anger and guilt I nurtured from the closure of GRC and for our collective failure to respond to the reproductive health needs that were left dangling. I felt we'd left so many women, men and children teetering on the edge.

'The UK government's been honouring Ebola responders with a special medal. Have you received yours?' Jill asked, placing her coffee cup down.

A moment passed as I lost myself in a rush of thoughts. I felt tiny in the leather sofa – an insignificant being thrown into the air, trying to reach out to anything so I could keep grounded. I allowed the bubbles of emotion to rise and leave. I exhaled. I had not taken any awards, the job was not over. I fought to hold back tears, as the months of underlying frustration pushed them painfully through.

'Looking back at everything, can you give me one word to describe how you feel?' Jill asked, prompting me for an answer.

'Ashamed.'

*

FREETOWN/MAGBURAKA, SIERRA LEONE

NOVEMBER 2015

The aeroplane juddered as it passed through the heavy storm clouds gathering like the furrowed eyebrows of a teenager over Lunghi. Humidity swept into the cabin as the doors opened and the tired human cargo unloaded. I breathed it in – an awakening, an arrival.

Waiting outside the terminal were pot-bellied men in dirty lab coats, with unnecessary stethoscopes hanging around their necks. They were checking each traveller: temperature, travel, contact with the bleeding, dying, bats or Ebola? The palpitations I had forgotten returned as the infrared thermometer pointed like a gun to my forehead and a number was shouted out at me.

I moved through immigration, officials leafing their way through my dog-eared passport and touts trying to sell me tickets into Freetown. Everything was familiar and comforting. Night had descended upon us by the time I got to the port. I looked out across the choppy sea, listening to the water crashing in on itself. I considered what the next few months might hold. An Australian man in his thirties stood next to me, having a smoke before the ferry arrived. He had been working in West Africa for several years, and was posted in Bo when the outbreak began. His company had evacuated him. This was his return journey, too.

The rain had begun to fall from the lofty clouds, and soon the full force of a West African storm rushed down. I recalled how I had imagined, and hoped, these downpours would wash the Ebola away. Now, in this new age of 'post-Ebola', perhaps the rain would wash away the memories and misery, revitalizing the land.

Through the rain, I struggled with my bags and the steep walk up from the jetty. I squinted to try to make out an MSF sign among the various NGO logos in the arrivals area. The flight had been delayed by several hours, and, though I had sent an email from the plane, I wasn't sure if the message had been received. I pushed my way through the congregating relatives, colleagues and drivers that were huddled under a shelter, and found the familiar red logo waving around on the end of a stick at the back.

'Doctor Benjamin?' asked the man holding the sign.

I was back.

It was after midnight by the time we pulled into the house. The rain continued to fall in a heavy torrent, the noise of it battering the tin roofs. A guard came running out in his trench coat and boots to let me in, but first the rigmarole of hand-washing and foot-spraying needed to be observed. He handed me an envelope with instructions, mobile phone and the key to my room. The house had a balcony on the top floor, overlooking the bay, and I sat there on a plastic chair, watching the storm flood the little streets and pound the sea. I pulled a cheese baguette I'd bought in the airport from my bag – stale, but edible enough – and washed down a malaria tablet with a Star beer I'd found in the fridge. Anticipation of the future built up within me as I allowed my mind to run as freely as the water below.

I'd arrived in Sierra Leone a couple of days earlier than planned, to join a multi-agency meeting on restarting sexual and reproductive health projects post-Ebola. My invitation was as a representative of the Royal College of Obstetricians and Gynaecologists, I attended with the medical coordinator for MSF in Sierra Leone. The meeting was made up of representatives from Voluntary Services Overseas, the Sierra Leone Ministry of Health and Sanitation and local NGOs, as well as religious leaders and independent consultants. There had already been several days of discussion and this was the finale, presenting their conclusions. Everyone gathered around a large circle of tables to share their critical reflections. The concerns for women were well founded. The WHO had released a report that morning confirming Sierra Leone as the country with both the highest maternal mortality rate and now also the highest lifetime risk of maternal death – an unenviable crown awarded to Chad and Somalia in the previous report of 2013. Unsurprisingly, not only was Sierra Leone considered the most precarious country to be a pregnant woman, it was worse now than it had been two years earlier.

The presentations were a mix of high hopes and dream chasers. There were plans to do everything: to get all the adolescent girls back into school, lobby for legalization and liberalization of abortion access, provide universal family planning and send teams around the country to fix the broken, remote health centres scattering the hills. It was all impressive and desperately needed, but the actual plans to make these monumental changes happen seemed absent. Yes, there needed to be better roads around the country and electricity into health centres – these were fundamental truths. Realizing them would be another issue altogether.

We discussed the many resources poured into the country as part of the Ebola response. Could the remaining donations and investments be utilized for improving the general health service? Hundreds of ambulances had been imported to assist with the safe transfer of the Ebola sick and dead; these would, apparently, be recommissioned as a paramedical service. If successful and strategically placed, this would mean a major reduction in the time it took patients to reach and receive emergency care.

A novice to these meetings, I preferred to listen and absorb rather than speak. The chairman of the meeting had other ideas. He watched me avoid his eyes, but this was not to be a free lunch.

'Benjamin,' he said, drawing the attention of the room towards me, 'as a representative of the Royal College, we would be pleased to hear your critical feedback'.

What could I say?

I suggested taking a more focused approach, rather than trying to do everything together. I reiterated what had been said on abortion care and contraceptive access, hoping this would spur other members into action, and I cautiously dropped the C-word. The country had an atrocious record of corruption. Just as some people had gained a profit during the emergency, there would be some who stood to benefit from its aftermath.

One third of Ebola funds remained unaccounted for, and, despite hazard pay being promised to front-line workers, it was suspected that lists of non-existent employees and duplications had been used to syphon off and divert money for personal gains.

Later in the day I met Sarah, the head of mission for MSF in Sierra Leone. She had been sitting in her office all afternoon, staring at her laptop. My briefings seemed like a welcome break for her. Sarah had worked for years in the Congo – Sierra Leone was a 'low security' context for her – and, having just completed a political degree in London, was ready to dive back into fieldwork. We sat out on the veranda of the office and she lit a cigarette. Overlooking the dramatic Freetown coastline, we chatted about the outbreak and the difficulties the team had faced in pushing to get the go-ahead to begin the maternity intervention from headquarters. Seagulls swooped down low, scouring for food between the small boats in the bay, a picture of tranquillity.

'Don't dwell on the struggles faced in getting this started,' Sarah said in her deep, smoke-rusted voice, as she blew smoke across the scene below. 'It's water under the bridge and the team needs to move forward. Focus on getting the project started.'

Her message was the same as had been relayed to me by colleagues in the Amsterdam office. I heard her loud and clear.

'A group of us are heading to Lumley Beach tonight. You going to join us?' she asked. With the outbreak declared over and social distancing restrictions lifted, the bars and restaurants were filling up again. It was Friday evening and the scene was open for business.

I had never experienced a night out in Freetown. I had never experienced a Sierra Leone where people could freely touch one another. Ruth was already stationed upcountry in Magburaka, where the new maternal and child health project would soon begin. She had been back in Sierra Leone for three months, pushing and fighting to get the project started. Her battle was the 'water under the bridge', where passions had turned bitter and exhaustion had taken the pride out of the win.

As I waited for the Land Cruiser to arrive, I called her phone, surprised at how nervous it made me. We had not seen one another in ten months, our relationship maintained through emails. I felt a sudden rush of uncertainty – what if we didn't get along? What if it all went wrong?

'Hey, brother.'

All those fears wilted away and I immediately wished I was already upcountry.

'We're just having a meeting,' she said. 'Can't talk now.' Then, to those she was with: 'Hey, ya'll, we have an obstetrician! This is happening, people!'.

I could hear voices in the background from the people at the meeting. 'See you in Magburaka!' I said.

I struggled to picture the scene at the other end of the phone line. There was a small international team in Magburaka. Their only clinical activity was providing healthcare for Ebola survivors. Recently, they had begun liaising with the governmental hospital to help put in place the correct infection prevention and control procedures. Although the outbreak had ended, marking forty-two days from the last recorded case of Ebola, the country was to continue ninety days of 'enhanced surveillance'. Liberia had also been declared free of Ebola; however, the Guinea situation remained active, and the porous borders exposed neighbouring countries to potential new, imported, cases.

I found it difficult to believe all corners of the country had been fully investigated, suspicious that, somewhere deep in the bush, remote villages with populations that had no reason to trust the outside world could be harbouring bastions of infection. There was political pressure to have the outbreak finished. Without any evidence, we pondered if undocumented chains of transmission could be passing below the radar of surveillance. If the meticulous attention required had been paid. Whether the victory of passing the arbitrary line that defines when an epidemic ends, might have been declared prematurely. With great animation, these conspiracy theories were beaten out over an evening beer in Freetown.

A couple of days later, I made my journey back to Magburaka. There was a tropical atmosphere I'd not appreciated previously, as if everything before this moment had been inscribed in my memory in grey. I stared at the long palm trees and the broad banana leaves bending over the road. The breeze carried the faint smell of gasoline – not overpowering, but present, like perfume when it's done right. Along the way, my mind flitted between Ebola and maternal healthcare. I had been obsessing for months over how safe maternity care would work in the context of low-level transmission or a fresh outbreak. I kept looking for lessons from the past eighteen months, hoping to identify the errors.

The Land Cruiser pulled up into the office of Magburaka Base. The last time I had been here it had been an empty shell, purchased in the days before I had left the country for administrative use of the ETC. I walked around now to find it buzzing and set up for action. Every corner I turned, someone did a double take: 'Dr Benjamin?'.

Ruth was out running errands and there was nothing pressing for me to do.

'We're going over to the government hospital – want to join us?' asked Otas, a German WatSan I had worked with before in the Bandajuma ETC. There had been long talks over how, once approved, MSF would reshape the maternity and child services in the existing hospital, improving infrastructure for healthcare with an emphasis on infection control, in preparation for further outbreaks.

'Patients will enter here and staff flow will be one-way, like this,' explained Otas, moving his arms to demonstrate the precise details. 'This area is for washing and here is for removing PPE.' He turned to a large space behind us, 'All of this can be turned into isolation'.

It was a thoughtful design, but all I heard was *Ebola*, rather than *maternal health*.

He was right to be cautious. High standards had to be maintained. But restructuring hospital departments to represent an ETC seemed disproportionately Ebola-centric. I felt disheartened. We were prioritizing Ebola over the practicalities of maternal and child health. We needed to find an equilibrium.

I kept these thoughts to myself, calculating how to shift the focus of the project towards general health activities. Ebola preparedness needed to be a foundation under us, not front and centre.

In the evening, the international team sat together in a large round hut, another tukul, a warm breeze blowing through as we ate bowls of thick groundnut soup. We all lived together in this compound, about a ten-minute walk from the government hospital, where we would all soon be working together too. Allan and Dennis had returned from Uganda to work in the project. I hadn't seen either of them since we were in Kailahun, over a year earlier. Their work focused on the Ebola survivor health aspects of the project, though this was declining and the future of their clinic looked uncertain. Sam, a Welsh public health doctor, had also joined us. He spoke with lyrical intonation and had a refreshingly positive outlook on pretty much everything. In the UK, there was rising discontent among junior doctors about their working hours and pay. Sam and I would switch between talking about the medical drama back home and the challenges in front of us in Sierra Leone. A conversation with Sam, though, no matter how serious, always resulted in smiles and laughter.

The sun did not rise till around 7 a.m., so it was dark when I got up at 5.30 a.m., creeping out of my room to percolate strong black coffee as the cool harmattan breeze blew in from the Sahara Desert. I inhaled the morning air, wrapped up in my hoodie as I meditated on the possible ways forward. The only light was the glow of Ruth's computer; she would rise before me, checking through emails, orders and lists. This became our daily moment, just the three of us – Ruth, me and our shared hopes.

Ruth and I began strategizing our vision for a maternal health service in the post-Ebola era. Months of talking without action had turned into urgency; we'd been like sports cars, revving our engines at the red light, and now we were flooring it, wanting to make up for lost time. We agreed we should assume we were working in a haemorrhagic fever 'low transmission' setting, rather than interpreting the WHO declaration as 'no transmission'. We needed to develop a way to meet our objectives and work safely within this new unknown context.

An agreement had not yet been signed between MSF and the Ministry of Health, and we would not have permission to provide clinical care in the government facilities until it was.

'So, we'll be in the hospital waiting for the paperwork to happen, but not intervening?' I asked Ruth, as we took our morning walk to the office. 'Even if we're standing right there?'

'Officially, no.'

An okada motorbike driver slowed down, beeping his horn for business as he passed us.

'But, I don't think we can engage like that,' Ruth continued. 'There's an ethical consideration. Like you say, we'll be right there.'

Smoke rose from the small fires of rubbish lit in the early morning at the roadside, tiny wafers of black ash floating down like macabre snowfall. Ruth shouted a greeting in Krio to a passer-by: '*Aw di mornin'?*'.

As we walked on, she said, 'The hospital isn't clean. There are needles discarded around the grounds and they reuse equipment which should be one-time use only. I worry about it.'

The solution, we decided, was to create 'grab bags' containing emergency protective equipment and essential supplies which we could use if present for an emergency.

'Our primary goal is to support the existing healthcare system. Work with the health teams to effect a positive outcome,' I said, as we arrived at the office. 'If we had our own supplies, we could take that support further, as and if necessary.'

Sam had been in Magburaka for several months, providing epidemiological and public health surveillance support to the District Health Management Teams. He attended weekly meetings, engaging in high-level discussions with public health officers. His natural charisma forged strong and mutually respected bonds between him and the Sierra Leonean officials. He was working to create an interactive map for infectious disease surveillance, alongside supporting vaccination programmes and preparedness for future disease outbreaks.

During the epidemic, there had been daily coordination meetings at District Ebola Response Centres. These were now weekly, bringing together the different hospitals, NGOs and health actors in the district to discuss case management of infectious diseases and surveillance strategies. I began attending these meetings with Sam; they were excellent opportunity to engage with the different actors in the region, to understand the challenges they were trying to overcome and brainstorm together on how to move forward. The emphasis remained on infectious disease surveillance, in particular how to make use of mobile phone technology to receive data from across the district, tracking illness clusters, patterns and developments. As we discussed the best ways to enhance the surveillance, we also advocated that maternal outcomes could be included. Politically, though, maternal deaths were contentious.

Home births, though widely practised, were illegal. The policy, which predated the Ebola epidemic, was an effort to reduce maternal deaths. The woman and her birth attendant risked penalty fines if delivery was attempted outside a healthcare facility. Though well meaning, the ruling acted as a disincentive for women, or their birth attendants, to seek assistance if there were complications. When a maternal death was reported, it triggered an investigation. These were often exercises in blame and reprimand, and were not necessarily welcomed by under-resourced and overworked peripheral health facility staff. These systems deterred women from attending and healthcare workers from reporting.

I had a mountain of tasks ahead of me. I felt impatient, wanting everything to happen immediately. I couldn't shake the idea that we were in the midst of another emergency. While many had taken a step back to unwind post-Ebola, I was obsessing over the maternal health situation. Disasters were happening around us, but out of sight. If you didn't look for it, you didn't see it, and if you didn't see it, then there was no emergency.

25: BOMB SCARE

'Bottom on the bed, please,' I said, as I laced the suture through the apex of the episiotomy. Blood dripped into a metal bowl between Stella's legs – slow, like the second hand of a clock, like her baby's heartbeat before birth.

She strained to twist her body round, to look at her son being rubbed and poked by the paediatrician.

'There'll be a little redness on his face from the forceps,' I told her and the man next to her. The colour in *his* face was only just beginning to return after the drama of birth.

All morning, I had been distracted, my mind returning to the email Ruth had sent. The emergency alarm had pulled me back to the labour ward, though.

'What's the story,' I'd asked the midwife as I entered the room.

'This is Stella. She's being induced for diabetes of pregnancy. She's been progressing and coping really well.'

I could see the printed fetal heart trace next to Stella; there had been a few dips, but now there was a profound change and it was staying slow. I heard the thump of the baby's heart on the monitor. *Thud.* Seconds of silence. Too long. We waited, looking at the monitor, as if looking would save the baby. *Thud.*

'We started pushing thirty minutes ago,' the midwife continued, as I washed my hands and asked for the emergency trolley. 'She's been doing really well – haven't you, Stella? – but the baby has been getting tired.'

I looked again at the printed heart tracing. *This baby needs to get out,* I thought. *Thud.*

'Stella, I'm just going to examine you, OK? Your baby is telling us he needs to be born. We're going to get him out together. OK?' I looked at Stella and the man next to her, who I assumed to be her partner.

'Is he ...? What happened? I don't understand.' Stella watched my face for a sign, looking at the midwife to throw her a raft.

'It's going to be fine,' she said, but the silence between each heartbeat was louder than anything else in the room.

The baby's head was not quite as low down as I had hoped. I let my fingers communicate between the baby, the pelvis and me. The space between each thud was getting longer.

'Stella, we need to deliver the baby. I'm going to use the forceps – the metal spoons we use to cradle the baby and lift him out. You'll still need to push. We'll do it together. OK?'

Stella agreed. What sort of agreement it was when faced with a non-choice was hard to ascertain.

The printout of the baby's heart trace was looking terminal – a wobbly downward line.

'Let's crash-call the paediatric team,' I said to the midwife as I picked up the first branch of the forceps.

'Don't push or anything for a moment,' I said to Stella, 'just breathe'. I felt the cold metal slip under my hand and around the baby's head. It was a precise movement, satisfyingly smooth.

I glanced at the monitor – it was flashing a red alarm.

'Stella, when the contraction comes, I want you to push right down.'

The midwife placed a hand on Stella's abdomen. The man, who was looking paler than before, leant in and kissed Stella on the forehead.

'Yes, I think we have one,' said the midwife. 'Stella, take a big breath and push!'

I clenched my hands and applied traction.

'Harder, Stella – you can push harder!' I shouted, as I felt the forceps moving outwards.

Stella's face had turned a deep red.

'I can't do it!' she shouted back.

'Yes, you can!' we all chanted back at her.

'You have to,' I said.

'OK,' said the midwife, 'here comes another one'.

'That's it, Stella,' I said, as I felt the change in direction of my pull. 'Don't let go. Keep doing exactly what you're doing.'

Her labia blanched as the head stretched them. I felt the tight resistance.

'Stella, I'm going to make a small cut, OK?' I said, as I released the bands of tissue with an episiotomy.

The forceps were almost out, the baby's black hair could be seen between the blades.

'Pant, Stella, pant!' said the midwife, as I eased the wide curve of the blade out. 'The next push and your baby will be delivered.'

As Stella prepared for the final push, I noticed the baby's chubby cheeks retract back inside her. I looked to the midwife and, in my calmest voice, said, 'Let's get her legs back'.

The midwife knew what I was really saying was, *This is a big baby and I'm worried about the shoulders.*

Stella filled her lungs and pushed down. Nothing moved. *At least the paediatricians are here,* I thought.

'Pull the alarm bell,' I said, feeling with my fingertip around the baby's head. 'Stella, the baby's shoulder is stuck; more people are going to come in to help.'

I tried to hold a poker face, attempting a smile to hide my fear. As a team we rehearsed this often, running through the drill.

I could see the baby's cheeks becoming blue and dusky in my hands. This baby needed oxygen, now.

'Everyone stop!' I shouted, then lowered my tone. 'Stella, stop pushing.'

I gathered my fingers together like the beak of a bird and entered the space between the head and vagina. *Fuck, it's tight,* I thought to myself, as I advanced, trying to find the baby's arm.

'Don't push, just breathe.'

I reached further inside, the tips of my fingers wriggling to grasp the hand, or hook an elbow. I could feel every eye in the room on me. Even the heart monitor was watching me. All of us were holding our breath – like the baby.

'Got it,' I whispered to myself. 'Don't do anything,' I said, as I carefully brought the hand forward. His arms extended out beyond his head, like a superhero preparing for flight. 'OK,' I said, as I rearranged my hands around the baby. 'Now, push!'

Everyone started shouting encouragement and Stella's cheeks puffed out hard as the baby's shoulder dropped, his body revolved and he delivered.

'Clamps and scissors!' I shouted, looking at his startled expression.

Now, Stella's baby was resting on her chest, searching for a nipple. 'How many stitches is it?' she asked.

'Just one,' I said. 'Like a shoelace running from one end to the other.'

I stepped out of the room, taking Stella's notes with me to the office opposite, where I would write down all the events of the birth. But I was still thinking about Salome Karwah and her family. I put the notes to one side and turned the computer on instead. Although I'd never met Salome, I couldn't get the picture of her face out of my mind. She was staring from the front cover of *Time* magazine, wearing an expression which said so little, and so much. I wondered if, in 2014, when the photo for 'Person of the Year' was taken, when she stood to represent the fallen, the survived and the fighting, she could have known that Ebola would be the death of her, three years later.

Ebola bombs, read Ruth's email to me. *The stigma lives on.*

Salome's death had just been reported, apparently caused by the complications of childbirth. Her mother, father, brothers and extended family had all succumbed to Ebola as it ravaged through Liberia. Salome too had been infected, but, alongside her sister and fiancé, had survived and then worked assisting others in the MSF ETC outside Monrovia.

Over two years after her survival, she gave birth to her fourth child in hospital. Shortly after going home she collapsed, having a seizure. The health workers refused to assist as she lay unconscious in the hospital car park. 'They did not want contact with her fluids,' said her sister. 'My heart is breaking.'

I imagined the scene. I imagined being one of those maternity staff. I wondered what rumours they had been told about Ebola survivors. What guidelines they could have read about pregnant women. I read the article again. All the adrenaline from Stella's delivery had dissipated. My heart beat, like her son's, had a weight upon it. I looked at Salome's photo. 'What a waste,' I said to the empty office, as I picked up my pen.

*

WEST AFRICA

NOVEMBER 2015

Jenny, the former GRC hospital manager, was now in Guinea, working with MSF in their last active ETC. It was her first time returning to an Ebola project since leaving Sierra Leone a year earlier. The context and global attitude towards Ebola had changed in that time. Now, international teams were trialling experimental drugs, using the antibody-rich plasma of survivors and vaccinations. A massive response had, although late to arrive, reversed the outlook and there was hope we were in the final days of the entire West African outbreak.

Severine and I had discussed our anger and frustrations that these experimental drugs and vaccines were being withheld from pregnant women. The ethics of giving a drug to pregnant women seemed clear: if the effect it will have on the pregnancy is in doubt, avoid it. But, the balance of possible benefit versus potential harm required measured objectivity.

With no known surviving baby born to an infected pregnant woman in any outbreak ever, and given the high mortality rate for pregnant women, it made no logical or moral sense to withhold access to potentially life-saving interventions. These were exceptional circumstances, yet, when it came to pregnant women, it was business as usual – and, ultimately, the denial of a fair chance at life.

Late in October, in the Forécariah province, Guinea, near to where Jenny was working, a woman who was seven months pregnant was confirmed to have Ebola. The woman was a known contact of a man who had recently died from the disease, and, while there was now a vaccine available, she was denied it. The vaccination was still considered to be experimental; however, early evidence had shown high effectiveness in protecting contacts of the infected. Ring vaccinations were being rolled out, creating a buffer between those infected, the exposed and the rest, with the intention of eliminating onward transmission of the virus.

Had she been included in the vaccinations, she might have been spared.

Once admitted into the MSF ETC, there was an effort to get her access to ZMapp. Guinea was partaking in a trial where patients could be randomly allocated to either receive or not receive ZMapp. Given the small trickle of Ebola patients and the fifty-fifty odds of receiving a potentially life-saving treatment, MSF declined to randomize patients on ethical grounds. Mortality rates without ZMapp were well documented; why flip a coin on the remaining patients' lives? MSF argued that she was one of the final patients of the outbreak and her pregnancy should have been considered an extenuating circumstance, but the plea was snubbed and access denied, unless randomization was accepted.

The woman did receive an experimental antiviral, favipiravir, which the WHO and the drug company had agreed for use in pregnant women. Several days after admission to the ETC, the woman went into spontaneous labour and delivered a live baby girl. But the woman then began bleeding. She bled till she died.

The newborn girl tested positive for Ebola. She was the last patient in the ETC and potentially the final case of the West African epidemic. Unlike her mother, the baby was granted access to ZMapp outside of trial conditions, having the first dose administered at one day old. She also received GS5734 (another experimental antiviral) and the white blood cells of an Ebola survivor. She was cared for by the whole ETC staff, and received specialized paediatric care from Jenny. She was named Nubia by her father, after one of the nurses.

Nubia went on to survive, a shining light and symbol of hope to us all. Her survival was unique for many reasons, but it also raised questions about our earlier assumptions. Nubia thrived as a young child, but she was also motherless. The lessons of her success were accompanied by the memory of our failures to her mother.

I corresponded with Jenny for updates on Nubia. I also asked if she had any contact details of our local colleagues from GRC, many of whom remained unemployed since the hospital's closure. Jenny didn't have any staff contact details herself, but she knew of someone who might. That person had the phone number of just one previous employee, but, when I made contact with him, I discovered he had contact details for everyone. The rumour mill, which had been so obstructive in the outbreak, now played right into our hands; soon, everyone knew MSF was back and planning to reopen a maternal and child health programme.

In those first days, we threw many balls in the air at once: connecting with local authorities, debating and writing procedures for future suspected or confirmed cases of Ebola, and developing a complete overview for the project. Ruth and I agreed, we wanted to think far beyond the hospital and out into the rural hills of Tonkolili District. In 2013, maternal deaths were reported to account for 36 per cent of all deaths in women aged between fifteen and forty-nine. According to official predictions, it was higher now. Much of this was out of sight from the cities, hidden in the mud huts and far-flung health posts in the countryside.

Each morning, the healthcare workers at Magburaka Government Hospital held a meeting to discuss cases from the previous shifts. I began attending the meetings and spent increasing amounts of time in the hospital, observing how the unit functioned, forging relationships and discussing how MSF would slot in with the existing Ministry of Health structures.

I sat in the small room. It was approaching 8 a.m. and the sun was up, a ceiling fan dangled above, frustratingly static. A handsome, muscular man in his twenties strode into the room.

'Good morning,' I said, standing to greet him.

'Morning, I'm Amara,' he said, putting his hand out to me, 'I'm a Surgically Trained Clinical Health Officer, I cover maternity with the doctor.' He flashed a broad smile and gave a firm handshake.

Gradually various paediatric nurses, midwives and health assistants of different cadres joined us. A tall and lanky doctor fell into the chair next to Amara. He covered his mouth as he gave a slow yawn. His eyelids hung heavily over his large brown eyes. Dr Kamara had been up most of the night, in and out of the operating theatre, performing caesarean sections.

The night midwife began summarizing the activity of the last twenty-four hours in a monotonous voice. The wards remained significantly underfilled. Healthcare centres and hospitals had been associated with the spread of Ebola and trust was slow to re-emerge. However, of the cases referred in from health centres, there seemed to be a high rate of caesarean deliveries. As the midwife moved on to the case of an eighteen-year-old woman, Dr Kamara's eyes opened.

'She arrived septic and in a bad condition,' he interrupted, his long fingers moving as if to dismiss the memory of her presentation. 'The labour had been happening for days. It was obstructed. The baby's head was visible from outside, but not coming. Her contractions had ceased and her bladder was distended. She had signs of a severe infection. The fetal heart

rate was rapid, alarmingly high.' He looked around the room, meeting the
gaze of his colleagues, then dipped his chin down and gave a small shake
of his head. 'I took her to the theatre.' Dr Kamara looked over to me. 'The
caesarean was very difficult. The uterus tore down to the cervix. Blood
was pouring from the arteries.' He spoke as if watching the surgery being
replayed. 'I struggled. The uterus was badly infected. It just kept tearing
through. It took me time to finish.' He paused to catch his breath. 'The
baby died minutes after delivery. The girl was bleeding a lot. She needs
blood, but we cannot find any.' Dr Kamara lowered his hands into his lap.

From around the room came many tuts, many heads shaking. 'She
came too late. Why do they come so late?' the nurses and midwives asked
each other.

Sam and I were planning an exploratory trip out into the more rural
areas of Tonkolili District the next morning. Sam wanted to gather GPS
coordinates for the map and collect information on possible disease outbreaks. I was piggybacking on his journey to survey how well equipped
the peripheral health units were to manage obstetric emergencies. We
would be visiting the health post the woman of Dr Kamara's night shift
had been sent from. I scribbled down her details, hoping to retrace her
journey and understand the pre-hospital events.

Like many women, she had begun her labour at home. Though pro-
hibited, home births accounted for roughly 50 per cent of all births. She
lived in an agricultural village, and her mother had given her 'native herbs'
to induce the labour. The contractions began, but, despite their force, she
did not give birth. The young woman walked several miles to the nearest
health post. At the peripheral health unit (PHU), she was assessed and
found to be in early labour still. Over the course of that day and night,
she progressed slowly through the labour. When she was ready to birth
her child, the contractions stopped. The health worker checked her and
found she had a full bladder, which can prevent the baby's head from
passing through the birth canal. She wanted to help the woman to pass
urine, but the simple equipment she needed had run out and not been
replaced. The health worker knew an ambulance would take too long
to get down the thin mud roads. She put the woman on the back of a
motorbike and sent her to another, larger, health centre.

The woman arrived just before sunrise. The baby's head was very low and could be seen. The midwife in the centre had had training on how to assist birth using a vacuum extractor, and the centre had a working machine, but she had never used it on a real patient and there was no one to supervise her.

On examination, she found the bladder to be distended and tense. The clinic had one urine catheter; it was supposed to be single-use only, but had already been repeatedly used as it was all they had. The baby's head was too low and was compressing the entry point for the catheter. Unable to pass the soft rubber tube, she called an ambulance and began antibiotics. Then they waited. And waited.

Her condition was deteriorating. The baby's head was at the exit to the world, and the mother's bladder was full. Eleven hours later, the ambulance arrived. It took another three to four hours to transport the patient down the potholed road to the main hospital.

She arrived at Magburaka Government Hospital in the evening, and a new story began with Dr Kamara.

And what was left for this eighteen-year-old patient? Possibly an obstetric fistula, like the other teenage girl on her ward who had been disowned by her family. And a scar on her uterus, leaving her at risk of other life-threatening complications in her future pregnancies, such as uterine rupture.

At every step of her journey, a simple intervention would have changed her (and her child's) personal history: access to safe delivery at the village; equipment and training in the various health units; ability to get to a place of safety in a timely manner; the knowledge and skills to avoid unnecessary and high-risk caesarean sections, and prevent obstetric fistula formation.

In one way, her story encouraged us. There had been highly motivated healthcare workers at every step. But the barriers to a safe birth made pregnancy a potentially critical condition. It illustrated that, to achieve genuine improvement, we needed to make changes along the whole journey. Not merely fixing the mess that arrived at the hospital, but tackling the backstory too. Not replacing, but supporting our colleagues to provide the care which any woman and her unborn child, anywhere in the world, deserve.

Sam and I spent three days driving around the Yoni Chiefdom visiting peripheral health units – usually single-storey buildings tucked off a road, varying in size and capability. Accessing some of them required driving for hours along mud roads, through dark green forests and over tumbling rivers and streams. We passed through small villages where women walked with carefully balanced fruit and vegetables atop their heads. These were our patients, the places they came from and the journeys they made. We would walk into the villages to find the local chairman or chief. Usually, he would be sitting with a small group of villagers, and we would request a short discussion about life after Ebola and their main concerns for maternal and child healthcare. Listening shaped an image of village life of which I had been embarrassingly unaware.

The healthcare workers spoke with passion about their work. They shared their stories of loss from the outbreak and their hopes for a better future. In each unit, we took a short tour, seeing the allocated area for childbirth and the equipment for a safe delivery. The more of these we saw, the more I understood why a woman might choose to stay at home.

What incentive was there to walk for several miles, pausing with each gut-wrenching contraction, to reach a dirty mattress on the floor, or a broken lithotomy bed?* One room had a hole in the ceiling above the delivery bed; water dripped down, mixed with the faeces of the bats which flew in and out. We could hear them squealing at one another, fighting for space in the rafters.

The PHU health workers often stayed in these small health posts. 'Look at how we live,' they would say, pointing to the disrepair as goats wandered in through open doors depositing their droppings on the clinic floor.

Although there is a 'free healthcare' policy for pregnant women and a list of essential items that should be available, the healthcare workers repeatedly told stories of long shipping delays. Often, there was nothing left, long before the next delivery arrived.

Every clinic we visited had posters stuck to their walls declaring the warning signs of Ebola. Behind doors we found unopened stockpiles of PPE, but in the clinical areas used needles lay on the table and latex gloves appeared to be washed for reuse. At one facility, there were rat droppings scattered across the porcelain scales used for weighing the newborns.

---

* A lithotomy bed is a bed with stirrups.

Despite all the events of the last eighteen months, all the training and health promotion, it felt like the switch that had been turned on for Ebola had been flicked back off. From the healthcare workers I got the distinct feeling of exhaustion and trauma. Ebola had been declared '*don don*'. It was over, consigned to history. Life and people were moving on. This also meant trying to forget that difficult time and all its associations, including the enhanced infection control.

The health workers told stories of challenging cases they had faced, but the most common grievance was the waiting time for assistance. Ambulances could take all day to arrive, while patients were bleeding or having seizures. There were sobering stories of women dying and health workers not understanding why. We discussed these cases together to see if a cause could be identified.

Rugiatu shared one such tale. Rugiatu's face was wrinkled with years of experience. She had a thoughtful, effective manner about her. I had the feeling she had seen it all and was unshockable, like the older, wiser consultants on the labour wards back in London. She complained of how she struggled to convince villagers of the benefits of using the health centre, rather than the traditional healers and their herbs.

'You come and hold a village meeting,' she said to us. 'They will listen to you, we can make it together.'

The table in front of us had discarded needles and empty glass medicine vials snapped open and spread over it. I resisted pointing out the hazard they posed, looked away and focused on the story she was telling.

'This fifteen-year-old girl last week, she had been at home in the village with the traditional birth attendant. I tell them to come here, but they won't listen; they say it is too far to come. The labour was long, and she had seizures and became unconscious. They called the traditional healer. He said there were demons inside the girl and he would call them out. The exorcism was long and the seizures did not stop.' Rugiatu adjusted herself on the wooden stool, her lappa skirt pulled tight between her knees. 'They waited a day before bringing her here. The village men brought her through the forests and fields, carried her all the way. I diagnosed eclampsia immediately.' Rugiatu patted her knees. 'I have seen it many times before in these young ones.'

With only candles for light, she treated the girl, inserting an intravenous line, beginning to reduce the blood pressure and administering life-saving magnesium sulphate. Rugiatu gave an oxytocin drip and delivered a healthy baby boy. The girl awoke and began talking.

Rugiatu had saved her life.

'But then she was so tired,' Rugiatu continued. 'So tired and sleeping so much. She needed energy, so I gave her more fluid in the drip.'

Rugiatu looked at me in despair. She thought she had done everything correctly and yet still the girl had died.

We tiptoed around the story, unpicked the details, and delicately weaved in fluid management. Rugiatu, a low-level health worker, had done her best with what she had – limited physical resources and limitations of knowledge.

She blamed the villagers for coming so late and saw focusing on this as the solution to preventing another death. I agreed, but we also had to look at what had happened in the centre: fluid overload in an eclamptic girl.

Rugiatu's was not the only tale of fatal management errors. Each one came with heart-breaking testimonies of wanting to do right. Without a process to review and learn, these events were destined to be misinterpreted and repeated. As Sam and I travelled through the Chiefdom, the health workers asked me how to manage cases they had seen: how to safely deliver a baby presenting breech, remove a placenta that is not expelling itself or stop bleeding after birth. It had not been the intention of the trip, but we ran impromptu simulations. Sam proved to be an excellent and dynamic assistant. He would play the pregnant woman, as the health worker and I ran through manoeuvres.

On the journey back to Magburaka, Sam and I discussed the information we had gathered. How could it help guide the basis of the future MSF project? Together with Abu, the driver, we brainstormed out loud. It seemed delays, supply and training were the biggest barriers. The ambulance service wasn't working – if anything, reliance on the ambulance was leading to higher morbidity and mortality. The promise of recommissioning the Ebola ambulances was moving nowhere fast. We needed to consider empowering the community to find alternate strategies. We needed to find ways to reduce obstruction, corruption and time-wasting at all stages of the woman's journey. We needed a specific delays reduction strategy.

On returning, we were met with bad news from Liberia: a new case of Ebola had been confirmed in Monrovia. It had been six months since

Liberia had declared their outbreak over. This was a blow to all three countries. The diagnosis fed our paranoia of undocumented chains of transmission in Sierra Leone. We felt it was only a matter of time before the same happened here, and we needed to be prepared. The press suggested the new case had re-emerged from a survivor, but this theory had not yet been proved beyond circumstantial evidence.

Active Ebola virus had been cultured in certain body fluids of survivors, signifying potential for ongoing contagion. Surprisingly though, given the high number of survivors in the community, cases with compelling evidence of transmission were scarce and often inconclusive. The premises and predictions of survivor transmission, particularly sexual, were misaligned with the experience on the ground. But, still, best to be cautious.

The fifteen-year-old boy who had initially presented to a Monrovia hospital with a fever was isolated, and he went on to die. His family, as contacts, were also put into isolation, and a further two (his brother and father) became infected. His mother had recently given birth, and she and the newborn child remained Ebola-free. However, when tested for antibodies against the Ebola virus, both the mother and baby were positive – indicating survival from a previous infection. This raised uncomfortable questions.

Emily, one of the health promotors who I had worked with in Kailahun and Bandajuma, had reported on a similar case that occurred in Sierra Leone back in January. In that instance, a twenty-year-old woman had given birth to a stillborn baby at a rural health centre. According to national protocol, all dead bodies, including fetuses miscarried or stillborn babies, were tested for Ebola. The fetus returned a positive result. This created a flurry of excitement, as the woman herself had never been suspected or treated for Ebola. In-depth discussions with the woman and her relatives unearthed that she had been in direct contact with known Ebola-infected people, including her husband; this had occurred during the course of the pregnancy. The woman had been ill, but both she and her healthcare workers had attributed this to the symptoms of late pregnancy. The illness was self-limiting and she recovered. However, the antibody tests on her blood confirmed that, although she was Ebola negative, she had recently been infected with the virus. We had known for a long time that not all people with Ebola had life-threatening illness – this was evident from the ETCs. That this was the same in a pregnant woman was not surprising. However, the fetus was a concern. In this reported case, minimal PPE had been used during the birth. Interestingly though, despite the fetus having very high viral loads, neither the traditional birth attendant nor the midwife were infected, exposing the gap in our knowledge on whether the positive PCR of a dead fetus represented inert viral fragments or actively contagious disease.

The Liberian case was further complicated because their retrospective contact tracing led the investigators to believe the woman had been infected and survived months earlier, during the main outbreak, when she had miscarried another pregnancy. She was never suspected of having had Ebola. They hypothesized that, during this most recent pregnancy, the virus had been reactivated, creating the new cluster. The theory, while plausible and convincing, had the potential to awaken the stigmatization of pregnant women. 'Ebola bomb' had been a term coined to refer to an infected pregnant woman – her belly teeming with virus and danger. Now, whether or not these women had known infections, and whether or not there was an active outbreak, these cases risked unearthing those fears again.

Ruth and I sat together at a long wooden desk, a continuous flow of people around us. But we barely noticed the buzz of the communal office; we were in our own zone, entirely focused on the wider public health consequences for pregnant women in this new era. We knew the damage the stigmatization of pregnant women could make, the way fear clouded decisions, so we had decided to write our own guidance for these 'no or low Ebola transmission' times.

Ruth and I discussed our experiences from the outbreak, previous papers published and former guidelines. We merged our thoughts, fears and hopes for the management of pregnant women presenting to healthcare facilities. We developed an informed set of principles alongside universal precautions, which balanced the safety of healthcare workers with the provision of destigmatized, respectful care for the women.

As we progressed with our various standards and guidelines for the upcoming project, the Ministry of Health, supported by the WHO, released its own updated guidance for pregnant women.

'Have you read them?' I asked Ruth, as we sat once again at the desk, drinking coffee. 'They've taken individual reports and small case series and applied them as sweeping rules for everyone.'

The updated guidance took the complicated issue of triaging pregnant women during the height of the outbreak, and attempted to simplify it, applying general rules to the non-outbreak setting. In short, if the pregnancy deviated from normal; isolate, test and await the result.

'They're ignoring the country baseline,' Ruth said. 'Women with pregnancy complications come late. Every woman with a problem will be considered a suspect. They're creating additional unnecessary delays for urgent care. And, if there's no Ebola outbreak, there's no reason to apply these rules.'

'Look how it's written,'I said, pointing to the document. '"Any woman with bleeding or rupture of membranes is to be considered as suspected Ebola."These are the most common presentations in pregnant women, with or without Ebola. There's no leeway for sensible decision-making. Let's say a woman with a placenta praevia arrives, bleeding heavily. These guidelines would have us consider her an Ebola suspect, whereas logic would tell the clinician there's an adequate explanation. She needs treatment, not delay.'

'They're going to worsen the stigma,' said Ruth, tapping her long fingers on the table. 'It's going to create more barriers in getting maternity care when there's an emergency.'

We raised our concerns with the authors. While these were acknowledged, there was no meaningful discussion of improvement or actions to change. We rejected their guidelines, and advised our contacts to do the same.

The WHO ran training events around the country for their updated guidance. Sam and I joined the official training in Magburaka. The guidance was complicated and clunky. Participants struggled to grasp the most basic principles, let alone the more arduous pregnancy-specific details. After the session, I sat on the steps outside the classroom with the facilitators. They were from Uganda, easy going and sociable. We shared some stories, and I confessed my opinion of their guidelines. Despite being tasked with rolling out the training, they had come to the same conclusion. They had been asked to teach it, but they too doubted its practicality or benefit.

After much ranting, threatening and despair, Ruth and I concluded the likelihood of the flawed guidance being followed was low. If months of training and focus on infection control had not resulted in changes to practice, such as disposing of used hypodermic needles or dirty gloves, how likely was an intricate flow-chart to succeed?

In Freetown, there was more adherence to the guidance, and we heard stories of women dying while awaiting unnecessary Ebola tests. These had been common events a year earlier, but now, outbreak declared over, they flew in the face of reason.

In one case described to me, a woman had presented to a hospital that was fully capable of providing obstetric surgery. As with many women in Sierra Leone, her unborn baby had died prior to arrival. She had clear signs of a uterine rupture and, while the team suspected this diagnosis, they also followed the new guidelines in which fetal death was an 'Ebola associated complication'. She should have gone to the operating theatre. She should have lived. Her pointless isolation proved she did not have Ebola, and also proved to be her death sentence.

26: THE THIRD DELAY

MARCH 2017

My head rested down on the hospital bed hidden round the back of the gynaecology area. The date had not long changed from 9 March to 10 March 2017. Night-shift doctors in the large central London hospital were not provided with an area or time to rest, so we stole opportunistically and closed our eyes in any fitting place we could find, whether that be the floor of a changing room or a gynae bed with stirrups. At night, the hospital sings a slower song, long corridors stretch out like a yawn. The security of the night shift, the blanket of quietness, is an illusion. The emergencies are faster, and, against the dark around us, they shine brighter.

My heavy eyes closed, my mind was still thinking about the patients in our care. I was wondering how long it would be before the woman in labour with twins would be fully dilated. I would need to be around for the delivery. There were a few other early labourers and a fetal heart tracing I was not entirely reassured by, but it wasn't bad enough to justify an intervention either: the obstetric tightrope. I visualized the different scenarios that might play out overnight. Would the twins come head first or feet? Would we need to do a caesarean section? Would everything go smoothly? The only predictability of obstetrics is its unpredictability. Overall, though, the night was calm. My mind slowed down a gear, my thoughts spaced out, the gentle sound of the machines around me soothed me like a mother gently hushing a newborn baby. I drifted off.

'Major incident! Major incident! THIS IS NOT A DRILL.'

Standing on my feet, my mind still resting on the gynae bed, I scrambled for the pager in my pocket, which was vibrating and alarming. I wobbled, and listened again as the message was repeated. Grabbing my phone, I ran to the labour ward next door, but there was no alarm going off there. The midwives were sitting calmly, writing notes and sipping cups of tea. Eyes wide open, I looked at them, startled like a hare facing the hunt.

'Is everything OK?' I asked. 'I got a major incident alert.'

A collection of blank faces looked back at me.

'It must be the explosion,' said one of the midwives, pointing to a computer live-streaming the news. The screen showed a tower block with smoke billowing out from shattered windows. The sound was muted, but a rolling banner read: *Breaking: Large Gas Explosion in Residential Building.* 'I know that building,' she continued. 'It's always been overcrowded.' I scanned the labour ward board to see if there was any new trouble on the horizon, then went to make a cup of instant coffee and prepare for the twins.

No more than five minutes later, I received a page from the emergency department. 'We've got survivors from the explosion arriving. There's a pregnant woman,' said the coordinating doctor. The tone of his voice was one of controlled panic, like the slow release of a pressure cooker. He didn't know much, but he was passing the baton of responsibility.

The emergency department lay deep in the inner bowels of the hospital – down the long curling stairs, into the basement – a windowless, fluorescent land of the wounded and dispossessed. Before reaching the department, I could smell the explosion's aftermath: a dirty toxic scent flowed out from the area where survivors and their relatives were arriving. In preparation for mass casualties, other patients in the department had been moved, beds emptied and non-emergencies sent home, so it was eerily quiet. A bored-looking plastic surgeon sat behind a desk, fidgeting with her fingers. I scanned around till I found a nurse to tell me where the pregnant woman was. Though the department was not busy, there was a feeling of an impending rush – the silence before the tsunami.

Kelly was sitting upright on a trolley, her clothes falling loosely over her bulging abdomen. She made a sad picture, with three young children next to her, all with the same shell-shocked expressions of nothingness. Their little faces were speckled with soot and their hair singed. It was disconcerting to have them sitting there, staring vacantly ahead – no crying, no reaction, nothing at all.

Kelly was working hard to breathe, despite the oxygen mask over her nose and mouth. Her chest was scattered with wheeze. I called for help; Kelly's problems were not obstetric.

We got medications to help open her airways and repeated tests to check her oxygen levels. All the while, Kelly remained upright, looking over her children, who looked silently ahead. The youngest daughter had climbed onto her lap and Kelly stroked her long, tangled hair. Kelly did not look right. I knew we needed help and again sounded the alarm. As I went to the phone to dial the crash code, the paediatrician shouted for me to come. Kelly had collapsed. Her small child still sat on her.

'Is she breathing?'

There was nothing. No sign of life at all.

'Get the kid off her.'

I had not performed cardiopulmonary resuscitation on a pregnant woman since returning from Sierra Leone a year earlier, but the muscle memory in such situations is strong. Kelly's children did not flinch – not a murmur – as they silently watched me compressing their mother's chest under my tight fists. Help arrived, and soon the full strength of a high-income country's health system was behind us.

Walking home, I felt dazed and lost, somewhere between Camden and central Sierra Leone. Disorientated, my mind danced between the present and past – a past for me, but not for those I had left behind. As I processed the aftermath of the night shift, memories and emotions were unlocked. The thoughts I had buried deep returned to haunt me once again. A familiar feeling of anger bubbled under my skin.

The twins were born after my shift ended. Two operating theatres, sterile equipment and a team of medics were immediately available, had their mother required them. She had not. The birth was uncomplicated, mother and babies healthy.

Kelly's journey was more difficult, and she stayed in the ICU a long time. She survived. Her life, though, was forever changed.

*

MAGBURAKA, SIERRA LEONE

DECEMBER 2015

Early December, and the MSF maternal and child health project in Magburaka had not yet begun. As a team of humanitarian workers, it was challenging to be present without being clinically active. We were in an uncomfortable state of being. We were physically on site, but without the usual, powerful, MSF machine in full throttle behind us.

In the mornings I would go to the hospital to see how the preparations were progressing and check in with the maternity team, building important relationships with our future colleagues. Early one morning I wandered in with the project coordinator, a Dutch woman in her forties who was candid and purposeful. The hospital was quiet; it was the twilight time between night shift and day shift. A nurse must have heard us arrive, appearing at the door and saying, 'Can you come? We have serious case'.

Together, we walked over to the delivery room. A twenty-year-old woman was lying flat on the bed. She had delivered a healthy baby boy at home the previous evening – her firstborn. She then began bleeding. Luckily, she had made it to the hospital in time to get help. Drugs were given to make her uterus contract, a urinary catheter was inserted and intravenous lines placed to administer fluids. But she continued to bleed. Over the course of the night, doctors had been called, but could not be reached. Relatives were asked to give blood, but not enough could be found, and then the technician for taking blood could not be found. The night nurses were exhausted and angry, shouting rather than telling us what they had done overnight. The woman lay, gasping, with her baby sleeping on the bed beside her.

Being the time of 'enhanced Ebola surveillance', we needed to continue taking special precautions. I put on the protective clothing and examined her. She was incredibly pale, not responsive, and her blood pressure was very low.

'Can we get oxygen?' I asked, turning to the tired team. 'Someone needs to bring the concentrator. Does anyone know where it is?'

The patient gasped, as if hungry for the humid air. The pallor was setting in on her cool clammy skin.

'She needs blood. Can we get the blood?'

As they began explaining that neither were available, I continued to examine her. Large blood clots spilled out as I rubbed her uterus. I repeated again what she needed: oxygen and blood.

The hospital had oxygen concentrating machines, but they were not kept inside the maternity department. I asked a student nurse to run and find one. Another nurse was sent to collect the waiting relatives and call the blood bank technician again. Incredibly, the technician appeared within minutes, as did the oxygen concentrator.

We sent the relatives to give blood, and began discussing how we could get oxygen for her. There were plug sockets in maternity, but they did not receive any electricity. The project coordinator began working on a solution, shouting frantic messages into her radio set. Generators were found and she scrambled to call for backup. As this was happening, I continued to squeeze and massage the woman's uterus to maintain its contraction.

Another Sierra Leonean colleague arrived and, seeing the desperate scene, came over to help. He took a careful, studied look at her pale face.

'She will not make it,' he stated.

'She's not dead yet. She needs oxygen. She needs blood,' I said.

'I think we have lost her,' he repeated.

'She is still breathing,' I argued.

The plug for the oxygen concentrator did not fit the size of the socket on our generator. More frantic talk. More shouting and confusion.

The project coordinator paced, talking into her radio and making calls on her mobile.

'There must be a way!' she shouted. I heard her asking the logistics team, 'Can you get here now? Yes, right now'.

As I continued rubbing the young woman's abdomen, her gasping stopped. Her eyes fixed.

Together, we began cardiopulmonary resuscitation.

The nurses couldn't find the basic breathing bag we needed, so we used one for a newborn baby till the adult size arrived.

'Run to the blood bank,' I called across the room to a student nurse. 'Find out how long it will be till we get blood.'

While he was gone, we continued, together, fighting, though we all knew we had lost the battle.

The nurse returned and looked upon us from across the room. Sierra Leonean and international medics were taking turns to pump the woman's heart, open her airway and push air into her lungs, asking what else we could do, what we could be overlooking.

'Well?' I called to the student nurse.

'They have not begun the blood donation yet. They are preparing now.'

Each of us looked at one another, and, together, we stopped. We wrapped her body in her colourful shawl and closed her young eyes.

Her baby, hours old, slept through the most important event of his life. His chances of surviving past his first birthday were bleak without his mother to protect and care for him.

The 'third delay' is when a patient gets to a health facility, but deteriorates because the care they need cannot be delivered – or, worse, it can be delivered, but comes too late.

The broken system had failed a healthy young woman, her newborn child, her family and a dedicated team of health workers that night. There were many reasons for failure – social, economic, political, medical and logistical – but there was no excuse.

When I heard people saying the *emergency* in Sierra Leone was over, I cringed. I wanted to show them, and say, *This is the emergency.*

At that time, we were one foot in. We were there, but not there. We were observers. I couldn't know how life would look a month from that point, but I hoped we would never feel a young mother's life turn to death in our hands again.

Joining the morning briefings each day brought familiarity with the team in the hospital, and the challenges they were working against. There were continual complaints of missing or exhausted supplies, patients who presented too late, the mobile phones that stopped working when help was needed and the electricity that did not exist.

Following the morning meetings, I sat with Dr Kamara and Amara in a small office tucked behind the operating theatre. There was a bed and desk, and a window covered with a thick mesh of metal wire to trap mosquitos. A pot of rice and another pot with a stew of cassava leaf or dried fish with potato leaf would be delivered, and they would heap food into bowls. Between the two of them, they managed to stretch themselves to provide twenty-four-hour cover every day. Their families lived in other parts of the country, and both had young children and aspirations for career development. The sharp smell of the stew rose in the steam from their bowls as we discussed their more challenging clinical cases in greater detail. Together, we deliberated on what we agreed was, and was not, acceptable management; when a decision for caesarean section had come too late, and when it was rash; whether their long hours ever clouded their decisions; how their colleagues could share the workload, and when the responsibility was fully theirs.

These breakfast sessions became training, quality improvement and relationship-building exercises. We all agreed caesarean sections should be reserved for cases where no alternative existed. But we differed in our opinions of which alternatives should be performed, and by whom.

I increased my daily presence in the hospital, eventually taking an unused room and putting a desk and a few chairs inside, so I could be in the hospital all day. In the back of the room, we built up an emergency supply of equipment and drugs, so, if there was a critical case we could respond effectively.

When not working on the future project's protocols and orders, or reviewing cases with Amara and Dr Kamara, I would sit in the maternity ward and chat with the government healthcare workers. I observed how their day evolved, and tried to understand what MSF's presence could add. The shifts were usually covered by a midwife or a lesser qualified maternal and child health aide, a traditional birth attendant (who also doubled-up as cleaner) and a nursing assistant. Kadiatu, a skilled and experienced maternal and child health aide, was highly regarded by the team. She had been working in Magburaka since after the civil war and recalled when MSF had previously worked in the hospital, before withdrawing in 2007.

'When they left, we still had so much equipment and so many drugs. MSF left a big donation,' she said, her eyes magnified by her thin-framed glasses. On her head was a piece of blue crêpe paper wrapped into a pointed hat. As a bishop wears his mitre, Kadiatu wore her conical paper hat, looking oddly distinguished and professorial. 'Then it finished,' she continued. 'There was nothing. No drugs, all the equipment broken, no money and nothing replaced. We had an ultrasound scanner, so we hid it away – locked it in a room. You know what happened? Someone cut a hole in the ceiling and stole it.' Kadiatu shook her head. 'Very bad, very difficult. So, I am very pleased to see MSF again.'

Kadiatu's words troubled me. MSF had disrupted the system here before; now, a decade later, we were re-engaging. I knew, as did Kadiatu, MSF would leave again. It was vital this project did not create a dependency or leave a vacuum on its departure. The exit plan needed to be considered before entry – how to leave better systems in place, rather than absent supply chains, income and support.

Kadiatu and the majority of the government-employed staff had continued working in the hospital throughout the Ebola epidemic. They had watched patient numbers decline as the population avoided health centres. Still, the wards were half empty. They had watched their colleagues, family and friends become infected. However, they had achieved where we in GRC had failed. Their work had never stopped.

Amara and Dr Kamara told me about performing caesarean sections with ice packs stuffed under their protective clothing to try to make the high temperatures bearable. They had tales of surgery on women who went on to die from Ebola, meaning the whole department had to be quarantined: all the staff, locked in together, for twenty-one days. And, when released, they continued working all over again.

'What was it like?' I asked Kadiatu.

'This woman was on the ward with all the others. Opposite my daughter. Imagine!' Kadiatu widened her already large eyes. 'We had all been looking after her and then she died. It was a shock. No one had thought of Ebola.' Under the enthusiasm of Kadiatu's retelling, I heard sadness – regret, perhaps. 'We were all kept in here,' she said, pointing to the main maternity ward. 'I was so frightened. And my daughter, with her baby . . . Awful.' She threw her hands dramatically into the air.

As the day drew on and the sun began to settle below the horizon, Kadiatu and her colleagues continued tending to their labouring women, but no lights came on. The hospital generator was only used when the operating theatre was required. There were solar-powered rechargeable batteries that could be used, but these only lasted a few hours, if they weren't broken. The charge points, though, were most often occupied with mobile phones.

Each time Kadiatu had a free moment, she would return to tell me more about hospital life during the epidemic. 'Mr Bangura, from the finances, came here to check on our books. He forgot his glasses, so I said, "Here, take mine, Mr Bangura; use them".' Kadiatu touched the chrome frame over her temple. 'I put them on again after. The next day, he got a fever. It was Ebola. I thought, *These glasses on my face were on his face.*' She paused to catch her breath. 'I threw them. I was so scared – and never let anyone use any of my things after.'

As my eyes adjusted to the evolving darkness inside the maternity ward, I asked, 'How do you see at night? How can you deliver a baby?'.

Kadiatu picked up her mobile phone from the table and stuck it in her mouth. At the end was a little torch light.

'Like this,' she said, sounding as if her mouth was full of boiled sweets.

I imagined providing clinical care, supporting the birth of a baby, with a mobile phone inside my mouth. And, on top of it all, in a place only recently free of Ebola, and with the ever-present risk of Lassa fever. While Kadiatu understood my horror, this was nothing out of the ordinary for her.

That evening, we had an international staff team meeting to discuss the plans for the opening of the project. These meetings were often tense. Ruth and I would push hard to move tasks forward. We had the history of the outbreak behind us, and, while the Ebola emergency was declared over, we agreed there was still a public health emergency. Newer team members had mostly arrived at the end of the outbreak, and were predominantly non-medical. We would summarize numbers of maternal and child deaths in the area, cases that had come into the hospital, challenges at the coalface, but, without directly witnessing these events, they remained abstract details to our new recruits. Ruth and I were the old nags in the project, trying to inspire through painting a picture of what existed in the hills around us.

The electricity situation was deeply troubling. We could not leave the hospital functioning in that way; we urgently needed to bring light and make it available at all times. Naively, I thought this would be a no-brainer. As an international humanitarian organization with health at its core, it seemed obvious we would ensure safe working conditions. MSF had been present in the town for over a year. We had generators (and could source more) and the expertise. It surprised me we had not intervened already. The request, however, was considered outside our remit.

The donation and maintenance of a generator would demand fuel supply, which in turn came with the responsibility for its consumption and continuation. The decision, though it felt black and white to me in the moment, was another blurring of the lines between NGO and governmental responsibility. Just as the existence of GRC had impacted on the accountability of the Free Health Care Initiative, our actions, however well intended, would have side effects and consequences.

'You are expecting nurses, doctors, cleaners to work in the dark with sharp instruments and bodily fluids. The biosafety risks are unacceptable,' I argued within the team of medical, logistical and coordination members.

'We are not taking responsibility for the generator,' replied a colleague firmly.

'What about if I'm called in to an emergency overnight? Will you leave me to work in the dark? What if I stick a scalpel in my hand? What if I trip and fall on to a used needle?'

'OK, we'll install an emergency generator and send a logistician to turn it on if an expat is called in overnight.'

'Right, so when an expat is in the hospital, the lights go on, and, when they leave, they're turned off. What message is that giving? It's OK for you to be at risk, but not me? No way.' I turned to others in the group. 'Remember the girl who died? How can this be allowed, on our watch? What would the people donating money want us to do?' I was playing all my cards.

Ruth had been listening intently. She was a woman of dignified composure, but a passion for the work ran in her veins. 'What the fuck is wrong with you all?' she snapped. 'How is this hard to understand? The hospital needs electricity. Health workers need to see. Patients need oxygen.' She was shaking with anger, tears spilling down her face. This was no longer about the hospital. It was personal. It was the memories and the promises. She stood and walked off.

Emails flew around furiously between team members, and from those in the field to management in Freetown. Eventually, a compromise was agreed on generator usage. A guard would be placed alongside a generator to ensure fuel wasn't stolen and to stop it being abused for non-clinical activities.

We ran simulation scenarios to practise getting an oxygen supply to different areas of the hospital, ensuring the correct adaptors were present and each person understood how the equipment worked. Ruth and I had wanted electrical supply for the whole hospital; we managed to negotiate it for maternity, paediatrics and the operating theatre. It seemed illogical to us that the adult wards would be left in the dark. The biohazard risks existed there too, and if there was a disease outbreak, the whole hospital would need to be secure.

We took what we got, but continued to advocate for better. We were stuck between extremes: on the one hand, headquarters were suffocating us with Ebola-related topics, despite the epidemic being declared over; on the other, we had colleagues behaving as if none of the previous eighteen months had ever happened.

The dichotomy created a dual reaction within Ruth and me: we remained hot on PPE and infection control precautions, while simultaneously keeping persistent focus on the current health needs of the population.

It felt pragmatic. It became exhausting.

27: CHRISTMAS

MAGBURAKA, SIERRA LEONE

DECEMBER 2015

The team had all been working flat out getting the project ready for activities to begin in January. Complicated construction plans kept everyone busy, creating occasional tensions within the team. Opinions on the core priorities and the right ways to achieve the project objectives differed, as did the sense of urgency.

The shadow of Ebola hung over us like a threatening storm cloud. Every action was guided by the premise that transmission could resume. A forgotten pocket of disease. A dragon moving in the shadows. A frustrating pre-occupation.

Late one night, I was called into the hospital. I wandered alone through the unlit corridors that led to the operating theatre. Inside, Amara was beginning a caesarean section for an obstructed labour with breech presentation. I would often hang around during surgeries, observing without scrubbing. If assistance was needed, I was present; if not needed for the mother, I would act as the paediatrician, as we did not have one. I observed Amara from the foot end of the bed. Only one light worked in the theatre and it shone down on him in a single beam, as if he were an actor on stage. Though not formally trained as a doctor, he was a most graceful and proficient surgeon. His fingers danced over the skin as he made the initial incision. At first, I thought my eyes were tricking me, but as he continued working his way through the layers of the abdomen I was sure I could not see a scalpel.

'No scalpel,' Amara confirmed afterwards, as he washed his forearms and hands.

'That's not possible. How can you operate without a scalpel?'

'There are no handles that fit the blades, so we just hold the blade between our thumb and fingers.'

I had no immediate answers. There were high personal risks to operating with a blade without a handle. But, if someone needed an emergency operation, what else could he do? I called a doctor working at another hospital, who agreed to send us a small supply of correctly fitting blades and handles; it was enough to tide us over till MSF began operations and got its act together.

Every day it seemed the hospital was missing the most basic items. At the same time, I was receiving emails about expensive high-tech PPE suits and special equipment we didn't need. We were being asked to jump past the basics to grasp at the shiny and sexy.

Christmas Day had been a hot topic of conversation for several weeks. It was to be a day off for everyone in MSF – international and local staff. The most important subject was who would cook Christmas lunch and what it would be. The field psychologist was taking the lead and had big plans for our team family dinner. A Christmas tree had been improvised out of the ETC's disused boot-stands, transformed by colourful dangling decorations and fairy lights. It stood in the tukul out front, next to our meeting area.

Ruth and I had planned to go to the hospital early on Christmas Day morning. It may have been a day of rest, but the hospital continued to operate. In the days leading up to Christmas, the doctors and community health officers had left, one by one, for their family homes, leaving one doctor available for the whole hospital.

Christmas Eve had been busy. Among the drama of birth and bleeding, a young woman who could neither speak nor hear had arrived. Zainab was approximately twenty weeks pregnant, with light vaginal bleeding. On examination, there was no fetal heartbeat. She was not in pain and showed no sign of imminent miscarriage. We tried to find ways to explain to Zainab that her baby had died, but none of us, local or international, could be sure she understood. We gave her tablets to prepare her body for the delivery. Ideally, these alone would begin the body's own natural processes in recognizing the pregnancy wasn't continuing. As with all deaths, the fetus would be swabbed for Ebola after birth.

Our predictions of low staffing levels were a vast underestimate. Kadiatu, the maternal and child health aid, was the only member of the maternity team to arrive at work on Christmas Day. She was undeterred.

'They will come after lunch,' she said. She looked ready for battle, relishing the prospect of having the maternity unit to herself.

The morning remained calm, and Ruth and I took the opportunity to continue preparing the department for the opening of the project. A few of the other expats had volunteered to come and join us later in the morning, to help set up and stock the new pharmacy. We planned to all return together to the base for a festive lunch.

A teenage girl arrived at around 11 a.m., having been in labour since the day before. She walked with a stoop and moaned quietly to herself in exhausted tones. Kadiatu got an intravenous line into her and began resuscitating her with fluids. On examination, the baby's head was low; we broke the bag of waters and a dark green fluid dribbled out – meconium. The sign of meconium is ominous, indicating the fetus has passed stool before birth. Meconium can be a signal the baby is struggling with the labour, but can also be a normal part of birth. Either way, there is a risk the baby will swallow or breathe in the sticky fluid, causing an airway obstruction or pneumonia. There is much debate about what to do in these situations. There is no way to know if the baby has already aspirated the meconium – in which case, performing an emergency caesarean section may be futile, causing more harm than benefit to the woman. Thankfully, once the membranes were broken, her labour began progressing. Ruth and I decided we would stay with Kadiatu till the girl had given birth, then join the team for the festive meal.

The teenage girl murmured to herself, but whenever her eyes caught mine, she would shout, 'Doctor! Oh Doctor!'.

Zainab, the deaf girl having a late miscarriage, walked into the delivery room. She pointed to her small belly and made a sound to indicate pain. The contractions had begun. She got on to the bed next to the other girl. We gave her some analgesia and awaited the miscarriage.

The fetal heart rate was being monitored in the teenage girl leaking thick meconium, using a handheld device pushed against her belly. As the labour progressed, the girl made the noises of an uncontrollable urge to bear down. The heart rate changed with each contraction, dropping to a slow beat, then gradually climbing back to where it had been before. Each time the heart rate went down, it took longer to return up, as if the baby's head was being dunked below water a little longer each time, forcing it to hold its breath, before letting it resurface.

Kadiatu re-examined the girl and found she was fully dilated, but the baby was tiring. We put together the apparatus for vacuum extraction as the girl grunted with exhaustion. Ruth told her in Krio the baby would come vaginally, but she needed to push. The poor girl just wanted the pain to stop. I placed the cup on to the baby's head; it was looking to the sky, but as she pushed and I applied traction, it turned and slid down. Kadiatu held the bicycle pump in her hand, sweating as she worked hard to maintain the vacuum. All together, we urged the girl to push down. The baby delivered with the second contraction – pale, floppy and covered in thick green meconium. I cut the cord and swapped my role, from obstetrician to paediatrician.

The baby was positioned to allow his airway to open. Kadiatu took the squeezy rubber sucker, removing meconium from his nose and mouth. I held the small mask over his chubby face as Ruth squeezed the little bag of air into his lungs. Watching his chest rise up, I counted the seconds out loud. His colour began returning and his heart rate raced up to normal. We wrapped the little boy in a shiny space blanket to keep him warm, his young mother watching as we continued helping him breathe.

Zainab watched on silently, trying to understand the events unfolding before her.

Each time the baby appeared to be making effort, we'd stop breathing for him. After a few minutes he would begin turning blue and stop moving his chest, and so we would resume manual ventilation. The cycle continued for almost an hour.

The young mother fell asleep as Zainab continued watching intently, every now and then pointing to the baby and making gestures to indicate she thought the baby had died. As this went on, a commotion from outside burst into the delivery room. A seventeen-year-old girl was having a violent eclamptic seizure. Kadiatu pounced on her to hold her shaking body down, and, together with Ruth, she got the magnesium sulphate drawn up and into her. Once on the eclamptic protocol, they gave her a drug to begin the labour. As they settled her and I continued to breathe for the meconium baby, Zainab began making exaggerated sounds and gestures.

Ruth gently parted Zainab's legs; the fetus had delivered. Ruth made reassuring noises and gestures, but it soon became clear that Zainab had not understood she was experiencing a miscarriage. The incoherent noises of shock and horror fell from her mouth as she looked at the poorly formed figure being wrapped in a lappa cloth. Zainab looked at me with accusing eyes: *Why try so hard for that baby, but nothing for mine?* The noises she made were a clear indication of her distress, and were distressing to hear.

The baby born through meconium continued to pink up, and then go floppy and blue again within moments of trying to step down manual ventilation. Together, Ruth, Kadiatu and I agreed we could do no more. We had no facility to be able to continue resuscitating the baby for a prolonged period. The exhausted mother gave a slow nod as Kadiatu explained, then closed her eyes as we stopped, moved away, and apologized.

The girl with eclampsia began contracting and writhing around in pain, while the girl whose newborn had died was half-sleeping. As we sat back to take stock of the events, Zainab began making noises again. We looked up at her and she pointed between her legs, where large clots of blood were pooling on the bed. I pushed firmly on to her uterus and they spilled out like slabs of liver. She was haemorrhaging. The difficulty we had communicating made managing anything incredibly challenging. I suspected there were small pieces of placenta left behind, causing the bleeding – a recognized complication of late miscarriages. She was rapidly developing a major haemorrhage, though, and if we did not do something to stop the bleeding she would be in serious danger. It was a terrible combination of events, non-communication and spiralling anxieties. I went to find the equipment for manual vacuum aspiration, as Ruth and Kadiatu drew up some diazepam to help calm her down.

Upon returning, I could see the blood clots gathering on the floor below Zainab's delivery bed. Ruth and Kadiatu had managed to reassure her and get her legs up into stirrups, and the diazepam was beginning to kick in. I cleaned and anaesthetized her cervix, inserting a curette into the womb to begin aspiration. The retained bits of placenta rushed into the syringe and her uterus clenched down around the suction curette. My shoulders dropped down; the bleeding had stopped, and so had Zainab's shrill screams.

'She's unconscious!' Ruth shouted from the head end of the bed.

I jumped up from my stool between Zainab's legs, looking at her still body and expressionless face. I checked her pulse – it was fast, but strong. Her chest gave a gentle rise. We cleaned her up and repositioned her so she could sleep off the diazepam in comfort. I could not begin to understand how Zainab would have interpreted the events of the day; it must have seemed an absolute horror show.

Ruth and I stayed with Kadiatu as more patients arrived: there were three women being induced into labour; a woman in her sixth pregnancy, with twins and severe pre-eclampsia; and a woman whose baby had died and we suspected had had a placental abruption. When the night shift arrived, having eaten their Christmas dinners, I gave instructions for each patient and made sure they could contact my mobile phone. Late in the evening, Ruth and I left.

The festivities were over, the plates washed and over half the team were in bed. I felt like a teenager returning home past curfew, receiving a cold look from my mother and a raised eyebrow from my father. Today, Ruth and I were outsiders – the black sheep of the family, who had missed Christmas lunch. Although we apologized, I couldn't help feeling there was a loss of perspective given the activity in maternity. I would've shared the events, but nobody asked.

We ate in silence, then I checked my phone was charged and headed to bed. My mind was fixated on the women we had left in labour, all with potentially life-threatening conditions, and the government-employed staff we relied on to deliver care through the night, knowing none of them had rested during the day.

I woke early and headed back to the hospital, nervous of what I might find. All three women had delivered normally, and safely. They were being transferred to the postnatal wards, making room for the next round of patients.

As time passed, the official commencing of the MSF project drew closer. There was still a lot to organize. How would we integrate the new staff employed by MSF with those already working in the hospital for the Ministry of Health? We were keen to avoid any bullying or intimidation brought on by group rivalry. Ruth and I stayed up late into the evenings, planning induction meetings and training. We wrote introductory guidelines and reviewed hospital plans, from how infection control procedures would work, to managing consumption of equipment and safeguarding against theft.

We had now managed to reconnect with each of the former anaesthetic nurses from GRC. They all applied to work again with MSF, at the new project in Magburaka, and, after interviews, we employed them all.

The anaesthetic nurses had a combined knowledge of Sierra Leonean obstetrics and years of familiarity with MSF. Their job interviews were a reunion. Abu Bakar, who had worked my first night shift back in GRC, and Suma, who had coordinated Bandajuma ETC activities, joined us. John, who had worked at Magburaka Government Hospital when MSF was there in the early 2000s, before GRC, had an immediate connection and knowledge of the place and staff. Alongside Thomas and Aminu, both wise to navigating the systems and resources available.

I had seen in GRC how these anaesthetic nurses were mentors to the clinical team, supervising complex care in critical patients, supporting infection control during Lassa fever and suspected Ebola cases, maintaining the operating theatre and liaising with sterilization services to ensure we were always prepared for whatever came through the door. We needed their attention to detail and local understanding.

They agreed to begin working with us before MSF activities were officially running in the hospital, and we could not have got everything in order without their guidance and wisdom. Together, they helped build the operating theatre team into a professionally organized group, with a functional roster and support network for the most difficult cases. Each day, we walked around the hospital complex together, identifying how we could improve standards to an acceptable level and discussing our visions for the future.

There were rooms in the paediatric and maternity blocks which were locked, and we had not managed to get access to the keys. We were predicting a rapid increase in patients, once the project opened and word spread of MSF's presence, so we wanted to maximize space. Ruth and I asked around, and each person told us of another person who would have the keys. We spent weeks going around in circles, frustrated we could not find a way in.

Our persistence paid off, and we finally gained entry to these empty wards and offices. Inside, piled from floor to ceiling, we found boxes of essential medications and surgical equipment. There were several boxes containing hundreds of scalpel handles. There were copious amounts of intravenous fluids, cannulas and equipment for maternal and neonatal resuscitation. I felt sick. Some of these rooms were directly adjoining the maternity block, where we had watched women die from a supposed lack of the very supplies we now found stockpiled. Most of the medication boxes had been ripped open, with a few packets taken from each.

As we began redistributing the medications and equipment to the clinical areas, nurses and midwives came over to Ruth and me, beaming. 'Thank you, MSF!' they said. 'God bless you, MSF.' But this stuff had all been there long before MSF pitched up. All we had done was open the door.

It was clear from their reactions, the staff had been unaware of the Aladdin's caves surrounding them. I wondered if these rooms had been locked to prevent items from going missing, perhaps out of concern the medications and equipment would be wasted, squandered or stolen, but the cynic in me suspected the open boxes were evidence of items being held back to increase demand, then resold at inflated prices. Either way, the denial of these commodities had led to avoidable disabilities and deaths. It was a disheartening couple of days. We took an inventory of everything in the rooms; the amount of supply hoarded was breathtaking.

'This place doesn't need MSF,' Ruth vexed. 'It needs management systems, supply chains and accountability.'

The official opening of the project was days away, and we were not ready. Ruth and I were in full emergency mode, but we felt alone. Despite assurances, the basics were not yet in place. The use of the generator for electricity remained controversial, running water was not available, waste bins had not arrived and the operating theatre still had only a single working light. I had been staying up at night, reading about how hospital systems operated to try to get my head around what needed to be in place as a minimum.

We began holding daily meetings, reviewing which tasks needed completing, who was responsible and what was needed. The tension in the international group crept up as other members felt Ruth and I were pushing them too hard. Five days before we were due to go live, we still did not have hygiene or sanitation systems in place. Late into the night, I would sit, staring at the sky. Over forty-five new healthcare workers were due to start working in the hospital, employed by MSF, but within the government system. How could we employ them to work in a hospital if it did not have minimum hygiene standards? What responsibilities did we have to them? After the consequences of internal infections of healthcare workers during the outbreak, it was paramount we started right.

I made a short list of seven standards that needed to be in place before the project could begin. I wrote them on a whiteboard in the general meeting area, with a big sign above: *BIOSAFETY*. The ghost of Ebola was still within me and I was being haunted.

Team members looked at the short list which had appeared overnight as they sipped their morning coffee. 'What is that?' I heard one asking another.

'Minimum standards to open the project,' I interjected. 'If they are not in place by Tuesday afternoon, no new clinical staff will be permitted to enter the hospital. The project will not open until it is safe to do so.'

It was a gamble, but it paid off.

28: A NEW YEAR, A NEW PROJECT, ANOTHER CHANCE

NORTH LONDON

26 DECEMBER 2020

Midnight was approaching when my phone vibrated with the ping of Jane's message: *It sounds like the whole of London is closed. Wait time for an ambulance is 600 minutes and there are currently seventy ambulances waiting to offload patients outside emergency departments across London, but there is nowhere for them to go. Let's hope our ladies stay well and improve.*

Merry Christmas! I replied, with a rolling-eyes emoji. There was little else to say. I'd booked into a hotel room, as staying next to the hospital felt safer then risking a journey home overnight, given the surge of COVID-19 and general Christmas on-call anxieties. I was almost halfway through the seventy-two-hour shift and I was already crawling. The torrent of patients washing up to the hospital had been unrelenting. It made the first COVID wave feel like it had been the practice run.

Happy Christmas to you too! Jane replied. I saw she was still typing and so I continued to stare at the screen. The day's events were running through my mind – the flurry of activity in maternity, met by the unending calls to the intensive care unit.

The neonatal unit has no cots left. The staffing levels tonight and tomorrow are atrocious. It's going to be really stretched.

Before I could reply, my phone flashed with a call from the hospital coming in – too bright and too loud for my tired senses.

'Mr Black, connecting you to delivery suite.'

'Hi – it's Benjamin, here,' I said, as I heard the click of lines switching.

'Hi!' Tamica's voice came over the line. She was one of the junior doctors covering the night shift, and eminently capable; I was glad to have her with me over the weekend. 'Sorry to disturb you, just an update,' she said.

'Go for it,' I said, as I began pacing up and down the room.

'Well, you know the unit is full. Too many premature babies delivered during the day and no cots left. The COVID-positive women across in intensive care are managing, for now, but one of them looks very bad. I'll go back to her, soon as I can get there. We also had a call from the coordinator in the emergency department. There are a couple of pregnant women with COVID, stuck in the back of ambulances. They want us to begin seeing them in the car park. What do you think?'

'Tell me more about ICU,' I said. Between all the births and emergencies of the day, it was ICU my mind kept returning to.

There were four pregnant women who needed support with their breathing, occupying beds uncomfortably far from the maternity unit. Each one was at a different stage of prematurity.

All weekend, we had been negotiating between the different specialties. Should we give more oxygen? Begin a life-support machine? Deliver the baby? All weekend, we had questioned which intervention would be wisest – what would make a difference? Or, should we hold tight and hope the drugs would work and the body would fight back? Each woman looked terrified. We felt the fear too, as they heaved to pull air into their scarred lungs, forcing oxygen through to themselves and their unborn child.

'I think you should do a caesarean now,' one of the women requested, between her gasping breaths.

I nodded, in deep contemplation, observing the numbers on the monitor behind her and eyeing the scalpel stuck behind her bed, in case she stopped breathing and needed an immediate caesarean delivery, right there.

All day, pregnant women had been calling to tell us they had tested positive for COVID. Every patient who came into hospital was now being tested as routine. The list of women who had come in to give birth was gradually turning red, as more brought back a positive result, most with no symptoms. Each result twisted the tension in the air a little more, like a guitar string, and I was waiting for the snap – the twang, when we might all fall down.

'Samira, who's thirty weeks pregnant – she looks the worst,' Tamica said. 'I'm going to go back to see her with the anaesthetist. Do you want me to call you afterwards?'

'Sure, you can call me for anything. But, yeah, if there's any change in the women in ICU, I'll come back, no problem at all.'

The hospital was once again overrun with COVID patients, and our staffing levels had plummeted with sickness, isolation and fear. And yet, maternity was bursting with activity. Life went on. The women and their companions increasingly brought COVID in with them. We had already tried diverting ambulances. We had already tried transferring the sickest, in case a cot was urgently needed. We had already asked for faster testing capability. All impossible. We were discussing how to ration oxygen usage to avoid a crisis like the one in the first wave.

I lay back on the bed in the Premier Inn. I could see the soft glow of the hospital outside the window, looking so calm from that distance. I closed my eyes, but all I could see was the ICU, and all I could hear were the echoes of coughing around me.

*

MAGBURAKA, SIERRA LEONE

JANUARY 2016

Months of talking, over a year of reflecting, and finally, on Wednesday, 6 January 2016, MSF officially entered into Magburaka Government Hospital. We brought forty-five additional healthcare workers into maternity and paediatrics, an immediate boost to the clinical teams, supporting their life-saving activities.

During the recruitment process, we had been meticulous in checking and cross-checking to ensure we did not employ anyone who already had a government contract. We aimed to be true to our word of not repeating the mistakes of the past. We wanted to boost existing services, not deplete them.

The medical part of our international team remained skeletal. Though we were expecting the arrival of new expats to join the project, bottlenecks and differing priorities had meant they would not be with us till later in the year. Nonetheless, with excitement and pride, we integrated the new MSF teams with those already working for the Ministry of Health. I took personal satisfaction and comfort in being reacquainted with many of my former Sierra Leonean GRC and ETC colleagues. There was a bond between us all, perhaps our shared recent history.

Alongside maternal and child health, MSF also had joint responsibility with the Ministry of Health for infection prevention and control in the hospital. Suma had been employed to oversee this critical aspect of the project. Though an anaesthetic nurse by training, he had been working in supervisory roles since before my arrival in Sierra Leone. When I first met Suma in GRC, he had been part of the background. I would see him or hear him, but I did not *know* him, nor did he know me. Our paths had crossed again in Kailahun, where we would occasionally stop and exchange pleasantries coming in or out of the High Risk area of the ETC. When our journeys had collided a third time, in Bandajuma ETC, it felt as if we had always been the closest of colleagues. Suma was respected by everyone who worked with him and, though he was softly spoken and understated, he had a very natural way of appealing to all levels of the hospital hierarchy. He was a safety net for us all.

Suma led a small team of nurses. We would joke that they were the 'infection control police' – and, in a way, they were. They were responsible for asking all who entered the hospital to wash their hands, checking temperatures and asking brief questions about people's reasons for attending. This was our early recognition and alert system. Each day, they would also inspect the wards, observing the doctors and nurses for hand-washing and wearing the correct protective equipment. Ebola was officially over, but we worked to make sure the basics remained in place from the start, avoiding slipping backwards, so we could focus our attention on treating patients with confidence.

I was most content being in the hospital, among the new and previous staff, observing how they worked together and how they managed the patients arriving. I aimed to be at the handover of each shift, as well as popping in late in the evening and calling early in the morning. This became my favoured activity – sitting and listening, being a colleague and a friend. Looking back, it exposed my arrogance and immaturity of eighteen months earlier, when the distinction between *us* and *them*, *international* and *local*, was pronounced and obstructive.

Those first days were hectic and magnificent. Patient numbers began increasing, particularly in paediatrics. We established a neonatal room, where newborn babies presenting with tetanus and other complications were treated. Their tiny wrinkled faces scrunched-up in pain as their muscles spasmed in response to any stimulation. The Sierra Leone team delivered medicine and analgesia, caring for the babies in the dark and quiet room.

Over the weekend, the ambulances kept coming, and in maternity we began receiving more critical patients. Sometimes, two patients would be squeezed in the back of an ambulance together, with their respective families too, as if the ambulance were a bus, collecting obstetric emergencies on its way round the district. We'd open the doors and try to judge which passenger was the most urgent on arrival. There were several women with ruptured uteruses. One needed an emergency hysterectomy, and another had taken so long to arrive at the hospital her womb had already become necrotic inside her.

On the Saturday, as I watched my new colleagues managing the patients arriving, a girl of slight frame walked in, propped up by a stooped elderly female relative. Memuna had come from one of the distant villages, having been in labour for days. She was dehydrated and exhausted, and, as she climbed on to the delivery bed, the scalp of her baby could be seen protruding from her vagina.

On examining her, we found that appearances deceived us. The head, having been stuck for at least two days, had drawn fluid, which collected like a cushion between the scalp and skull, pulled in by gravity and pressure. Though the skin and hair could be seen at the entrance of Memuna's vagina, the head itself remained wedged up in the pelvis. Memuna's vulva had swollen and her bladder distended. Her uterus had created a tight ring, as if every part of her young body protested to birthing. This combination of features allowed no space for the baby to come down. We knew the baby was dead; we needed to ensure Memuna did not follow her.

A team spread around her. Kadiatu commanded the younger nurses to collect equipment and help her insert intravenous lines, while reassuring Memuna about what was happening.

As the resuscitation continued, I turned to Amara and asked what his next move was going to be. We were standing at the end of the bed, both of us draped in light yellow gowns over our scrubs, wearing heavy wellington boots and face shields to protect our eyes from body fluid splashes. Sweat dribbled down our faces as Amara carefully ran over the assessment and we considered the options.

'Vacuum delivery?' he asked, his face giving away a lack of conviction.

'The head is too high. It's stuck. If you pull, it will fail.'

Amara looked at me thoughtfully. 'But the fetus is dead; shouldn't we try, before a caesarean?'

'You're right,' I said. 'Putting a scar on her uterus would be a shame. She's young and she took days to reach the hospital. Next time will be worse.'

Amara looked uncertain. Was I saying do the vacuum or not?

'There's another way,' I said, as Memuna rolled her small, stretched body on to its side. 'Another way for the fetus to come out without touching her uterus.' I urged Amara to complete the puzzle.

The midwives and nurses around Memuna looked at us, waiting for an answer.

'Destructive delivery?' Amara offered to the room.

Kadiatu explained to Memuna and the old lady that we would take her to the operating theatre, and how we intended to deliver the baby; they agreed.

Ruth had performed destructive deliveries in South Sudan. She joined Amara and me as we scrubbed for the operation. We all agreed, this was the correct way forward.

Memuna needed proper analgesia for both her physical and psychological comfort, and, with this, she soon fell into a deep sleep. I was able to drain her bladder of urine, and then we set about choosing our instruments. We did not have the specialized equipment designed for the procedure. I lay a sterile green cloth over a metal table and placed the surgical instruments available in neat rows. We surveyed what tools we had.

Ruth picked up the heavy curved hysterectomy clamps. 'These will work,' she said, placing them next to the scalpel and speculums already set aside.

'First, you'll need to find the fontanelle,' I explained to Amara. 'The intention is to allow the skull to collapse, then the baby can pass through the pelvis and deliver.'

Amara nodded as he listened.

'It is not risk free,' I said, 'but it's safer for her than cutting the uterus open'.

Ruth and I stood to the side as Amara slid his fingers over the protruding scalp. The swelling made it difficult to find the usual landmarks. He looked to me as he pushed deeper inside.

I recalled the words of my senior registrar from my first year of obstetric training. In a London operating theatre, I had been where Amara was now, assessing the fetal position before a forceps delivery. The registrar, seeing the confusion on my face, had leant in and whispered to me, *Imagine she has a glass pelvis – visualize.*

Amara stepped aside and, remembering her words, I closed my eyes, letting my fingers do the seeing. The soft fontanelle, where the skull bones come together, was sitting downwards, the baby looking upwards, with her head stretched out, as if trying to sniff the morning air.

'It's here,' I said to Amara, my fingertips resting on the fontanelle. I showed him the angle of my fingers, like a path leading to the prize.

Amara tried again; I watched as the crease over his nose smoothed away, then I passed an instrument to his free hand.

'One moment,' I said, as I moved my hands to Memuna's abdomen. I felt for the circular form of the head under her muscles. Placing a palm on each side, I pushed firmly down, fixing it in place. 'All right, you can go.'

Ruth gave Amara encouraging instructions as he began opening the cranial vault. We knew he was in the correct place when the white and grey brain matter began spilling down into the bucket between Memuna's legs.

Several other midwives and nurses had come to observe the procedure, and they gathered around the end of the operating table, mesmerized as the delivery completed.

Amara and I felt inside the womb for any evidence of uterine rupture. There was none. The journey was not yet over for Memuna, though. The labour had been long and obstructed, and the tissue lying between the vagina and bladder had been compressed for days. With no blood able to reach and nourish it, it had sloughed away, leaving an open sore. Memuna was developing an obstetric fistula.

The weekend continued in a haze of maternity and paediatric cases, as this new team learnt to work together, overcoming the inevitable growing pains of the collaboration. By Sunday, though, we were starting to feel a little more settled. The rest of the international team had left to get some rest by the time I made my usual late-evening visit. I checked in with the outgoing day shift and incoming night team. Wandering in the dark between the paediatric and maternity departments, I couldn't help but feel a deep sense of fulfilment, not only because the project was flourishing, but also because of the ashes from which it was born.

Just as I was bidding goodnight to the team, another ambulance rolled up to the back gate. Stuffed inside were two women who had been referred from far away, each with various family members also cramped into the ambulance with them. They were both conscious and I assumed the peripheral health unit had referred one and then decided to offload the other opportunistically.

Antony, the CHO who had worked in the Magburaka ETC and wanted to become an obstetrician, had been employed by MSF to join the project, and he was dealing with the new arrival. I was keen to leave the team to it, but a niggling feeling made me wait. The women were placed on to beds next to one another, with an off-white dressing screen between them. Amara and Antony took one patient each and began formulating their opinions.

The woman to the left was pale and skinny, and her heartbeat was rapid and weak. Antony wasn't sure what the issue was, but had correctly diagnosed that the baby had died. No blood could be seen, but he assumed she must be bleeding somewhere. Amara examined the woman to the right. She had a hand over her large belly and made a deep groan of sadness. When Amara pulled up her brightly patterned lappa, we looked at each other knowingly. There was a long vertical scar stretching down from her umbilicus, signifying a previous caesarean section. We had another uterine rupture. Her baby, too, was no longer alive. If we were to follow the official guidance, both these women would need to be isolated as possible Ebola cases before surgery. Both had time-critical emergencies, where delay would cause harm or death.

We began assessing the women to decide whose state was the more perilous. Both needed urgent surgery, but one would have to wait. I could see we needed help. I called Ruth, deeply apologetic; I knew she needed to rest, but we needed more hands than we had. Ruth came with Carolin, a newly arrived nurse from Germany, and we called in an extra anaesthetic nurse, John. The woman on the left had a desperate blood count of just over 3 g/dL. We couldn't find any veins to cannulate and provide treatment. Her body was in shutdown. We decided to take her to theatre first, but, after some discussion, we changed our minds. Ruth, Carolin and John would continue trying to get intravenous access and blood for her, while the woman we suspected of having a uterine rupture would go to theatre first; she too had a low blood count, but was more stable.

I watched Amara perform an expert laparotomy. The uterus had opened like a clam shell. He swiftly extracted the freely floating fetus and repaired the rupture. Then, with her consent and that of her family, he removed her fallopian tubes to prevent further pregnancies. It was this procedure which would most likely save her life in the years to come.

It was after midnight when Amara closed the woman's abdomen. I ran back along the dark corridor to assess the other woman in the delivery room, my footsteps echoing around me. Small groups of patients and relatives sat outside, looking up as I sprinted past. The other woman was lying straight and motionless. John had managed to get an intravenous line into her foot and fluid was running through. When I had worked in GRC, I had often relied on John in precarious times. I would hear his voice reassuring the women in the operating theatre. 'Nothing to worry about', he would chant, as if a mantra. His presence comforted me.

The relatives had been sent from the back of the ambulance to the laboratory to donate blood; their blood group matched, but the donation was not ready yet. John and I wheeled her to the theatre. We would give her the blood while operating.

Amara and I decided to operate together. On entry, we found this woman had had a profound placental abruption. Her uterus was swollen and bruised, soaked with the blood from the detached fetus and placenta. Although we had both seen abruptions, we had never seen anything like this. The womb was peeling like a sunburnt child. Blood oozed out from any place we touched. We decided less was more, performed the caesarean section and did as little else as possible. We had created a special room for our sickest mothers next to the delivery room. After the surgery, we wheeled her in and checked her blood count: it was 2 g/dL after transfusion; it was incredible she was alive.

It was about 2 a.m. when I left the hospital to take some rest back at the base. The generator had been turned off long before I arrived. I sat outside in the silence, surrounded by the thick, black, star-studded sub-Saharan sky.

We made it, I thought to myself. First weekend done.

Despite the complex cases posed to a new team finding their feet, no woman in our care had died. It was with a heavy heart that I realized not one baby born had survived.

My eyes must have been closed for only a few hours when I was awoken by the ringing of my phone. Amara was back in the hospital, struggling with a patient.

'Sorry, but can I get some advice?' he asked. 'This girl is here – she's fifteen and full term. She's having eclampsia. We can't stop the seizures. The blood pressure is uncontrolled. We have given her everything. Maximum dose of every drug.'

'Right,' I said, sitting up under my mosquito net, trying to recall what the textbooks advised for such a situation.

'The baby is alive,' Amara added. 'We want to take her for a caesarean section.'

'Hold on,' I said, searching round my room for some clothes. 'Don't move her if she's unstable.'

We ran through what medication had been given. They really had thrown the book at her.

'And what's her blood pressure now?'

'Last one was 220 over 115.'

'Give another injection of hydralazine,' I said, doubting my own advice; this was uncharted territory for me.

'More?' Amara hesitated. 'According to the guide, she's had the maximum amount allowed.'

He was correct to question me. Hydralazine is a powerful blood pressure drug. If given too quickly or in the wrong amount, it can crash the blood pressure, causing other problems.

'Yes. And don't take her to theatre. I'm on my way in.' I threw my T-shirt on and ran out to get a car to the hospital.

I was met by an anxious team. The girl was thrashing around wildly, her blood pressure remaining stubbornly high.

'Let's push a little more,' I said, picking up the syringe of hydralazine.

The team was divided. Nobody wanted another stillbirth. We were all keen to get the baby out, but I was concerned that operating before the blood pressure and seizures were controlled could be lethal to the mother. I held steady, feeling the weight of my decision as I slowly injected the hydralazine into her vein.

The morning team began arriving. It was John, the anaesthetic nurse, who had the idea of sprinkling an alternative oral tablet under her tongue. 'We did this in GRC all the time,' he said, grinning as he crushed the tablet. I was sceptical, but had nothing else to suggest as the girl snapped in and out of seizures and slumber. John pinched her nose and, as soon as her mouth opened, dropped the white powder inside.

It worked like a charm. Her blood pressure began dropping to safer levels, though she was still very unwell. Her kidneys were making barely any urine and she remained agitated. We also knew that we needed to get the baby out while she was stable. She could have another seizure at any moment.

Watching the operating theatre that morning was beautiful. A calm and efficient team of five anaesthetic nurses, most of whom were not scheduled to be working, came together to give this young girl meticulous care. The baby's cry broke the shadow hovering over us – a healthy and strong boy, quickly united with his waiting grandmother as we continued caring for his mother.

That first weekend will stay etched in all of our memories – not only for the patients we saw, but for those we didn't see too.

While we were busy in the operating theatre with Memuna on Saturday afternoon, a twenty-two-year-old woman called Mariatu Jalloh had come to visit the outpatients' clinic. She had travelled from Bamoi Luma, a town in the north-western district of Kambia, bordering Guinea. MSF was not involved in general adult care and she was seen and treated by one of the Ministry of Health clinical health officers. Mariatu presented with vague and general flu-like symptoms, having already been to the traditional healer. She was seen, sent for some tests, and went home. She died three days later, at a family home in Magburaka Town, then had a traditional burial. As with all deaths (including stillbirths and miscarriages) during the ninety days of 'enhanced surveillance', she was swabbed for Ebola before burial.

On Thursday, 14 January, we had a team meeting in the evening. We all sat around a large plastic table inside the tukul, the mood good and jovial. One week into the project and the teams were working out well. We had further reason to celebrate: it was forty-two days since the last confirmed case of Ebola in Liberia or Guinea. The WHO was finally due to announce the entire Ebola outbreak of West Africa over. Sarah, our head of mission, was visiting from Freetown and made a short speech. We raised our bottles of beer and, remembering those colleagues who had fallen sick or died, toasted a bittersweet triumph.

Approximately ten minutes later, our phones began ringing with rumours that Mariatu Jalloh's swab was positive.

29: FAR FROM PERFECT

MAGBURAKA, SIERRA LEONE

THURSDAY EVENING, 14 JANUARY 2016

Suddenly, you are no longer just another NGO project in Africa; you are at the centre of the world and everyone is watching your next move.

One eye open, the dragon stirs again.

Among the international team, there were four of us – Ruth, Allan, Dennis and I – who had significant experience of working with Ebola. We all, also, had significant trauma. Ruth and I looked to one another from opposite ends of the long table, still clutching our bottles of Star beer. Communicating with eyes only, we understood we should show no sign of panic or fear. And we needed to get to the hospital. Casually, as if it were any other evening, we walked round to a car to make a visit. We were still unclear about the information, or whether Mariatu's test result was public knowledge. The sample was being sent to a second laboratory for confirmation. As it stood, all we had was a rumour through internal networks.

The hospital felt as it always did in late evening – subdued and sleepy. We didn't go to maternity or paediatrics, but headed straight to the adult outpatients' area. A small gathering of healthcare workers stood around, whispering to one another in rapid bursts. The clinical health officer who had treated Mariatu stood in the middle of the gathering with the triage paper in her hand. Her face was crumpled with disbelief and distress. She told us about the consultation and pointed at the paper demonstrating that Mariatu had not met the criteria for suspicion. The instincts of Ebola kicking in, I looked at the paper, sussing whether we should be handling it with gloves and caution.

Together, we traced Mariatu's steps. She had been in the waiting room, consultation area and laboratory. It was already several days ago;

decontamination would be more of a psychological exercise than of any real benefit, but we decided to sort it out nonetheless. The atmosphere was a tense calm, like when the temperature drops just before a thunderstorm begins. I wandered around the hospital, making subtle checks here and there, not wanting to raise suspicions. Amara and John, the anaesthetic nurse, were in the operating theatre, finishing off a caesarean section. I went in, pleased and relieved to see they were following infection control procedures. I took John to one side as Amara completed the surgery. But John had already heard the news, the Sierra Leone rumour mill as efficient as ever.

Ruth left with Sarah, the head of mission, to attend an impromptu meeting of the District Health Management Team, and we all met up back at the base, late in the evening. Though the result was not yet official, we knew tomorrow the announcement would come and the Ebola circus would begin. Ruth and I had discussed this scenario many times and had put together a basic contingency plan to ensure normal health services could continue.

'Now, we test it,' Ruth said.

We spoke late into the night, strategizing for the days ahead. When I finally lay down on my bed, my mind meandered around the memories of the last eighteen months: the faces in the Ebola treatment centres; the feeling of suffocation in the heavy PPE and dense face masks; my family. I rested the back of my hand on my forehead by reflex, asking myself, *Are we really about to do this again?*

At 5 a.m., Ruth and I got up and quietly left for the hospital in the dark. The confirmation had not yet come, but all the town knew. We made our way from ward to ward, checking on every single patient in the hospital, adults and children, regardless of whether they were part of the MSF project or not. We talked to all the staff in each area, hearing their concerns and reassuring them.

'We have all been through this before,' I said. 'We are in this together.'

We checked there were hand-washing facilities and sufficient protective equipment, making a note of what was needed where, and we retraced the flow of patients through the hospital, following their journey and planning the wisest place for isolation facilities. Finally, we reviewed the patient charts for any worrying signs of Ebola.

'What about this guy?' I said to Ruth, pointing to a patient's chart in the adult ward. 'Looks like he's had a fever for a few days; he's not responding to treatment, and there's no diagnosis.'

He was tucked in a bed at the back corner. We stood and observed from a distance. His prominent ribs stood out against his wrinkled skin, and an arm dangled from one side of the bed, swaying with his rapid breathing.

'He'll need testing,' said Ruth, both of us wondering how long he had been languishing in the ward.

As the morning light grew stronger, more members of staff began to arrive. Amara joined us as we continued surveying how and where isolation facilities could be rapidly set up. A small isolation tent at the hospital's front gate was expanded from a four-bed capacity to six, and over the following days we took over an empty car park next to the isolation area, creating seventeen beds for suspected Ebola patients. Separate isolation areas were created for pregnant women and children, thought out according to their needs. Before the sun had risen, before the world was told, we – MSF and the local government – were preparing and implementing. This time, we were not going to be behind Ebola. We were putting up defences and we were getting ready to fight.

When the official announcement finally came, it was of no surprise to any of us. People's reactions were mixed: some were thoughtful, lost in their memories of the past; others were motivated and pumped for action; and some just philosophically took it on board and continued with business as usual. I had assumed our fledgling project would suffer and the new staff would not come to work. I was wrong. Everyone came, enthusiastic to nip this in the bud.

The WHO identified around 150 contacts of Mariatu, spread across four districts. We all held our breath, expecting a resurgent epidemic. We focused our attention on keeping the hospital open, while other organizations began vital communications with the local population and community leaders.

Politics quickly resurfaced. The Vice President and Minister of Education visited Magburaka and declared that the new Ebola case was not real – an outrageous publicity stunt, with the potential to divide communities and reignite mistrust of the health sector.

A few of us had got wind of rumours spreading that MSF had invented the Ebola case to give us a reason to remain in the country. These, coupled with the brewing anxiety caused by the Vice President's comments, made for additional security concerns.

Prior to Mariatu's case, we had been screening and triaging all patients for signs which could indicate the disease. The definition of Ebola suspicion changes according to the context; the 'non-outbreak' setting accepts most people will not have Ebola and therefore focuses on non-response to treatment. Once a case is confirmed, the definition reverts to 'outbreak', which is wide and general. There is a fine balance between help and harm during the screening process. If patients and their symptoms are not scrutinized properly, this can result in the unnecessary isolation of many (easily treatable) conditions. We carefully questioned each patient, and used universal precautions for everyone. But this took time, delaying treatment. The Ebola state of mind insidiously resurrected itself.

We tweaked the already developed protocols for the project on the identification of Ebola-suspected patients. There was agreement that diagnosis of any suspect cases should be made in collaboration between MSF and the Ministry of Health, hence sharing the responsibility. Where there was uncertainty, an additional Ebola-experienced person would be called. In practice, this meant Ruth and I were permanently on call for any Ebola alerts that found their way to the hospital.

The government was quick to recreate 'voluntary quarantine' for the high-risk contacts of Mariatu in the home where she had died. Similarly, the healthcare workers who had been in contact with her during her visit to the hospital were quarantined in one of the empty adult wards within the hospital.

As active case-finding activities began, suspected Ebola patients were sent in to the hospital from all over the district. Often, these were poor individuals who'd had the misfortune of answering 'yes' to questions that, on paper, spelt out E-B-O-L-A. However, with a bit of nuance and contextualization, they were almost never true suspects.

The maternal and child health project continued to receive more and more patients. Despite our attention now being stretched to the evolving Ebola response, we were also achieving our objective of maintaining and expanding routine healthcare.

In the dark days of late 2014, hospitals had become abandoned no-go areas. In Magburaka, the last bastion of the West African Ebola epidemic, the hospital was a hive of life-affirming activity. Women and children were choosing to navigate the risks of attending hospital, for the benefits of available healthcare.

Each day, I would run back and forth from the hospital front gate to give opinions on uncertain suspect cases. Back in maternity, I watched the triage of women being brought in by ambulance, training colleagues to apply common sense and no blanket rules for bleeding or stillbirths. Ruth and I would roam around the adult and paediatric wards, and the laboratory, to check in on staff, lend moral support and identify problems.

On Monday, the maternity ward was full with labouring women. Simultaneously, the front gate had a queue forming, as more patients attended, each one needing to go through a detailed screening and triage process to check for Ebola symptoms. While helping clear the backlog at the gate with Suma, I got an urgent call to return to maternity.

'There's a girl in distress. It's breech presentation. The baby isn't coming out.'

I could hear screaming in the background. Maternity was at the opposite end of the hospital. I left Suma and his team to continue triaging the queue and ran across the hospital compound.

There were three women in the room together, all in labour. The young girl I had been called about rolled around the bed, yelling and crying. An older woman stood next to her. I put on a gown, surgical cap, face shield, wellington boots and gloves, and plodded over to her.

'Let her know I'm going to touch her abdomen,' I said to the midwives in the room, 'and ask her to try to come on to her back'.

Her pregnant belly felt like a stone, as if tense in a continuous contraction. The girl let out another wail of pain. I looked at her, then moved my gaze to the woman standing next to her like a sentry.

'Did she get peppa?' I asked the room.

'What, Doctor?' said Kadiatu, startled by the abrupt question.

'Injection. Did she have the peppa injection?' I said, my eyes fixed on the older woman. 'Ask her.'

Kadiatu spoke to the older woman, the patient's mother-in-law, nodding and shaking her head.

'Yes, Doctor,' she shouted over wailing from the girl. 'She was given it.'

Oxytocin, the drug used as treatment for haemorrhage, was also available in the community. Referred to as *peppa*, it was given to speed up the birthing process. I recalled, from GRC, it was also a major cause of ruptured uteruses.

'How much?' I shouted back.

'Two – they injected two bottles.'

'Tell her I need to check what is happening inside.'

Carefully, I parted the girl's labia, expecting the breech to be visible. She must've begun pushing too early, I thought to myself as I slowly placed my fingers inside to feel how high the breech was. If we did not deliver this baby soon, her uterus would rupture. But something inside felt wrong.

The baby was not breech. I felt a hard, bony head, poised for birth. The membranes were still intact, pulled tight, bulging like a water bomb about to blow. She was fully dilated, but the baby's head remained high up. I skirted my fingers around the edge of the head, my little hands reaching to places others could not. I could feel something else, behind the baby's head.

'Everyone just wait,' I said, still uncertain what I was feeling, but concerned, if the waters broke, we could be in trouble. 'Don't rupture the membranes here. We need to go to theatre, fast.'

As we dashed to theatre, I called Amara to join me. The girl had a spinal anaesthetic block in preparation for possible surgery. This time, I broke the membranes. Clear amniotic fluid poured out as I moved my hand up further behind the baby's head.

'What the—?' I looked at Amara. 'Scrub for caesarean.'

I felt the head of another baby stuck behind the one trying to come down. Twins, entangled in one another. The oxytocin-induced contraction was trying to squeeze both of them through a hole designed for one at a time.

We rapidly cut open her abdomen, her uterus moments from rupturing. A transparent window had formed where the muscle fibres were pulling away from one another. I cut through it, releasing the tension, and yanked the babies out. Their screaming filled the room.

When I returned to the front gate, a new patient of concern was waiting. A fourteen-year-old girl from a house on the street where Mariatu had died was in the triage tent, with a fever and lethargy. I went back over the history Suma's team had taken. She probably had malaria, but the location of her residence seemed like too much of a coincidence. We needed to get a blood sample to confirm if she was negative for Ebola. We decided that Allan and I, together with a member of the Ministry of Health, would get into full PPE to isolate her. We planned ahead how we would get her inside the isolation area and what we would each do after. As before, the key was to be efficient. The Ministry of Health member would take blood for testing, then Allan and I would immediately begin treating her for malaria. I had not worn full Ebola PPE since a year earlier. I felt like I was entering a time warp as I began selecting the boots, apron and yellow plastic suit. I had not imagined being back in this situation.

Together, we carried the girl on a stretcher to an area where she could be seen, from across an orange fence, by her family. Allan and I had not worked side by side like this since Kailahun, back in August 2014. In silence, we operated in orchestral proficiency. Despite the sad scene of returning to the days of isolation and PPE, we were able to provide her with all the care she would have got in the general ward – a step forward, at least.

On the evening of Tuesday, 19 January, Mariatu's aunt, who had cared for her niece during her sickness and death, developed a fever. She was to be transferred to the hospital from the quarantine house for assessment on Wednesday. We had been expecting, sooner or later, contacts of the first case to develop symptoms. The challenge would be making sure they could be cared for, while maintaining normal hospital services. We were acutely aware of the fascination Mariatu's aunt provoked in the general public, both from those who feared she signified onward transmission and those who did not believe Ebola was back. We discreetly admitted her into isolation, away from prying eyes and far from the other patients.

A combination of local staff and Suma's team began taking a history of her illness. Ruth and I hung back, watching them take charge.

'Do you smell it?' Ruth asked me.

We had both been around long enough to recognize the subtle changes that came with Ebola infection – the exhausted effort of moving and a haziness in the eyes. The test was taken, but we both knew what the result would be.

Ruth and I chatted with her from across the orange isolation fence. She reminded me of so many of the earlier patients, having the same look of resignation to whatever will be.

Before the aunt's test was returned positive, we had pre-emptively mobilized counsellors to get the news to her before the local gossip spread. We were concerned about community reactions and quickly sorted out transfer to the new national Ebola referral centre at 34 Military Hospital, in Freetown. The day was not over though, as four more maternity ambulances arrived. We were successfully isolating and testing for Ebola, while a stone's throw away we continued to perform emergency surgery and resuscitate mothers and babies.

Local and international responders piled into Magburaka to exert their influence as the outbreak-response machine revved back into gear. For us, getting an early handle on the situation inside the hospital was vital, and securing it was essential; we could not let it fall to Ebola. The community's trust in us depended on it.

Increasingly, women were travelling to stay in the hospital at the end of pregnancy to wait for a safe delivery. I found this astonishing and took it as evidence we had the confidence of the people.

I had gone back to the base on Friday evening, at the end of a long and tiring week. The one-year anniversary of my grandmother's death was approaching and my younger cousin, back in Manchester, had got engaged. My extended family were gathered, celebrating and remembering. Sitting on the doorstep of the kitchen, thick and spicy groundnut soup in my bowl, I called home. I soon found myself on loud speaker to a silent room – a correspondent from the field. I heard gasps from the room in Manchester as I ran through my week. Finally, I had to bring the call to an end, as three of the women who had been waiting in the hospital were contracting at the same time, and I needed to return to them. Apologizing to my family, I hung up to the sound of them all shouting, 'Go, go!'.

One of the women was from a remote village, carrying twins, and they were born just before my arrival. Another woman was still in labour, having her eleventh child. I sat at the back of the delivery room, observing as the team cared for her without complication. The third woman, Sia, was twenty-five years old, in her seventh pregnancy and had no living children. All of her previous six pregnancies had resulted in stillbirth or

early death. Sia had been with us for several days, and we decided with
her to induce the labour to avoid another late stillbirth. She was a petite
woman. Her gravid uterus bulged under her skin, as if a separate entity
altogether. I had assumed she would have already given birth; we had
given her the medication in the morning and her body should have been
sensitive to its potency.

In the delivery room, Sia avoided eye contact. Her round face looked
like a currant balanced on a watermelon. She made no noise, gave no
expression to give away what was happening inside. Her demeanour hid
everything, except her terror. The team was uncertain what to do.

'Let's check,' I said.

The baby's head was low down, waiting for birth. It may have been
waiting for some time, his mother too frightened to push him out, afraid
history would repeat itself a seventh time. United, we gently coached her
through the final stages as she whimpered between her short pushes.

The baby was born with the umbilical cord wrapped tightly round his
neck. He showed no effort to breathe, his body limp and floppy.

We took him over to a resuscitation area, and began squeezing air into
his tiny lungs. We watched the blue skin transform to pink. A beautiful
cry cracked the silence. We took the boy for her to see. A delicate smile
flickered from the corners of her lips. But she did not put her arms out
for the boy. Colour drained from her face and her head dropped back. On
the floor below the delivery bed, blood was pooling. The blood gushed
out from her small body, her uterus floppy and unresponsive. Amara
attempted to examine her, but the blood filled too fast to see anything.

'Let's go to theatre,' I said, watching the blood rush out. We knew her
slight stature did not have the reserves to cope with a massive blood loss.
I ran from maternity, down the long corridor to the operating theatre.

'We need to go, now!' I shouted to the resting theatre team.

Grabbing the stretcher and running back to maternity, all I could
think was, *What if Sia has finally birthed a live baby, only to die from a
haemorrhage?*

We transferred her to the operating theatre, while giving more drugs
to stop the bleeding, but, like wine from a bottle, blood continued to
flow out. I squeezed her uterus with two hands till they hurt, then Amara
took over, and we swapped again once he tired, both of us willing it to
contract, to close off the vessels bleeding out.

'I'm going to see if we have anything else in the pharmacy,' I said to Amara, as he stood between her legs, leaning his body forward to give extra weight to his manual compression of her womb.

The pharmacy was back down the corridor by maternity. I searched through the wooden shelves and unpacked boxes for any drugs which were unavailable in the theatre, and for a balloon to put inside her womb. I grabbed what I could find and ran back to the theatre. As I scrubbed again, I saw the blood still spluttering out of Sia. We were heading towards a hysterectomy.

'Let's give it five more minutes,' I said, as I injected another drug in the hope it would awaken her uterine muscles. 'Did we find blood? Have you got the laparotomy set?' I said to John, the nurse anaesthetist.

'I think it's getting firmer!' shouted Amara, his hands still squeezing her womb.

'Let me feel,' I said, placing my hand on to her abdomen, where his had been. Finally, strength had returned and the bleeding abated. We stood and watched, waiting to ensure this wasn't a transient pause, expecting this to be false hope. But the drugs were working and the bleeding was no more.

The intensive care room we had created next to the delivery room already had a patient inside – a woman with severe pre-eclampsia, who had given birth earlier in the day, but continued to show signs of organ failure. We put another bed in for Sia; both women needed intense care.

I checked up on the other areas of the hospital and headed home as the sun was beginning to consider another day. The week had been exhausting, and, while I wouldn't have wanted to be anywhere else, I was feeling the toll.

I woke a couple of hours later to a text message from Ruth. She had heard me coming in around 4 a.m. and suggested I have a late start. I desperately needed the rest, but I needed to know the patients were improving first. I made a brief hospital round and was pleased to see both Sia and the woman with pre-eclampsia were showing positive signs of recovery. Sia was still too weak to hold her baby, but she lovingly gazed at her mother, who held and rocked him at the end of her bed.

Late morning, I returned to my room. It felt incredibly luxurious to lie down during the day, allowing my eyes to close and my mind to drift off.

It didn't last long.

'Sorry – I know you just left, but we have a situation here,' Ruth said over the mobile. The line was unclear, but I gathered there was a difficult case at the screening tent. Ruth and a Ministry of Health colleague were already involved, but they needed another opinion.

I returned to find the team struggling with an isolation decision. A nine-year-old girl had been brought in by her mother, with a high fever, diarrhoea, weakness, difficulty breathing and not eating. She had enough symptoms to firmly meet Ebola suspicion. The girl was visibly very sick, but most probably with severe malaria. In her critical condition, isolating her would limit the care she could receive. If we did not isolate her, though, we would be risking a very precarious situation. We questioned the mother again, who sat across the orange plastic fence from us, her daughter in her lap. She looked at us, the defendant facing the judge and jury. We searched for a way to justify the decision to admit her to the general paediatrics, but we knew we were cornered.

Together, we agreed to isolate her and then immediately begin resuscitation, intensive antimalarial and broad antibiotic treatment. Ebola demands speed control; nothing happens fast. As we got prepared to isolate, putting the protective clothing on, the girl's breathing slowed, then stopped. The mother still sat opposite us with her daughter on her lap, face to face with us and our verdict. We could not touch her, we could only throw a cloth over for the mother to wrap her daughter's body as she murmured and sobbed. The child had been labelled a suspect and we needed to maintain cool clinical management. The body had to be treated as if Ebola positive and the whole area decontaminated.

The posthumous test was negative. Ebola's brutality stung, not only for the illness it caused, but for the collateral damage it forced us to participate in.

As the team prepared to go in and collect the body, I watched one of them posing for a photo on their phone. This was not unusual. The PPE was new to several of the team members and there was both novelty and pride in being fully dressed in the iconic suits. It was though, too much for me, given the ongoing scene of mother and daughter. The tiredness and raw emotional drama unfolding punched me in the gut. I had to get away from it all. I could feel a volcano of emotions surging upwards within me and wanted to be alone.

'Thanks for coming!' Ruth shouted after me.

While there is no weakness in crying, at that moment it was the opposite of how I wanted to be perceived by the team. I locked myself in the office, pulled the curtains and wept. Pacing the room, I swore out loud a litany of expletives, till there were no words or feelings left.

The tests of conscience, ethics and clinical judgement kept coming. Each patient we discussed, we relied not only on the pro forma in front of us, but on our professional acumen and personal experiences. We worked hard to individualize the system, recognizing that adults, children and pregnant women presented differently, and we put more emphasis on travel and contact history than symptoms alone. The focus had shifted from finding a reason to isolate a patient, to finding a reason *not to*. This change reflected that, though we were back in an 'outbreak', we were a long way from the circumstances of 2014. There is no perfect, but there is being human and trying to do the best that can be done in a far from perfect situation.

As the next week began, we welcomed the arrival of extra team members who were flown in by MSF to help support us. The familiar faces of Marcio, Hilde, Grazia and Tina were among those who arrived. The 'emergency' phase, though, was largely over in Magburaka. They travelled further north to support with outreach activities and the clinical trial of the Ebola vaccination in Kambia. Replacements for Ruth and me also arrived, alongside a greater international presence for the standard project.

There were no further cases of Ebola following Mariatu's aunt. On 4 February, we heard she had tested negative in Freetown, following treatment. She was now an Ebola survivor, and the dragon's final puff of smoke in the entire 2014 to 2016 Ebola epidemic of Sierra Leone. On her return to Magburaka, she visited the hospital and asked if she could work with us. There could be no greater endorsement than that.

30: NOT NORMAL

LONDON

MAY 2020

'Are you Stacy?'

A face-mask-clad woman looked up from a reclining chair. On her chalk-white pregnant abdomen were the two cylinders of a fetal heart rate monitor, held in place with blue elastic straps. The machine printed a long, jagged line, like an unending row of menacing little teeth.

'Yeah,' she said, looking up briefly, before looking back at her hands, inspecting their short, bitten fingernails.

'You came to the hospital because your baby stopped moving? It says here you haven't felt anything for –' I looked at the paper handed to me – 'six days?'.

'Yeah, he just went quiet.'

'Six days without feeling movements is a long time, Stacey. Is there any reason you didn't come in earlier?' I asked, wondering about domestic violence.

'I'm scared of the coronavirus. And I heard I couldn't come with anyone to the hospital. I didn't know.' She turned to look at the monitor. 'Is he OK?'

'Yes, he's fine,' I said, folding the printed heart rhythm. 'Are you OK if we talk a bit more about options, going forward?'

As I walked down the long hospital corridor, I scrolled through news apps on my phone. There was an article about increasing numbers of women opting to freebirth – a home birth without any trained birth attendant. There was another article about New York hospitals refusing entry of birth partners, and a series of interviews with women on how they were feeling about the sudden changes in protocol. A picture of a woman with long brown hair popped up. *Birth Under Lockdown*, it read. In the article, she told her story of labour and birth at another local hospital, claiming her partner was only allowed in at the moment of birth and was sent away shortly after. She said she was left to labour alone. I struggled to believe the story, but then, I wasn't there. *This is the opposite of community engagement*, I thought. *Actually, where is the community engagement?* I asked myself as I entered the staff room.

I made myself a coffee and watched my colleagues gathering for our meeting. We formed an irregular circle of chairs, awkwardly placed in an effort to maintain social distancing. I recalled sitting in a circle of community elders, back in 2016. Their faces had been marked with deep creases, their voices measured and low. They had shared their collective trauma with me. I remembered the feeling of surprise when their voices turned to anger.

We will not let the ambulance take our women. We watched as it came and took our people in that Ebola time. We never saw them again. If we hear the siren, we will throw stones.

Their concern and distress had been etched across their faces. Who to trust? What to believe? How to save a life?

'What do you think about letting partners come?' asked Jane, as I joined the meeting.

'Look, I think we have to work towards keeping the service appealing. If women and their partners fear the hospital, they'll delay coming. We'll see worse outcomes – not from COVID, but because of what they read in the news or assume to be the case.'

'But we need to protect ourselves,' interrupted Lauren. 'We're saying, "Keep people out of the hospital", "Protect The NHS" and all that, you know? How can we then say partners can waltz in and out?'

'We have to strike a balance,' I said, looking around the room at my colleagues. 'We have to avoid knee-jerk reactions. I understand our colleagues are frightened, but so are our patients. We need to listen to them all, hear the concerns of the staff and work with them to build confidence and safety. Communicate with the patients, engage with our communities and help them to continue accessing services. If a woman avoids the hospital because she's frightened of being alone, the risks of having a poor outcome are going to be higher.'

The conversation continued, ebbed and flowed. We talked ourselves around in circles, dissecting assumptions from reality, retrieving evidence-based practice from the media hysteria that had infiltrated our own perceptions.

'Are you OK?' Jane asked as we left the staff room and headed back towards the labour ward. I have known Jane since my first job as a junior obstetrician. She sensed my discomfort.

'I'm working on something else. I've been getting some messages from refugee camps overseas. How will they manage if their staff don't have the correct protection? If they can't get drugs? If the people can't travel? We're looking at a situation where the health service stops functioning. It's not COVID concerning me, it's the collapse of reproductive health-care. We're talking about handing out clean delivery kits to pregnant women. A bar of soap, a razor blade, some plastic sheeting. Distributing these kits for community usage, preparing for a worst-case scenario.'

Jane and I walked on to our labour ward, where the citrus and chlorine scent of detergent hit my eyes and nostrils.

'You know, Jane,' I said, 'when this is over, do you think we will have learnt anything? Surely, we can't go back to the way it was before?'.

Jane looked along the corridor – trolleys of PPE outside labour rooms. 'When this is over? When.'

*

TONKOLILI, SIERRA LEONE

FEBRUARY/MARCH 2016

The end of Ebola was not the end of the emergency, just as the start had never been the beginning. Women and children continued to face difficulties in accessing healthcare, and continued to die at unacceptable levels. With the boost in numbers of locally employed and international staff at the project, and as the most recent Ebola outbreak dwindled away, we were able to divert our energy towards the community.

The epidemic had taught us the importance of listening and engaging with all the community. The same was true for understanding the underlying factors leading to poor health outcomes. As we spent more time out in the surrounding villages, it became increasingly apparent that the complex backdrop of issues dictating how and when a community decided to seek healthcare for a pregnant woman were paralleled with those which had exposed the country to the spread of Ebola.

Together with colleagues from the hospital, we travelled out to villages and peripheral health units across Tonkolili District. Our aims were multiple: for the hospital workers to see and understand the villagers' perspectives, and for us to investigate the main barriers faced by the people and their health workers. Then, to begin discussions on how to work together to overcome them.

Early one morning in February, I sat in the compound before the others had risen, drinking my usual strong coffee and listening to the birds and the occasional buzz of a motorbike passing outside the gate. The cool air washed over my skin and I breathed it in, tasting the scent of burning from the nearby villages. My mobile phone abruptly flashed with Kadiatu's number on the display screen.

'Good morning, Kadiatu,' I said, taking another slurp of coffee.

'Good morning, Doctor. No, no – it is not a good morning.'

I looked over to where the guards slept and wondered if the driver was in there. I could see the car was parked near the gate.

'We have started this day in the worst way, Doctor. An ambulance arrived from Yoni Cheifdom with a thirty-two-year-old mother. She has six living children. She is in late pregnancy with this one. At her farming village, out in Yoni, she had bleeding – no pain, Doctor. Bleeding, but not in labour. It started early yesterday morning.' Kadiatu spat this last detail, her voice jumping in tone and force. 'She told her husband. They did not wait. They walked together, six miles, to the health centre. She was clever. She knew something was wrong. The staff were not at the clinic, so he waited to be seen. When the clinic staff came, they saw she was having a haemorrhage. Thirteen hours, Doctor. Thirteen hours they waited for the ambulance to come. They arrived here an hour ago.' Kadiatu stopped.

I waited a moment for her to catch up with herself. 'Kadiatu, what happened when she arrived?'

'She was in the back of the ambulance with her husband. She was very pale and gasping. We tried to find a vein. I called for another to come and help me. We searched, but it took time. Her heart rate was high, but we could not find the blood pressure. Then, I got the vein, but she stopped breathing. We tried, but she was already gone.'

The woman and her husband had done everything that could have been asked of them. They recognized there was a problem and sought medical help early. But still she died. A personal disaster, with tragic repercussions for her husband, children and village.

After a few weeks, a small group of us travelled to her village. It was far in the hills of Yoni. Our journey, the reverse of hers, took us through cassava plantations, the star-shaped leaves bristling in the harmattan breeze. We passed rural settlements with houses made of solid red bricks, and others of timber and mud. Villagers watched us drive past from their doorsteps, rice grains spread outside on the red dust floor, drying in the sun. Small groups of women pounded rice with long heavy wooden pestles, bashing the husks off the grains. I wondered about pregnant women, the placental abruptions we saw and the vigour of their work. Chickens and goats ran out of the car's way as we juddered along the mud road from village to village. My anger at the life lost was challenged by my ignorance of the starting point – its distance, the difficulties. As we arrived, a young child, dressed only in dust, ran out shouting '*Opoto! Opoto!*' with excitement and fear. As we disembarked he darted back out of sight.

A crowd gathered around the vehicle and we asked where we could find the husband. A tall, wrinkled man pointed up a slope, off the road, to a row of mud houses. A man in his forties was sitting outside. I hesitated for a moment, wondering if he would direct his grief at us. But he was welcoming. We walked together to pay our respects at her grave. I felt overcome with emotion. I swallowed down as I thought, *Here lies a mother we could have, should have, saved.* The husband and his neighbours told their story.

'What is the point of a hospital if you can't get to it?' he asked me.

We followed the woman's journey to the health centre and listened to the staff there too. My mind had created a set of events which did not reflect the reality. We returned to the hospital in Magburaka to relay what we had learnt, all the while taking note of the geography. At every interaction, we came back to a single premise: there must be a better way.

As we collected the realizations shared from these meetings, we began formulating ways to overcome the barriers to healthcare. The stories coming from the villages were sombre: taxi drivers who would triple the price if a woman was bleeding; ambulance drivers who refused to drive unless receiving backhanders; traditional birth attendants who were afraid of penalty fines if a woman needed transferring from home. There were multiple tales of disrespectful care inside facilities. In some instances, the village feared the hospital, not only because of Ebola, but because it was far from familiar faces and familiar food. They feared not being able to afford the journey home – or, worse, if they died, their family would suffer financially to bring their body home. Some concluded it was better to die in the village. This was the choice pregnant women were making.

'It is a self-fulfilling argument,' I said to Ruth, after returning from a day of visiting outlying villages. 'All these barriers – the imagined and the real – they lead to late decision-making and very late arrivals to the hospital. By the time she gets here, we are already in a losing battle. If you think you will die at the hospital, then you avoid going there. The idea alone terrifies you. You wait, till finally no other option remains. Death in the village, or try the hospital. You arrive in extremis and die. You prove the point, and your corpse reinforces the message to the other women.'

Ruth looked out to the hills. 'We need to hear and connect,' she said. 'Understand their thought process. The rationale behind the decisions. We must learn from them, re-evaluate the role we play in their journey.'

Some of the villages we went to had been hit hard by Ebola. There were houses boarded up, no-go areas left for the ghosts to wander. I wondered if I had treated some of those who had once occupied these eerie spaces.

In one village, with the abandoned houses looming behind us, we held a group meeting. Men, women and children gathered in a circle. The last time they had seen MSF vehicles was at the height of the epidemic. Antony and Kadiatu led the discussions. They spoke the same local dialect and were excellent at engaging with those sitting before us. The villagers' concern, as was often the case, was that Ebola was thought to be back inside the hospital. Antony was honest and open. He confirmed there had been Ebola, and explained how the hospital was safe. He worked hard to impart the gains of coming early when there were complications. He invited their responses, listening and reflecting on their specific worries. His closing words, spoken like a commandment, took everyone's breath away:

'It is not normal for your sister to die giving birth.'

The crowd stared in silence. A few women lowered their heads into their hands. Every person knew a woman who had died from pregnancy complications. It was a moment of respect for those departed, and a realization that change was, and continues to be, possible.

Ruth, Sam and I left Magburaka together at the start of March. Over twenty-one days had passed with no further Ebola cases, and, though we were still shy of the forty-two days to officially declare the outbreak over, we knew it was our time to go. Loic, a free-spirited Dutch doctor, was sent as my replacement. He had been in the project for several weeks already, and my continued presence, rather than supporting his transition, now risked undermining him. It was time for new blood, without the baggage and history Ruth and I shared, to inject a different energy and emphasis into the project. Maura, an American midwife who had worked in Yemen and South Sudan, arrived and dedicated herself to the peripheral health units, while finally a paediatrician also joined the international team. In the week running up to our departure, I spent my time being present, soaking up the company of my local colleagues, reminiscing with them about the different projects we had worked in together and the life-changing times we had shared.

It was a charged goodbye. The days of GRC hung heavily on my mind, as they always had. The closure of the facility and ethical conundrums to which I never found answers or peace.

As I passed through Freetown, I was debriefed by Sarah, who asked what this mission had meant to me. I thought for a moment, but the truth stung: I wanted absolution – to find a small way to repair our failings to women and their communities over the previous years. I knew we never could, but I hoped we had planted a seed that would grow into something stronger for the future.

AFTERWORD

LONDON

JANUARY 2019

> *Dear Dr Benjamin, I received your letter. I was thinking, how can you remember all these things? I was so happy. Fatmata.*

> *Dr Benjamin! I will be a happy man the day I lay my hands on a copy of that book. We need a documentary of all the events which happened during those years. My best regards, Suma.*

I read the WhatsApp messages again. As if in a bottle on the seashore, each time I opened them, the aroma of Sierra Leone escaped. The testimony we shared, the lives we remembered.

'I want to call it *Belly Woman*,' I told Suma, a year later.

'A book for the *be'len''uman dem*,' he reflected. Suma flipped the words on his tongue, feeling out the syllables, making judgement. 'Yes, *The Belly Woman Book* – they should have their story told. It is our legacy.'

*

LONDON

APRIL 2021

The warmth of the sun heated my back as I jogged up the slope of the north London park. Small crowds gathered together, their music playing and drinks flowing. There was a holiday feeling. I took deep breaths as I climbed the steepest part of the hill. The air was pungent with dope. I thought how it smelt as green as the grass below my feet, and laughed to myself as I continued my usual route round the summit and back down into the village.

Pictures of rainbows decorated the sash windows facing out to the street. *Thank You NHS*, was written below one. *Heroes*, claimed another. Walking towards me were a young couple, deep in conversation, wearing surgical face masks around their necks, like a fashion accessory. The woman pushed a ringlet of hair behind her ear with her hand. The blue latex glove made me shudder as she went on to scratch the corner of her mouth. I heard Juli's voice in my head: *If you have gloves on your hands, it means they are dirty.* The thought transported me to GRC and the struggle to spread the message of infection control, that it's not only the gloves protecting you, but your behaviour too. Our inability to have a consistent approach to preventative measures and our fear of hospital-acquired Ebola infections had tipped us over the edge.

Would our actions have been different, knowing what we know now? I believed they would.

COVID-19 is very different to Ebola. But still, we have all lived in an epidemic now and the parallels are startling. The spreading and belief of rumours and fake news. The difficulty the public and health professionals have with grasping infection control principles. The struggles to recognize the disease, test for it and trace the exposed. The emptying of health facilities, loss of access to services and increase in demand. The battle of politics over lives. The feeling of a tsunami cresting in freeze-frame – bit by bit, waiting for the crash, watching, hypnotized, expecting the tide to turn.

'Us' and 'them' is an illusion. He who is 'them' today, can be 'us' tomorrow. That is not to say we are all the same – we are not. The playing field is not level. We each have our own struggles, coping strategies and resilience. The participation and opinions of the most affected populations should be central to informing actions, yet these are often side-lined or overlooked. There are divisions of power, culture and wealth; these, though, should not be mistaken for divisions of capability, knowledge and wisdom.

Medical and social advances over the years from where this story began have been astonishing. The last epidemics of Ebola have pushed forward innovations in isolation facilities, allowing for more human interaction and less PPE. Large multidrug trials have demonstrated treatments which can significantly increase survival rates, and ZMapp was not proven to be one of them.

The development of Ebola rapid diagnostic tests, also known as 'antigen' or 'lateral flow' tests, offer hope for quicker and earlier results, without requiring transfer to an ETC first. There are safe and effective Ebola vaccines available. Pregnant women have been included in studies, providing precious knowledge on how to care for them. Infected women have survived and birthed surviving infants. But the overall survival rate for all people infected has remained elusively unchanged. The collision of medical science, human nature and the mysteries of the natural world builds a house of mirrors. The way out is not as clear as we may first think, but, from above, we are less lost than we had assumed.

The progress riddles me with guilt. I reside in a world built out of the decisions from the past, judged by the knowledge of the future. *If only*, I say to myself, *we had known then what we know now*. I've learnt *medical facts* are not to be taken at face value; they are to be questioned. Within objective measurements are layers of hidden detail and subjective influences. Mortality from Ebola at the start of the West African outbreak was generally thought to be 70 per cent; for pregnant women, it was thought to be between 80 and 90 per cent. As community knowledge improved, case management developed and international and local efforts picked up pace, the mortality rate declined. Infection with Ebola remained a very serious diagnosis, but, rather than a probable death, there was roughly a fifty-fifty survival ratio. Pregnant women were found no less likely to survive; given the same opportunity for care as their non-pregnant counterparts, they had the same survival rate. Which begs the question, what is the greatest risk factor for a pregnant woman? Pregnancy, or the expectations of the health-care systems on which she relies? In February 2020, the WHO replaced its guidance for managing pregnant women and Ebola, removing the damaging and dangerous guidance which had given credibility to stigmatization.

We have been on another journey with COVID-19. The WHO were proactive, outspoken and direct in advocating for a response. The reaction of each nation state and the repercussions of their decisions will be reckoned for generations to come.

As was the case in West Africa, organizations are only as good as the people working within them. I truly believe no person or organization entered the Ebola response without good intentions. The depth of those intentions, though, can be eclipsed by the shadow of the ego. The door to the world of new and emerging infections swung open with COVID-19.

There's a danger when everyone is an expert. When everyone is shouting for attention, it is harder to hear those who speak sense. Epidemics, like any emergency, are developing and dynamic situations; all of us should remain grounded, open to being corrected and re-evaluating the truths we understood yesterday. Truth can change. Egos can kill.

No person, organization or institution is beyond criticism. Neither are we immune to praise. The physical and emotional exhaustion of being immersed in an emergency can tempt us to focus on the negative. The intensity reminds us of a universal objective – to reduce suffering. After all, this is what it means to be a humanitarian.

The siren of a passing ambulance broke my internal monologue. I stopped jogging for a moment and watched the florescent yellow box on wheels continue its journey. I took deep breaths, filling my lungs and holding down the air. My heart pulsated, banging against my ribs. I felt life hitting me. I looked at my phone for the time, and a series of WhatsApp messages from Sierra Leone greeted me. *Dr Benjamin, we have a serious case.* I swiped the screen, my mind switching to obstetrician. Wherever I am, Sierra Leone is never far away.

Pregnancy and birth outcomes are the most divergent of all global health survival statistics. Yet this is the cord connecting us all; everyone was born. In January 2020, I returned to Magburaka. The drama, despair and deaths continue, as does the survival. The project which began in 2016 continues to work all hours of all days to fight for a woman's right to life. More women come now than ever before. The Sierra Leone National Emergency Medical Service began in October 2018; if functional, the coordinated system of ambulances has a huge potential for reducing the delays women face. The Ministry of Health and Sanitation, together with partner organizations, continue to strive for better, aspiring for gold standards and hoping for the resources to achieve their goals. There are still many hurdles, but for each woman who returns home alive and healthy, she takes with her a message of hope. *It is normal to live.*

As an obstetrician, I meet many women and their partners as they navigate their pregnancy journey. I often never know how those journeys end. I get a flash of the story, one angle only: an antenatal visit, the moment of birth, the post-partum haemorrhage – a single chapter in a book, closed before I can read on. The Mr and Mrs Johnsons of my world come and go with their pre-eclampsia and expectations, as do I from theirs. It is not possible to remember them all, but I am thankful to each of them. Every interaction brings a new lesson, or refreshes learning forgotten. Walking to and from work, I reflect on the patients I have seen. My mind often wanders back to the Ebola camps of 2014; the haunting images evoke a visceral reaction within me. The two young brothers and my whispered promise to them still blows through me. Those days, those promises, I will carry with me for all my life – as will my colleagues working today in the most modern hospital intensive care units. They too will remember a time of death, a time when all we could do as health workers was support the body and hold the hands of the dying when their families could not. They will remember a time when demand outstripped nurses, ventilators and hospital beds; the impossible decisions faced when resources are rationed. They too will ask questions: *Could it have been different?*

The warning alarm was sounded early on how the COVID-19 pandemic could impact women's access to healthcare. As with Ebola, devastating predictions of an apocalypse on reproductive health arrived: between 12,000 to over 56,000 additional maternal deaths in low- and middle-income countries; an extra 49 million women without access to contraception; 15 million more unintended pregnancies; 3 million more unsafe abortions and over 160,000 newborn deaths. It is thought these worst-case scenarios did not materialize, however the disruption to women's healthcare remained staggering. We may never know the full extent or scale of the consequences.

COVID-19, like Ebola before it, has been declared 'unprecedented', 'unchartered territory' and we've been told 'lessons need to be learnt'. These are meaningless excuses, pre-emptive of failure. The alibi should fool no one. Lessons have been identified repeatedly, and ignored repeatedly. Though the spread and scale have been overwhelming, they have overwhelmed *because* we did not heed the precedent set by epidemics and emergencies of the recent past.

As with pregnancy-related deaths, catastrophe was avoidable in the West African Ebola epidemic. In time, the same may be said for the COVID-19 pandemic. Until we respond to global inequalities, ignored abuses, corrupt systems and the arrogance of the powerful, these tragic events will persist.

The dragon will continue to move among us.

ACKNOWLEDGEMENTS

Among other things, *Belly Woman* is the story of a journey. To all those who travelled alongside me and to my friends in Sierra Leone, this is your story as much as it is mine. Thank you for your friendship, comradery and light humour in dark times. I hope I have remembered well and shared correctly.

To my parents, Lida and Malcolm, without you I'd be no one. Thank you for your infinite support, listening to my endless worries and sharing every page of this story in life and literature. I hope I have made you as proud to be my parents, as I am to be your son.

The effort to get *Belly Woman* to publication has been another journey, albeit of a different nature. I have been incredibly fortunate to have encountered much selfless generosity from people who owed me nothing and asked for nothing in return.

Thank you to Archna Sharma at Neem Tree Press for giving a home to *Belly Woman* and believing in sharing the story as much as I do. Your trust in this book and what it has to offer has been everything I needed to get past the finishing line. Thanks to Jade McGrath and all the Neem Tree family. Thanks to Penelope Price for her expertise and forensic eye, and to James Jones for creating a cover with thought and meaning.

Thank you to Michela Wrong for your unwavering support, advice and excellent company on crisp autumn walks, and to Niraj Shah for always listening, even when I was bored of my own voice. Don't go thinking publication gets either of you off the hook; there's plenty more drinks, dinners and debates to be had.

Thanks to all those who gave their time, thoughts and honesty by reading part or all of the developing manuscript. Special thanks to Arieh Doobov for reading the very first draft, rolling-up your sleeves and diving right in. Thank you to Mez Aref-Adib, Rosamund Southgate, Jane Laking, Geraldine O'Hara, Gillian McKay, Alice Janvrin, Emily Paul, Alexandra Singer, Charlotte Foley, Shelley Lees, James Smith, Sam Hoare, Donald Campbell, Leah Deutsch, Silje Lehne Michalsen and

Jane McKenzie for being generous with your time and opinions. Thanks to Carolyn Paul for your obstetric and literary wisdom, and for the introduction to the wonderful Sara Patel. Sara, thank you for your detailed review and guidance, it has been invaluable.

I entered the world of book writing ignorant of its complexities, pitfalls and peculiarities. My thanks for the guidance and wisdom of Cristina Whitecross, Leah Hazard, Aminatta Forna, Jonathan Conway, Clare Bullock, David Godwin and family, Angela and Mikaela Lee, Francesca Segal, Ross Russell, Jen Christie, Debbie Owen, Damien Brown, Richard Arcus, Maria Carter and Aisha Fofana Ibrahim. Thank you to Jana Sommerlad for your confidence in *Belly Woman* from the outset, and helping me cut through the crap.

To Regina Spektor, thank you for your generosity in giving me permission to use a lyric from your beautiful song *Laughing With* as a chapter title. Your support means a lot.

Belly Woman would not exist had MSF not offered me my first position in Sierra Leone. Thank you to Brigitte Daubeny for getting me in and pushing me forward. MSF is an inspirational and dynamic organisation; everyday countless peoples' lives are better because it exists. There are too many colleagues and friends to mention, but I extend special thanks to Severine Caluwaerts for her mentorship and voice of reason. I also want to thank colleagues Daphne Lagrou and Eva De Plecker for their patience with me when I was in at the deep end. Ruth Kauffman, without your determination this would have been a much shorter story, thank for all you have taught me.

Thank you to Lindsay West for validating my desire to take a different career path. To all my friends and colleagues at The Whittington, Royal Free and Homerton University Hospitals: thank you for shaping me into the doctor I am today.

To my big, loud family in Manchester, London and Tel Aviv: thank you for accepting me as I am, never asking me to be anyone else and making me proud of where I come from. This book is for you too.

Thanks to Fareed Shiva for sharing several years' worth of evenings, weekends and holidays with *Belly Woman*. Thank you for your patience, hospitality and making me laugh when nothing and no one else could.

Finally, thank you to every person who has taken the time to read or listen to *Belly Woman*. As we all know now, the end of this book is far from the end of the story.

Médecins Sans Frontières (MSF) is an international, medical humanitarian organization working in more than seventy countries around the world. Their medical teams act fast to save people's lives in conflict zones, natural disasters and epidemics. To find out more, or to donate, visit: www.msf.org.uk.

CapaCare is a non-profit humanitarian organization dedicated to medical education and training. Their work includes the surgical training of community health officers in Sierra Leone and life-saving maternal healthcare. To find out more, or to donate, visit: www.capacare.org.

END NOTES

Author's note: Person, Position and Purpose

An advocacy paper for sexual and reproductive health rights to be integrated into epidemics: McKay G, Black B, Mbambu Kahamba S, Wheeler E, Mearns S, Janvrin A. *Not All That Bleeds is Ebola: How has the DRC Ebola Outbreak Impacted Sexual and Reproductive Health in North-Kivu?* (Rescue Committee, New York, 2019).

For each death, approximately thirty women are severely or permanently disabled through complications of pregnancy: Firoz T, Chou, D von Dadelszen P, Agrawal P, Vanderkruik R, Tunçalp O, *et al.* 'Measuring maternal health: focus on maternal morbidity.' *Bulletin of the World Health Organization* 91(10), 2013, 794–96 (doi: 10.2471/BLT.13.117564).

The spread of the disease is symptomatic of the status quo: Milne A. 'UK under fire for suggesting coronavirus "great leveller"' (Reuters, 9 April 2020). Available at: https://www.reuters.com/article/us-health-coronavirus-leveller-trfn/uk-under-fire-for-suggesting-coronavirus-great-leveller-idUSKCN21R30P [cited 18 May 2020]. And: Timothy R. 'Coronavirus is not the great equalizer – race matters' (*The Conversation*, 6 April 2020). Available at: https://theconversation.com/coronavirus-is-not-the-great-equalizer-race-matters-133867 [cited 18 May 2020].

Chapter 1: Birth Complications

A woman dies every two minutes from a pregnancy-related complication: *Maternal Mortality* (WHO, 19 September 2019.) Available at: https://www.who.int/news-room/fact-sheets/detail/maternal-mortality [cited 5 December 2021].

Her death will be tragic, not only for herself and her children: Moucheraud C, Worku A, Molla M, Finlay JE, Leaning J, Yamin A. 'Consequences of maternal mortality on infant and child survival: a 25-year longitudinal analysis in Butajira Ethiopia (1987–2011).' *Reproductive Health* 12(Suppl.1), 2015, S4 (doi: 10.1186/1742-4755-12-S1-S4).

It will be the loss of all the functions she, as a woman, brings to society: Gill K, Pande R, Malhotra A. 'Women deliver for development.' *The Lancet* 370(9595), 2007, 1347–57 (doi: 10.1016/S0140-6736(07)61577-3).

Almost all maternal deaths occur in poor countries: *Maternal Mortality* (WHO, 19 September 2019). Available at: https://www.who.int/news-room/fact-sheets/detail/maternal-mortality [cited 5 December 2021].

If this is Ebola, it changes everything: Black B, Caluwaerts S, Achar J. 'Ebola viral disease and pregnancy.' *Obstetric Medicine* 8(3), 2015, 108–13 (doi: 10.1177/1753495X15597354).

Ebola virus disease: Kadanali A, Karagoz G. 'An overview of Ebola virus disease.' *Northern Clinics of Istanbul* 2(1), 24 April 2015, 81–86 (doi: 10.14744/nci.2015.97269).

The risk of infection for healthcare workers: *Health Worker Ebola Infections in Guinea, Liberia and Sierra Leone* (WHO, 21 April 2015). Available at: https://www.who.int/hrh/documents/21may2015_web_final.pdf [cited 20 November 2018].

There had been rumours of suspicious deaths for months: Sack K, Fink, S, Belluck P, Nossiter A. 'How Ebola roared back.' *New York Times*, 30 December 2014. Available at: https://www.nytimes.com/2014/12/30/health/how-ebola-roared-back.html [cited 8 November 2021].

First confirmed cases of Ebola in the country: Wauquier N, Bangura J, Moses L, *et al.* 'Understanding the emergence of Ebola virus disease in Sierra Leone: stalking the virus in the threatening wake of emergence.' *PLoS Currents* 7, 20 April 2015 (doi: 10.1371/currents.outbreaks.9a6530ab7bb9096b34143230ab01cdef).

Female traditional healer from Kailahun: *Sierra Leone: A Traditional Healer and a Funeral* (WHO, 1 September 2015). Available at: https://www.who.int/news/item/01-09-2015-sierra-leone-a-traditional-healer-and-a-funeral [cited 20 November 2018].

West African Ebola epidemic reported 28,616 cases, including 11,325 deaths: Ohimain EI, Silas-Olu D. 'The 2013–2016 Ebola virus disease outbreak in West Africa.' *Current Opinion in Pharmacology* 60, 2021, 360–65 (doi: 10.1016/j.coph.2021.08.002). And: *2014–2016 Ebola Outbreak in West Africa* (Centers for Disease Control and Prevention, 8 March 2019). Available at: https://www.cdc.gov/vhf/ebola/history/2014-2016-outbreak/index.html [cited 5 December 2021].

Resulting deaths from the loss and fear of healthcare: Wilhelm JA, Helleringer S. 'Utilization of non-Ebola health care services during Ebola outbreaks: a systematic review and meta-analysis'. *Journal of Global Health* 9(1), 2019, 010406 (doi: 10.7189/jogh.09.010406). And: Parpia AS, Ndeffo-Mbah ML, Wenzel NS, Galvani AP. 'Effects of response to 2014–2015 Ebola outbreak on deaths from malaria, HIV/AIDS, and tuberculosis, West Africa.' *Emerging*

Infectious Diseases 22(3), 2016), 433–41 (doi: 10.3201/eid2203.150977. And: Mæstad O, Shumbullo E. *Ebola Outbreak 2014–2016: Effects on other Health Services* (CMI Chr. Michelsen Institute, 2020); available at: https://www.cmi. no/publications/7212-ebola-outbreak-2014-2016-effects-on-other-health-services [cited 1 March 2022].

Chapter 2: Pre-Departure Planning

Sierra Leone had the highest ratio of women dying to live births: *Trends in Maternal Mortality: 1990 to 2013.* Estimates by WHO, UNICEF, UNFPA, The World Bank and the United Nations Population Division (WHO, 2014).

60 per cent decrease in women dying from childbirth: *Safe Delivery: Reducing Maternal Mortality in Sierra Leone and Burundi* (Médecins Sans Frontières, 2012).

A fifth of all caesarean sections: Email to author from S. Caluwaerts (26 February 2016).

Initial suspicions and identification of the disease: Baize S, Pannetier D, Oestereich L, *et al.* 'Emergence of Zaire Ebola virus disease in Guinea.' *New England Journal of Medicine* 371(15), 2014, 1418–25 (doi: 10.1056/NEJMoa1404505).

Chapter 3: Gondama

One fifteen-year-old girl out of every twenty-one in Sierra Leone: *Trends in Maternal Mortality: 1990 to 2013. Estimates by WHO, UNICEF, UNFPA, The World Bank and the United Nations Population Division* (WHO, 2014).

Chapter 4: So Many I Stopped Counting

One fifth were carrying babies that had already died: Garry R. 'An obstetrician reborn.' *Journal of Obstetrics and Gynaecology* (*BJOG*) 120(8), 2013, 911–14 (doi: 10.1111/1471-0528.12131).

Women would shave their heads: Described by Peter Piot, one of the doctors who originally identified the Ebola virus in his book *No Time To Lose: A Life in Pursuit of Deadly Viruses* (New York: W. W. Norton & Co, 2012).

Chapter 5: Medical Roulette

Harrowing reports of ghost towns: Nossiter A. 'At heart of Ebola outbreak, a village frozen by fear and death.' *New York Times*, 11 August 2014. Available at: https://www.nytimes.com/2014/08/12/world/africa/at-heart-of-ebola-outbreak-a-village-frozen-by-fear-and-death.html [cited 21 November 2018].

Unsafe, illegal 'backstreet' abortions were estimated to account for over 10 per cent of all maternal deaths in the country: Paul M, Gebreselassie H, Samai M,

Benson J, Sas K. 'Unsafe abortion in Sierra Leone: an examination of costs and burden of treatment on healthcare resources.' *Journal of Women's Health Care* 4(2), 2015, 1–6 (doi: 10.4172/2167-0420.1000228).

Chapter 6: No One Laughs at God in a Hospital

No one laughs at God in a hospital: Chapter title taken from the lyrics of Spektor R, *Laughing With* (Sire Records, 2009).

The Sierra Leone Free Health Care Initiative had been launched by the government in 2010: Maxmen A. 'Sierra Leone's free health-care initiative: work in progress.' *The Lancet* 381(9862), 2013, 191–92 (doi: 10.1016/s0140-6736(13)60074-4).

Delays in recognizing, reaching and receiving treatment have long been accepted as the underlying reason for high maternal deaths: Thaddeus S, Maine D. 'Too far to walk: maternal mortality in context.' *Social Science & Medicine* 38(8), 1994, 1091–10 (doi: 10.1016/0277-9536(94)90226-7).

In the UK, a woman would not be left fully dilated: *Intrapartum Care for Healthy Women and Babies* (National Institute for Health and Care Excellence (NICE), 3 December 2014). Available at: https://www.nice.org.uk/guidance/cg190/resources/intrapartum-care-for-healthy-women-and-babies-pdf-35109866447557 [cited 15 October 2018].

Over twenty fewer than the WHO recommends for basic healthcare: Chen L, Evans T, Anand S, Boufford J, Brown H, Chowdhury M, *et al.* 'Human resources for health: overcoming the crisis.' *The Lancet* 364(9449), 2004, 1984–90 (doi: 10.1016/S0140-6736(04)17482-5).

Facilities themselves were often not fit for purpose: Abdullah I, Kamara AB. 'Confronting Ebola with bare hands: Sierra Leone's health sector on the eve of the Ebola epidemic.' In: I. Abdullah and I. Rashid (eds) *Understanding West Africa's Ebola Epidemic: Towards a Political Economy* (London: Zed Books, 2017), pp. 112–36.

Chapter 8: Below the Surface

Ethically, we were in no-man's-land: Black B. 'Obstetrics in the time of Ebola: challenges and dilemmas in providing lifesaving care during a deadly epidemic.' *British Journal of Obstetrics and Gynaecology* 122(3), 2015, 284–86 (doi: 10.1111/1471-0528.13232).

The official toll had surpassed 400 confirmed cases in Sierra Leone: *Ebola virus disease, West Africa – update 18 July 2014* (WHO, 18 July 2014). Available at: https://web.archive.org/web/20140725195212/http://www.afro.who.int/

en/clusters-a-programmes/dpc/epidemic-a-pandemic-alert-and-response/outbreak-news/4225-ebola-virus-disease-west-africa-18-july-2014.html [cited 7 December 2021].

Amniocentesis, removing a sample of amniotic fluid to test it for Ebola: Baggi F, Taybi A, Kurth A, van Herp M, Di Caro A, Wölfel R, *et al.* 'Management of pregnant women infected with Ebola virus in a treatment centre in Guinea, June 2014.' *Euro Surveillance: Bulletin Europeen sur les Maladies Transmissibles (European Communicable Disease Bulletin)* 19(49), 2014, 20983 (doi: 10.2807/1560-7917.es2014.19.49.20983).

Chapter 9: Unprecedented

Michel had worked in every major Ebola outbreak since 2000: van Herp M. 'Exclusive: A Médecins Sans Frontières specialist on how the unprecedented spread of the Ebola virus in West Africa makes the work of medics tougher than ever' (*Independent*, 12 April 2014). Available at: https://www.independent.co.uk/life-style/health-and-families/health-news/exclusive-a-m-decins-sans-frontires-specialist-on-how-the-unprecedented-spread-of-the-ebola-virus-9256670.html [cited 21 November 2018].

First confirmed Ebola case in Freetown: *Sierra Leone Hunts Ebola Patient Kidnapped in Freetown* (BBC News, 25 July 2014). Available at: https://www.bbc.co.uk/news/world-africa-28485041 [cited 24 November 2021].

MSF continued sounding the alarm: Press release: *Race Against Time to Control the Ebola Outbreak* (Médecins Sans Frontières, 11 July 2014). Available at: https://www.msf.org/sierra-leone-race-against-time-control-ebola-outbreak [cited 20 November 2018].

Samaritan's Purse: Dennis B. 'Ebola crisis provides glimpse into Samaritan's Purse, SIM' (*Washington Post*, 20 August 2014). Available at: https://www.washingtonpost.com/national/health-science/ebola-crisis-sheds-light-on-controversial-samaritans-purse/2014/08/20/0b9d670a-27b5-11e4-86ca-6f03cbd-15c1a_story.html?utm_term=.84959cbf870a [cited 20 November 2018].

Samaritan's Purse were willing, if done with support from MSF: Hurum L. 'A few days in July.' In: M. Hofman and S. Au (eds) *The Politics of Fear* (New York: Oxford University Press, 2017), pp. 51–59.

Kenema Government Hospital had high rates of internal Ebola transmission: Senga M, Pringle K, Ramsay A, *et al.* 'Factors underlying Ebola virus infection among health workers, Kenema, Sierra Leone, 2014–2015.' *Clinical Infectious Diseases* 63(4), 2016, 454–59 (doi: 10.1093/cid/ciw327).

Approximately 25 per cent of the patients in the Kenema ETC were staff:
O'Dempsey T. 'Failing Dr Khan.' In: M. Hofman and S. Au (eds) *The Politics of Fear* (New York: Oxford University Press, 2017), pp. 175–86.

Chapter 10: Kailahun

Police shot tear gas to disperse the crowd: Fofana U. *Ebola Center in Sierra Leone Under Guard After Protest March.* (Reuters, 26 July 2014). Available at: http://www.reuters.com/article/us-health-ebola-africa/ebola-center-in-sierra-leona-under-guard-after-protest-march-idUSKBN0FV0NL20140726 [cited 20 November 2018].

Through treating an infected pregnant woman: Bah C. 'Eurocentric epistemology: questioning the narrative on the epidemic's origin.' In: I. Abdullah and I. Rashid (eds) *Understanding West Africa's Ebola Epidemic: Towards a Political Economy* (London: Zed Books, 2017), pp. 47–65.

An experimental treatment called ZMapp: Crowe K. *Dying Sierra Leone. Dr Sheik Umar Khan Never Told Ebola Drug was Available* (CBC News, 18 August 2014). Available at: http://www.cbc.ca/news/health/dying-sierra-leone-dr-sheik-umar-khan-never-told-ebola-drug-was-available-1.2738163 [cited 20 November 2018].

The team was locked in a debate of medical ethics ... Every argument was convincing and every argument was flawed: O'Dempsey T. 'Failing Dr Khan.' In: M. Hofman and S. Au (eds) *The Politics of Fear* (New York: Oxford University Press, 2017), pp. 175–86. And: Pollack A. 'Opting against Ebola drug for ill African doctor.' *New York Times*, 12 August 2014. Available at: https://www.nytimes.com/2014/08/13/world/africa/ebola.html [cited 10 October 2021].

The team treating the Samaritan's Purse patients grappled with many of the same dilemmas: Mobula L. 'When potentially lifesaving drugs are both experimental and in very short supply: a clinician's story from the front lines of the battle against Ebola.' *American Journal of Tropical Medicine and Hygiene* 93(2), 2015, 210–11 (doi: 10.4269/ajtmh.15-0302).

Chapter 11: State of Emergency

WHO announced a Public Health Emergency of International Concern in the Democratic Republic of Congo: *Ebola Outbreak in the Democratic Republic of the Congo Declared a Public Health Emergency of International Concern* (WHO, 17 July 2019). Available at: https://www.who. int/news/item/17-07-2019-ebola-outbreak-in-the-democratic-republic-of-the-congo-declared-a-public-health-emergency-of-international-concern [cited 7 December 2021].

Emirates airline banned all flights to Conakry: Withnall A. 'Ebola outbreak: Emirates becomes first major international airline to suspend all flights to virus-affected region' (*Independent*, 3 August 2014. Available at: https://www.independent.co.uk/news/world/africa/ebola-outbreak-emirates-becomes-first-major-international-airline-to-suspend-all-flights-to-virusaffected-region-9644770.html [cited 22 November 2021].

Further international airlines followed suit: Anderson M. 'Ebola: airlines cancel more flights to affected countries.' *Guardian*, 22 August 2014. Available at: https://www.theguardian.com/society/2014/aug/22/ebola-airlines-cancel-flights-guinea-liberia-sierra-leone [cited 22 November 2021].

Where access was needed most: Agence France-Presse 'Ebola outbreak: airlines stop flights as US expert warns outbreak will "worsen"' (*Telegraph*, 28 August 2014). Available at: http://www.telegraph.co.uk/news/worldnews/ebola/11060487/Ebola-outbreak-Airlines-stop-flights-as-US-expert-warns-outbreak-will-worsen. html [cited 20 November 2018].

Chapter 12: Invisible Insurgents

Over forty healthcare workers from Kenema were infected with Ebola: Kilmarx PH, Clarke KR, Dietz PM, *et al.* 'Ebola virus disease in health care workers – Sierra Leone, 2014.' *Morbidity and Mortality Weekly Report*, 63(49), 2014, 1168–71.

At least twenty-two hospital staff dying: Nossiter A, Solomon B. 'T hose who serve Ebola victims soldier on'. *New York Times*, 23 August 2014. Available from https://www.nytimes.com/2014/08/24/world/africa/sierra-leone-if-they-survive-in-ebola-ward-they-work-on.html [cited 10 December 2021].

Ebola patients were able to walk freely in and out of isolation: Kratz T. 'The international aid response in Sierra Leone.' In: M. Hofman and S. Au (eds) *The Politics of Fear* (New York: Oxford University Press, 2017), pp. 85–100.

WHO had declared the Ebola epidemic to be a Public Health Emergency of International Concern: *Statement on the 1st meeting of the IHR Emergency Committee on the 2014 Ebola Outbreak in West Africa* (WHO, 8 August 2014). Available at: https://www.who.int/news/item/08-08-2014-statement-on-the-1st-meeting-of-the-ihr-emergency-committee-on-the-2014-ebola-outbreak-in-west-africa [cited 7 December 2018].

Over four months after accusing MSF of being 'alarmist': 'Ebola: pushed to the limit and beyond' (Médecins Sans Frontières International, 2015). Available at: https://www.msf.org/ebola-pushed-limit-and-beyond [cited 7 December 2018].

93 per cent and 89 per cent of women had died: Mupapa K, Mukundu W, Bwaka M, Kipasa M, De Roo A, Kuvula K, *et al.* 'Ebola hemorrhagic fever and pregnancy.' *Journal of Infectious Diseases* 179(Suppl.1), 1999, S11–12 (doi: 10.1086/514289). And: Report of an International Commission: 'Ebola haemorrhagic fever in Zaire, 1976.' *Bulletin of the World Health Organization* 56(2), 1978, 271–93.

Chapter 13: Two Young Brothers

Walking through the deserted wards to the area being used for Ebola isolation: Nossiter, A. '"Don't touch the walls": Ebola fears infect an African hospital.' *New York Times*, 7 August 2014. Available at: https://www.nytimes. com/2014/08/08/world/africa/dont-touch-the-walls-ebola-fears-infect-hospital.html [cited 21 November 2018].

The lack of ETC beds in the country: Beaubien J. *Tom Frieden's Ebola Assessment: The Risk is Increasing* (National Public Radio, 28 August 2014). Available at: https://www.npr.org/sections/goatsandsoda/2014/08/28/344017921/tom-friedens-ebola-assessment-the-risk-is-increasing [cited 12 November 2021].

The epidemic was out of control: Wolz A. 'Face to face with Ebola – an emergency care center in Sierra Leone.' *New England Journal of Medicine* 371, 12 (2014), 1081–83 (doi: 10.1056/NEJMp1410179).

Chapter 15: Exodus

Ebola viral load and survival: Fitzpatrick G, Vogt F, Moi Gbabai O, Decroo T, Keane M, de Clerck H, *et al.* 'The contribution of Ebola viral load at admission and other patient characteristics to mortality in a Médecins Sans Frontières Ebola Case Management Centre, Kailahun, Sierra Leone, June–October 2014.' *Journal of infectious Diseases* 212(11), 2015, 1752–58 (doi: 10.1093/infdis/jiv304).

Never had they known Ebola to visit their world before: Schoepp RJ, Rossi CA, Khan SH, Goba A, Fair JN. 'Undiagnosed acute viral febrile illnesses, Sierra Leone'. *Emerging Infectious Diseases* 20(7), 2014, 1176–82 (doi: 10.3201/eid2007.131265).

Senegal's refusal to allow flights from the most affected countries to land: Frankel T. 'Alarm grows as Ebola outbreak spurs more flight cancellations, border closures' (*Washington Post*, 25 August 2014). Available at: https://www.washingtonpost.com/world/africa/alarm-grows-as-ebola-outbreak-spurs-more-flight-cancellations-border-closures/2014/08/25/87e6d020-2c66-11e4-994d-202962a9150c_story.html [cited 1 February 2022].

Brussels Airlines' decision, alongside Royal Air Maroc, to maintain flights: Worland J. 'Why one airline flies to West Africa despite Ebola.' *Time*, 10 October 2014. Available at: http://time.com/3490961/brussels-airlines-ebola/ [cited 20 November 2018].

Chapter 16: Life in Limbo

Another American got infected: Jones A. 'Third American contracts Ebola. CDC warns epidemic "is out of control"' (*Gawker*, 2 September 2014). Available at: http://gawker.com/third-american-contracts-ebola-cdc-warns-epidemic-is-1629678249 [cited 20 November 2018].

All the Zmapp is gone: McCarthy M. 'US signs contract with ZMapp maker to accelerate development of the Ebola drug.' *British Medical Journal* 349(4 September 2014), g5488 (doi: 10.1136/bmj.g5488).

Doctor didn't treat Ebola patients yet still caught the virus: Poon L. 'US doctor didn't treat Ebola patients yet still caught the virus' (National Public Radio, 3 September 2014). Available at: http://www.npr.org/sections/goatsandsoda/2014/09/03/345535069/u-s-doctor-didnt-treat-ebola-patients-yet-still-caught-the-virus [cited 20 November 2018].

Recent financial cuts made to WHO: Fink S. 'Cuts at WHO hurt response to Ebola crisis.' *New York Times*, 3 September 2014. Available at: https://www.nytimes.com/2014/09/04/world/africa/cuts-at-who-hurt-response-to-ebola-crisis.html [cited 7 January 2019].

The conviction and heart of a genuine humanitarian: *Norwegian Aid Worker Recovers from Ebola* (Médecins Sans Frontières, 22 October 2014). Available at: https://www.doctorswithoutborders.org/what-we-do/news-stories/story/norwegian-aid-worker-recovers-ebola [cited 20 November 2018].

Chapter 17: Same, But Different

The entire 200-bed facility had closed down: Press release: *Sierra Leone: MSF Suspends Emergency Paediatric and Maternal Services in Gondama* (Médecins Sans Frontières, 15 October 2014.) Available at: https://www.msf.org/sierra-leone-msf-suspends-emergency-paediatric-and-maternal-services-gondama [cited 20 November 2018].

MSF International President, told the United Nations: Liu J. *United Nations Special Briefing on Ebola* (Médecins Sans Frontières, 2 September 2014). Available

at: https://www.doctorswithoutborders.org/what-we-do/news-stories/research/
united-nations-special-briefing-ebola [cited 20 November 2018].

Liberian President Ellen Johnson Sirleaf to US President Barack Obama:
Flynn D. *Liberian President Appeals to Obama for U.S. Help to Beat Ebola*
(Reuters, 13 September 2014). Available at: https://www.reuters.com/article/
health-ebola-usa/liberian-president-appeals-to-obama-for-u-s-help-to-beat-
ebola-idUSL5N0RE12I20140913 [cited 20 November 2018].

UK, US and France had announced ambitious responses: O'Grady S. *Colonial
Lines Drawn Again for Ebola Aid* (Foreign Policy, 22 September 2014.) Available
at: https://foreignpolicy.com/2014/09/22/colonial-lines-drawn-again-for-ebola-
aid [cited 20 November 2018].

MSF team leader, Jackson Naimah, addressed the Security Council: Naimah
J. *Statement to the United Nations Security Council Emergency Session on Ebola*
(Médecins Sans Frontières, 18 September 2014). Available at: https://www.
msf.org/msf-addresses-un-security-council-emergency-session-ebola [cited 1
December 2021].

**United Nations Mission for Ebola Emergency Response (UNMEER) was
established the following day:** *UN Announces Mission to Combat Ebola, Declares
Outbreak "Threat to Peace And Security* (UN News, 18 September 2014). Available
at: https://news.un.org/en/story/2014/09/477762-un-announces-mission-com-
bat-ebola-declares-outbreak-threat-peace-and-security [cited 1 December 2021].

Tasked with leading and coordinating the multitude of UN agencies: *UN Mission
for Ebola Emergency Response (UNMEER)* (United Nations, 2015). Available at:
https://ebolaresponse.un.org/un-mission-ebola-emergency-response-unmeer
[cited 1 December 2021].

Though there were concerns: Lupel A, Snyder M. *Reimagining Crisis Response:
Lessons from the UN's Ebola Mission'* (IPI Global Observatory, 28 February 2017).
Available at: https://theglobalobservatory.org/2017/02/ebola-unmeer-unit-
ed-nations-sierra-leone-liberia [cited 1 December 2021].

Sierra Leone began a three-day lockdown: Mark M. 'Ebola lockdown in Sierra
Leone: nationwide three-day curfew.' *Guardian*, 17 September 2014. Available at:
https://www.theguardian.com/society/2014/sep/17/ebola-three-day-shut-down-
sierra-leone [cited 1 December 2021].

Team of health workers and journalists . . . found murdered: Mark M. 'Bodies
found after Ebola health workers go missing in Guinea.' *Guardian*, 18 September
2014. Available at: https://www.theguardian.com/society/2014/sep/18/ebo-
la-health-workers-missing-guinea?CMP=twt_gu [cited 1 December 2021]. And:

Belluz J. *Ebola Health Team Found Dead* (Vox, 19 September 2014). Available at: https://www.vox.com/2014/9/18/6430563/ebola-virus-health-team-found-dead-in-guinea [cited 1 December 2021].

Returning New York doctor from an MSF project: Santora M. 'Doctor in New York City is sick with Ebola.' *New York Times,* 23 October 2014. Available at: https://www.nytimes.com/2014/10/24/nyregion/craig-spencer-is-tested-for-ebola-virus-at-bellevue-hospital-in-new-york-city.html [cited 20 November 2018].

Kaci Hickox was detained in a tent and quarantined against her will: Hanna J, Fantz A. *Maine Nurse Won't Submit To Ebola Quarantine, Lawyer Says* (CNN, 29 October 2014). Available at: https://edition.cnn.com/2014/10/29/health/us-ebola/index.html [cited 20 November 2018].

Five new infections were occurring each hour: Weaver M, Boseley S. 'Ebola infecting five new people every hour in Sierra Leone, figures show.' *Guardian,* 2 October 2014. Available at: https://www.theguardian.com/world/2014/oct/02/ebola-infecting-five-every-hour-sierra-leone [cited 20 November 2018].

As is done with Himalayan communities: Rushwan H. 'Misoprostol: an essential medicine for managing postpartum hemorrhage in low-resource settings?' *International Journal of Gynaecology and Obstetrics* 114(3), 2011, 209–10 (doi: 10.1016/j.ijgo.2011.06.006).

Risk of transmission from breastmilk: Bausch DG, Towner JS, Dowell SF, et al. 'Assessment of the risk of Ebola virus transmission from bodily fluids and fomites.' *Journal of Infectious Diseases* 196(Suppl. 2), 2007, S142–47 (doi: 10.1086/520545).

Chapter 18: Belly Woman

The standard test being used in the outbreak was a form of polymerase chain reaction: Broadhurst MJ, Brooks TJ, Pollock NR. 'Diagnosis of Ebola virus disease: past, present, and future.' *Clinical Microbiology Reviews* 29(4), 2016, 773–93, (doi: 10.1128/CMR.00003-16).

Chapter 19: Bandajuma

Daily ward round: Black B. *Fear, Hope Mark Life Inside Ebola Center in Sierra Leone: Witness* (Reuters, 9 December 2014). Available at: https://www.reuters.com/article/us-health-ebola-witness-idUSKBN0JN10G20141209 [cited 31 October 2021].

Separating a mother from her children: Black B. 'Christmas appeal 2014: Benjamin Black on Ebola through his eyes' (*BMJ Opinion,* 5 December 2014). Available at:

https://blogs.bmj.com/bmj/2014/12/05/christmas-appeal-benjamin-black-on-ebola-through-his-eyes [cited 31 October 2021].

£225 million would be spent on curbing the epidemic: Freeman C. 'British Ebola clinic opens for patients in Sierra Leone.' *Telegraph*, 5 November 2014. Available at: https://www.telegraph.co.uk/news/worldnews/ebola/11212080/British-Ebola-clinic-opens-for-patients-in-Sierra-Leone.html [cited 20 November 2018].

UK response had one ETC partially open: O'Carroll L. 'British-built Ebola hospital in Sierra Leone only partly operational.' *Guardian*, 20 November 2014. Available at: https://www.theguardian.com/world/2014/nov/20/british-ebola-hospital-sierra-leone-partly-operational [cited 20 November 2018].

Eleven treatment beds were available, and a total of twenty-eight patients had been treated: O'Carroll L. 'World's Ebola response slow, patchy and inadequate, MSF says.' *Guardian*, 2 December 2014. Available at: https://www. theguardian. com/global-development/2014/dec/02/ebola-medecins-sans-frontieres-west-africa [cited 20 November 2018].

ETCs were providing only 60 per cent of the beds needed: Michaels-Strasser S, Rabkin M, Lahuerta M, *et al.* 'Innovation to confront Ebola in Sierra Leone: the community-care-centre model'. *The Lancet Global Health*, 3(7), 2015, e361–62 (doi: 10.1016/S2214-109X(15)00045-5).

Immediate strike of over four hundred staff: *Sierra Leone Ebola Nurses on Strike* (BBC News, 12 November 2014). Available at: https://www.bbc.co.uk/news/world-africa-30019895 [cited 20 November 2018].

Chapter 21: Pregnancy Prevention

Without access to emergency obstetric care, a potential 120,000 pregnant women could die: *Ebola Wiping Out Gains in Safe Motherhood* (UNFPA, 16 October 2014). Available at: https://www.unfpa.org/press/ebola-wiping-out-gains-safe-motherhood [cited 20 November 2018].

ActionAid claimed one in seven pregnant women could die in childbirth: Alexander S. *Giving Birth in an Ebola Epidemic: 1 in 7 Women Could Die* (ActionAid UK, 11 November 2014). Available at: https://reliefweb.int/report/sierra-leone/giving-birth-ebola-epidemic-1-7-women-could-die [cited 20 November 2018].

A twenty-fold increase from pre-Ebola levels: Boseley S. 'One in seven pregnant women could die in Ebola-hit countries, say charities.' *Guardian*, 10 November 2014. Available at: https://www.theguardian.com/world/2014/nov/10/ebola-one-in-seven-pregnant-women-could-die [cited 20 November 2018].

No different from the risks in other humanitarian emergencies if no assistance arrives: Black B, Bouanchaud P, Bignall J. *et al.* 'Reproductive health during conflict'. *Obstetrician & Gynaecologist* 16(3), 2014, 153–60. Available at: https://doi.org/10.1111/tog.12114.

Over 90 per cent drop in women accessing their services: Stopes M. 'Family planning uptake.' In: *Ebola Outbreak: Impact on Reproductive Health and Proposed Mitigation Strategy* (UNFPA, Freetown, Sierra Leone, 2014).

There was a 44 per cent to 172 per cent increase in unplanned pregnancies during the epidemic: *Rapid Assessment of Ebola Impact on Reproductive Health Services and Service Seeking Behaviour in Sierra Leone* (UNFPA, Freetown, Sierra Leone, March 2015). Available at: https://reliefweb.int/sites/reliefweb.int/files/resources/UNFPA%20study%20_synthesis_March%2025_final.pdf.

This would lead to an increase in unsafe pregnancy terminations: Mitchell H. 'Sierra Leone: teenage girls are dying from unsafe abortions and risky pregnancies.' *Guardian*, 20 July 2017. Available at: https://www.theguardian.com/global-development-professionals-network/2017/jul/20/teen-pregnancy-sierra-leone-involve-men [cited 20 November 2018].

Door to door antimalarial campaigns: Press release: *1.5 Million People in a Country Affected by Ebola Receive Drugs to Prevent Malaria* (Médecins Sans Frontières, 10 December 2014. Available at: https://www.msf.org/sierra-leone-15-million-people-country-affected-ebola-receive-drugs-prevent-malaria [cited 11 December 2021].

Chapter 22: The Cavalry Arrives

Accusations of flouting medical ethics: Sprecher A. 'Finding an answer to Ebola's greatest challenge.' In: M. Hofman and S. Au (eds) *The Politics of Fear* (New York: Oxford University Press, 2017), pp. 187–201.

Fighting a forest fire with spray bottles: Watson-Stryker E. *Ebola: 'Fighting a Forest Fire With Spray Bottles'* (Doctors Without Borders USA, 2 September 2014). Available at: https://www.doctorswithoutborders.org/what-we-do/news-stories/story/ebola-fighting-forest-fire-spray-bottles [cited 20 November 2018].

Total number of cases could have been halved: Kucharski AJ, Camacho A, Flasche S, Glover RE, Edmunds WJ, Funk S. 'Measuring the impact of Ebola control measures in Sierra Leone'. *Proceedings of the National Academy of Sciences of the United States of America* 112(46), 2015, 14366–71 (doi: 10.1073/pnas.1508814112).

Suffered a staff infection, and they'd been accused of opening when unprepared: Kitamura M, Gbandia S. *UK Faces Criticism for Ebola-Containment Steps in Sierra Leone* (Swissinfo, 8 December 2014). Available at: https://www.swissinfo. ch/eng/bloomberg/u-k--faces-criticism-for-ebola-containment-steps-in-sierra-leone/41157490 [cited 11 December 2021].

Marred by negative press attention: Connor S. 'Sierra Leone criticises Save the Children's running of Ebola centre' (*Independent*, 9 December 2014). Available at: https://www.independent.co.uk/news/world/africa/sierra-leone-criticises-save-the-children-s-running-of-ebola-centre-9913438.html [cited 11 December 2021].

A letter written by British medics volunteering with Emergency: Confidential communication: *Undisclosed Sources: Report from UK-Med Recruited NHS Health Workers Contracted to Emergency* (December 2014).

WHO had published a list of potential treatments eligible for 'compassionate' use: *Potential Ebola Therapies and Vaccines: Interim Guidance* (WHO, 5 November 2014). Available at: http://apps.who.int/iris/handle/10665/137590?locale=ar [cited 20 November 2018].

Both had the potential for worsening organ failure and unappealing side effects: Gupta-Wright A, Lavers J, Irvine S. 'Concerns about the off-licence use of amiodarone for Ebola'. *British Medical Journal* 350(20 January 2015), h272, (doi: 10.1136/bmj.h272).

News of Emergency and their experimental treatments did hit the UK press: Boseley S. 'Untested Ebola drug given to patients in Sierra Leone causes UK walkout.' *Guardian*, 22 December 2014. Available at: https://www.theguardian.com/world/2014/dec/22/ebola-untested-drug-patients-sierra-leone-uk-staff-leave [cited 20 November 2018].

Emergency released a vigorous declaration of denial: Press release: *Facts, Lies and Tales About Ebola – Sierra Leone* (Emergency, 5 January 2015). Available at: https://reliefweb.int/report/sierra-leone/facts-lies-and-tales-about-ebola [cited 20 November 2018].

Threatened legal action against the 'slanderous' press, though none was taken: Emails to author from S. Boseley (24 October 2018) and R. Pailey (24 October 2018).

Other times when medical studies had been carried out on populations without due consent: Pailey R. *Treating Africans with an Untested Ebola Drug* (Al Jazeera, 3 January 2015). Available at: https://www.aljazeera.com/opinions/2015/1/3/treating-africans-with-an-untested-ebola-drug [cited 31 October 2021].

Chapter 23: Tonkolili

Patients continued being sent across the country: O'Carroll. 'Ebola cases surge in Sierra Leone.'. *Guardian*, 1 December 2014. Available at: https://www. theguardian.com/global-development/2014/dec/01/ebola-cases-surge-in-sierra-leone [cited 02 December 2018].

Decided to provide care closer and build a new one-hundred bed ETC in Tonkolili: Theocharopoulos G, Danis K, Greig J, *et al.* 'Ebola management centre proximity associated with reduced delays of healthcare of Ebola virus disease (EVD) patients, Tonkolili, Sierra Leone, 2014–15.' *PloS One* 12(5), 2017, e0176692 (doi: 10.1371/journal.pone.0176692).

WHO reported there were now 615 beds available: *Ebola Response Roadmap Situation Report: 17 December 2014* (WHO, 2014). Available at: https://apps.who. int/iris/bitstream/handle/10665/145679/roadmapsitrep_17Dec2014_eng.pdf?sequence=1&isAllowed=y [cited 3 February 2022].

It *was* a technical triumph: Film: *Construction of Magburaka Ebola Treatment Center, Sierra Leone* (Médecins Sans Frontières, 14 January 2015). Available at: https://www.youtube.com/watch?v=zcvYMEnrh6A [cited 20 November 2018].

Chapter 24: Full Circle

Pregnancy-referral ETC: Press release: *Sierra Leone: MSF Opens Maternity Unit for Pregnant Women with Ebola* (Médecins Sans Frontières, 29 January 2015). Available at: https://www.msf.org/sierra-leone-msf-opens-maternity-unit-pregnant-women-ebola [cited 9 December 2021].

Judeo-Kashani, a dying language: Mansour I. 'Preserving endangered Jewish languages before they go extinct' (*Tablet Magazine*, 22 July 2013). Available at: https://www.tabletmag.com/sections/community/articles/endangered-jewish-languages [cited 7 October 2021].

ETC teams were fighting over who got to admit the remaining patients: Walsh S, Johnson O. *Getting to Zero* (London: Zed Books, 2018), pp. 294.

Ruth wrote to me in exasperation: Email to author from R. Kauffman (5 June 2015.)

Sierra Leone was declared free of Ebola: *Statement on the End of the Ebola Outbreak in Sierra Leone* (WHO, 7 November 2015). Available at: https://afro.who.int/media-centre/statements-commentaries/statement-end-ebola-outbreak-sierra-leone [cited 20 November 2018].

Sierra Leone's maternal mortality was predicted to rise by a further 74 per cent: Evans DK, Goldstein M, Popova A. 'Health-care worker mortality and the legacy of the Ebola epidemic.' *The Lancet Global Health* 3(8), 2015, e439–40 (doi: 10.1016/S2214-109X(15)00065-0).

Chapter 25: A New Beginning

The highest maternal mortality rate and now also the highest lifetime risk of maternal death: *Trends in Maternal Mortality: 1990 to 2015. Estimates by WHO, UNICEF, UNFPA, World Bank Group and the United Nations Population Division* (WHO, November 2015).

It was worse now than it had been two years earlier: Jones S, Gopalakrishnan S, Ameh C, White S, van den Broek N. "'Women and babies are dying but not of Ebola": the effect of the Ebola virus epidemic on the availability, uptake and outcomes of maternal and newborn health services in Sierra Leone.' *BMJ Global Health* 1(3), 7 October 2016, e000065 (doi: 10.1136/bmjgh-2016-000065). And: Kassa ZY, Scarf V, Fox D. 'The effect of Ebola virus disease on maternal health service utilisation and perinatal outcomes in West Africa: a systematic review.' *Reproductive Health* 19(1), 35, 4 February 2022, (doi: 10.1186/s12978-022-01343-8).

Hundreds of ambulances had been imported: Inveen C. *The Case of Sierra Leone's Missing Ambulances* (Al Jazeera, 26 November 2015). Available at: https://www.aljazeera.com/indepth/features/2015/11/case-sierra-leone-missing-ambulances-151116115001872.html [cited 20 November 2018].

Atrocious record of corruption: Chêne M. *Overview of Corruption and Anti-corruption in Sierra Leone* (Transparency International, 22 September 2010). Available at: https://knowledgehub.transparency.org/assets/uploads/helpdesk/256_Corruption_and_anti_corruption_in_Sierra_Leone.pdf [cited 20 November 2018].

One third of Ebola funds remained unaccounted for: O'Carroll L. *Auditors Report: Sierra Leone has Failed to Properly Account for a Third of Ebola Funds Between May and October 2014*. Available at: https://www.scribd.com/document/255896806/Auditors-report-Sierra-leone-has-failed-to-properly-account-for-a-third-of-Ebola-funds-between-May-and-October [cited 20 November 2018]. And: O'Carroll L. 'A third of Sierra Leone's Ebola budget unaccounted for, says report.' *Guardian*, 16 February 2015. Available at: https://www.theguardian.com/world/2015/feb/16/ebola-sierra-leone-budget-report [cited 20 November 2018].

Rising discontent among junior doctors: Tran M, Morris S. 'Urgent talks set to resume to head off junior doctors' strikes.' *Guardian*, 30 November 2015. Available at: https://www.theguardian.com/society/2015/nov/30/urgent-talks-set-to-resume-to-head-off-junior-doctors-strikes [cited 31 November 2018].

Chapter 26: Bomb Scare

Salome death had just been reported: Baker A. 'Liberian Ebola fighter: a *TIME* person of the year, dies in childbirth.' *Time*, 27 February 2017. Available at: https://time.com/4683873/ebola-fighter-time-person-of-the-year-salome-kar-wah [cited 12 May 2020].

International teams were trialling experimental drugs, using the anti-body-rich plasma of survivors and vaccinations: Giahyue J. 'Untested Ebola drugs begin trials in West Africa.' *Scientific American*, 6 January 2015. Available at: https://www.scientificamerican.com/article/untested-ebola-drugs-begin-trials-in-west-africa [cited 20 November 2021]. And: van Griensven J, De Weiggheleire A, Delamou A, *et al.* 'The use of Ebola convalescent plasma to treat Ebola virus disease in resource-constrained settings: a perspective from the field.' *Clinical Infectious Diseases* 62(1), 2016, 69–74(doi: 10.1093/cid/civ680).

While there was a vaccine available, she was denied it: Caluwaerts S. 'Nubia's mother: being pregnant in the time of experimental vaccines and therapeutics for Ebola.' *Reproductive Health* 14(Suppl.3), 14 December 2017, 157 (doi: 10.1186/s12978-017-0429-8).

Early evidence had shown high (vaccine) effectiveness in protecting contacts: Henao-Restrepo AM, Longini IM, Egger M, *et al.* 'Efficacy and effectiveness of an rVSV-vectored vaccine expressing Ebola surface glycoprotein: interim results from the Guinea ring vaccination cluster-randomised trial.' *The Lancet* 386(9996), 2015, 857–66 (doi: 10.1016/S0140-6736(15)61117-5).

Ring vaccinations were being rolled out: Ebola ça Suffit Ring Vaccination Trial Consortium. 'The ring vaccination trial: a novel cluster randomised controlled trial design to evaluate vaccine efficacy and effectiveness during outbreaks, with special reference to Ebola.' *BMJ Clinical research* 351, 27 July 2015, h3740 (doi: 10.1136/bmj.h3740).

The plea was snubbed and access denied, unless randomization was accepted: Caluwaerts S. 'Nubia's mother: being pregnant in the time of experimental vaccines and therapeutics for Ebola.' *Reproductive Health* 14(Suppl.3), 14 December 2017, 157 (doi: 10.1186/s12978-017-0429-8).

She bled till she died: As above.

Unlike her mother, the baby was granted access: As above.

Nubia went on to survive: Dörnemann J, Burzio C, Ronsse A, *et al.* 'First newborn baby to receive experimental therapies survives Ebola virus disease'. *Journal of Infectious Diseases* 215,(2), 2017, 171–74 (doi: 10.1093/infdis/jiw493).

Nubia thrived as a young child: Gulland A. 'Meet Nubia: the only baby to ever have survived Ebola' *(The Telegraph,* 1 June 2018). Available at: https://www. telegraph.co.uk/global-health/science-and-disease/meet-nubia-baby-ever-have-survived-ebola [cited 20 November 2021].

Maternal deaths were reported to account for 36 per cent of all deaths in women aged between fifteen and forty-nine: *Sierra Leone Demographic and Health Survey 2013* (Statistics Sierra Leone (SSL) and ICF International, 2014). Available at: https://dhsprogram.com/pubs/pdf/fr297/fr297.pdf.

Home births accounted for roughly 50 per cent of all births: Sharkey A, Yansaneh A, Bangura P.S, *et al.* 'Maternal and newborn care practices in Sierra Leone: a mixed methods study of four underserved districts.' *Health Policy and Planning* 32(2), 2017, 151–62 (doi: 10.1093/heapol/czw104).

Ebola had been declared '*don don*': Bah AL. *Ebola "Don Don" in Sierra Leone: Celebration, Tears and Reflection* (Sierra Express Media, 11 November 2015). Available at: https://sierraexpressmedia.com/?p=76377 [cited 15 December 2018].

A new case of Ebola had been confirmed in Monrovia: Giahyue J. *Liberia Monitors Over 150 Contacts as Virus Re-Emerges* (Reuters, 22 November 2015.). Available at: https://www.reuters.com/article/us-health-ebola-liberia-idINK-BN0TB0GV20151122 [cited 11 December 2021].

This theory had not yet been proved beyond circumstantial evidence: Crozier I. 'Ebola virus RNA in the semen of male survivors of Ebola virus disease: the uncertain gravitas of a privileged persistence'. *Journal of Infectious Diseases* 214(10), 2016, 1467–69 (doi: 10.1093/infdis/jiw079.) And: Christie A, Davies-Wayne GJ, Cordier-Lassalle T, *et al.* 'Possible sexual transmission of Ebola virus – Liberia, 2015.' *Morbidity and Mortality Weekly Report* 64(17), 2015, 479–81.

His family, as contacts, were also put into isolation: Dokubo EK, Wendland A, Mate SE, *et al.* 'Persistence of Ebola virus after the end of widespread transmission in Liberia: an outbreak report.' *The Lancet Infectious Diseases* 18(9), 2018, 1015–24 (doi: 10.1016/S1473-3099(18)30417-1).

Emily . . . had reported on a similar case in Sierra Leone: Bower H, Grass JE, Veltus E, *et al.* 'Delivery of an Ebola virus-positive stillborn infant in a rural community health center, Sierra Leone, 2015.' *American Journal of Tropical Medicine and Hygiene* 94(2), 2016, 417–19 (doi: 10.4269/ajtmh.15-0619).

Ministry of Health, supported by WHO, also released updated guidance for pregnant women: *Diagnosis and Management of Suspected Ebola and Acute Haemorrhagic Fever in Health Facilities and Isolation Units for use in Normal*

(Non-Epidemic) Circumstances (Freetown: Sierra Leone Ministry of Health & Sanitation, 2015). And: *Diagnosis and Management of Ebola Virus Disease in Screening and Isolation Facilities and Ebola Treatment Units During an Epidemic* (Freetown: Sierra Leone Ministry of Health & Sanitation, 2015).

We raised our concerns: Email to author (from undisclosed), 23 November 2015.

No meaningful discussion of improvement or actions to change: *Ebola Virus Disease in Pregnancy: Screening and Management of Ebola Contacts, Cases and Survivors* (WHO, 2018). Available at: http://apps.who.int/iris/bitstream/handle/10665/184163/WHO_EVD_HSE_PED_15.1_eng.pdf;sequence=1 [cited 20 November 2018].

These had been common events a year earlier: Hayden EC. 'Maternal health: Ebola's lasting legacy.' *Nature* 519(7541), 2015, 24–26 (doi: 10.1038/519024a).

Chapter 27: The Third Delay

His chances of surviving past his first birthday were bleak without his mother: Moucheraud C, Worku A, Molla M, Finlay JE, Leaning J, Yamin A. 'Consequences of maternal mortality on infant and child survival: a 25-year longitudinal analysis in Butajira Ethiopia (1987–2011).' *Reproductive Health* 12(Suppl.1) , 2015, S4(doi: 10.1186/1742-4755-12-S1-S4).

They had achieved where we in GRC had failed: Drevin G, Mölsted Alvesson H, van Duinen A, Bolkan HA, Koroma AP, von Schreeb J. '"For this one, let me take the risk": why surgical staff continued to perform caesarean sections during the 2014–2016 Ebola epidemic in Sierra Leone.' *BMJ Global Health* 4(4), 19 July 2019, e001361 (doi: 10.1136/bmjgh-2018-00136).

Chapter 29: A New Year, A New Project, Another Chance

Not only for the patients we saw, but for those we didn't see too: MacDougall C. 'World Health Organization says Ebola is over in Sierra Leone – for now' (*Newsweek*, 17 March 2016). Available at: https://www.newsweek.com/2016/04/08/sierra-leone-ebola-free-world-health-organization-438123.html [cited 20 November 2018].

Mariatu had travelled from Bamoi Luma: Fofana U. *Dozens Feared Exposed as Sierra Leone Confirms New Ebola Death* (Reuters, 15 January 2016). Available at: https://www.reuters.com/article/us-health-ebola-leone-idUSKCN0UT0Q3 [cited 11 December 2021].

WHO was finally due to announce the Ebola outbreak of West Africa over: *Latest Ebola Outbreak Over on Liberia; West Africa is at Zero, but New Flare-Ups*

are Likely to Occur (WHO, 14 January 2016). Available at: https://www.who.int/
news/item/14-01-2016-latest-ebola-outbreak-over-in-liberia-west-africa-is-at-
zero-but-new-flare-ups-are-likely-to-occur [cited 11 December 2021].

Chapter 30: Far From Perfect

Spread across four districts: 'Sierra Leone puts more than 100 people in quarantine
after new Ebola death.' *Guardian*, 17 January 2016. Available at: https://www.
theguardian.com/world/2016/jan/15/ebola-victim-in-sierra-leone-feared-to-
have-exposed-27-others-to-virus [cited 16 March 2018].

The government was quick to recreate 'voluntary quarantine': 'Sierra Leone
identifies more than 100 contacts in Ebola case.' *Africa Times*, 19 January 2016.
Available at: https://africatimes.com/2016/01/19/sierra-leone-identifies-more-
than-100-contacts-in-ebola-case [cited 11 December 2021].

Active case-finding activities began: *Fear and Suspicion as Ebola Returns to Sierra
Leone* (Al Jazeera, 21 January 2016). Available at: https://www. aljazeera.com/
news/2016/1/21/ebola-in-sierra-leone-new-case-spreads-community-fear [cited
11 December 2021].

Maintaining and expanding routine healthcare: Black B. 'Sierra Leone: we save
lives of women in childbirth – while fighting Ebola.' *Guardian*, 23 February
2016. Available at: https://www.theguardian.com/global-development/2016/
feb/23/ebola-sierra-leone-save-lives-women-childbirth-msf-hospital [cited 11
December 2021].

Mariatu's aunt had developed a fever: *Ebola Situation Report – 3 February 2016*
(WHO, 2016). Available at: https://apps.who.int/iris/handle/10665/204285
[cited 20 November 2018].

There were no further cases of Ebola following Mariatu's aunt: *Sierra Leone
Discharges Last Known Ebola Patient* (Reuters, 8 February 2016). Available at:
https://www.reuters.com/article/uk-health-ebola-leone-idUKKCN0VH1ZX
[cited 11 December 2021].

Chapter 31: Not Normal

Women opting to freebirth: Summers H. 'Expectant mothers turning to freebirth-
ing after home births cancelled.' *Guardian*, 5 April 2020. Available at: https://
www.theguardian.com/lifeandstyle/2020/apr/05/expectant-mothers-turn-to-
freebirthing-after-home-births-cancelled [cited 18 May 2020].

New York hospitals refusing entry of birth partners: Kusisto L, West M. 'New
York hospital systems ban partners from delivery room.' *Wall Street Journal*,

24 March 2020. Available at: https://www.wsj.com/articles/new-york-hospital-system-bans-partners-from-delivery-room-11585004655 [cited 18 May 2020].

She said she was left to labour alone: Kale S. "'I started shouting at the midwives": the stress of giving birth under lockdown.' *Guardian*, 10 April 2020. Available at: https://www.theguardian.com/lifeandstyle/2020/apr/10/i-started-shouting-at-the-midwives-the-stress-of-giving-birth-under-lockdown [cited 18 May 2020].

What do you think about letting partners come?: Black B, Laking J, McKay G. 'Birth partners are not a luxury.' *BMJ Opinion,* 24 September 2020. Available at: https://blogs.bmj.com/bmj/2020/09/24/birth-partners-are-not-a-luxury [cited 24 September 2020].

The complex backdrop of issues dictating how and when a community decided to seek healthcare for a pregnant woman: Elston JWT, Danis K, Gray N. *et al.* 'Maternal health after Ebola: unmet needs and barriers to healthcare in rural Sierra Leone.' *Health Policy and Planning* 35(1), 2020, 78–90 (doi: 10.1093/heapol/czz102).

Afterword

Innovations in isolation facilities: Devi S. 'FRONTLINE: a new treatment facility for Ebola virus disease.' *The Lancet* 392(10163), 2018, 2428 (doi: 10.1016/S0140-6736(18)33118-0).

Treatments which can significantly increase survival rates: Mulangu S, Dodd LE, Davey RT Jr, *et al.* 'A randomized, controlled trial of Ebola virus disease therapeutics.' *New England Journal of Medicine* 381(24), 2019, 2293–303 (doi: 10.1056/NEJMoa1910993).

ZMapp was not proven to be one of them: Davey RT Jr (and the Multinational PREVAIL II Study Team). 'A randomized, controlled trial of ZMapp for Ebola virus infection.' *New England Journal of Medicine* 375(15), 2016, 1448–56 (doi: 10.1056/NEJMoa1604330).

Development of Ebola rapid diagnostic tests: Mukadi-Bamuleka D, Bulabula-Penge J, De Weggheleire A, *et al.* 'Field performance of three Ebola rapid diagnostic tests used during the 2018–20 outbreak in the eastern Democratic Republic of the Congo: a retrospective, multicentre observational study.' *The Lancet Infectious diseases* S1473-3099(21)00675-7, 14 March 2022 (doi: 10.1016/S1473-3099(21)00675-7).

Safe and effective Ebola vaccines available: *Ebola Vaccine: Information about ERVEBO®* (Center for Disease Control and Prevention (CDC), 8 November 2012). Available at: https://www.cdc.gov/vhf/ebola/clinicians/vaccine/index.html [cited 11 December 2021].

Pregnant women were found no less likely to survive: Caluwaerts S, Van Herp M, Cuesta J, *et al.* 'Pregnancy and Ebola: survival outcomes for pregnant women admitted to MSF Ebola treatment centres in the West Africa outbreak.' *F1000Research*, 27 June 2018 (doi: 10.7490/f1000research.1115707.1) Available at: https://f1000research.com/documents/7-945 [cited 20 November 2018].

Greatest risk factor for a pregnant woman: Gomes MF, de la Fuente-Núñez V, Saxena A, Kuesel AC. 'Protected to death: systematic exclusion of pregnant women from Ebola virus disease trials.' *Reproductive Health* 14(Suppl.3), 14 December 2017, 172 (doi: 10.1186/s12978-017-0430-2).

WHO replaced its guidance for managing pregnant women and Ebola: Guidelines for the Management of Pregnant and Breastfeeding Women in the Context *of Ebola Virus Disease* (WHO, 2020). Licence: CC BY-NC-SA 3.0 IGO.

The most divergent of all global health survival statistics: Ronsmans C, Graham WJ. 'Maternal mortality: who, when, where, and why.' *The Lancet* 368(9542), 2006, 1189–200 (doi: 10.1016/S0140-6736(06)69380-X).

The Sierra Leone National Emergency Medical Service: Caviglia M, Putoto G, Conti A, *et al.* 'Association between ambulance prehospital time and maternal and perinatal outcomes in Sierra Leone: a countrywide study.' *British Medical Journal Global Health* 6(11), 2021, e007315. (doi: 10.1136/bmjgh-2021-007315).

Predictions of an apocalypse on reproductive health: Roberton T, Carter ED, Chou VB, *et al.* 'Early estimates of the indirect effects of the COVID-19 pandemic on maternal and child mortality in low-income and middle-income countries: a modelling study.' *The Lancet Global Health* 8,(7), 2020, e901–08 (doi: 10.1016/S2214-109X(20)30229-1. And: Riley T, Sully E, Ahmed Z, Biddlecom A. 'Estimates of the potential impact of the COVID-19 pandemic on sexual and reproductive health in low- and middle-income countries.' *International Perspectives on Sexual and Reproductive Health* 46, 16 April 2020, 73–76 (doi: 10.1363/46e9020).

These worst-case scenarios did not materialize, however the disruption to women's healthcare remained staggering: *Technical Note: Impact of COVID-19 on Family Planning: What We Know One Year into the Pandemic* (UNFPA, 11 March 2021). Available at: https://www.unfpa.org/sites/default/files/resource-pdf/COVID_Impact_FP_V5.pdf [cited 22 December 2021].

We did not heed the precedent set by epidemics and emergencies of the recent past: Black B, McKay G. 'Covid-19 and reproductive health: What can we learn from previous epidemics?' *BMJ Opinion* 19 March 2020. Available at: https://blogs.bmj.com/bmj/2020/03/19/covid-19-and-reproductive-health-what-can-we-learn-from-previous-epidemics [cited 18 May 2020].